The Alternative Dictionary
of Symptoms and Cures

By the same author

Overcoming the Menopause Naturally by Dr Caroline M. Shreeve (Century Arrow, 1986)

The Alternative Dictionary of Symptoms and Cures

*A Comprehensive Guide to Diseases and
Their Orthodox and Alternative Remedies*

Dr Caroline M. Shreeve

CENTURY
LONDON MELBOURNE AUCKLAND JOHANNESBURG

This book is dedicated, with love, to my husband David,
to my mother, and to Rupert.

First published in 1986 by Century Hutchinson Ltd
Brookmount House, 62–65 Chandos Place, Covent Garden,
London WC2N 4NW

Century Hutchinson Australia Pty Ltd
PO Box 496, 16–22 Church Street, Hawthorn, Australia, Victoria 3122

Century Hutchinson New Zealand Ltd.,
PO Box 40–086, Glenfield, Auckland 10, New Zealand

Century Hutchinson Group SA (Pty) Ltd.,
PO Box 337, Bergvlei 2012, South Africa

British Library Cataloguing in Publication Data
Shreeve, Caroline M.
The alternative dictionary of symptoms and
cures: a comprehensive guide to diseases
and their orthodox and alternative remedies.
1. Therapeutic systems – Dictionaries
I. Title
615.5   R733
ISBN 0-7126-1292-0

Photoset by Rowland Phototypesetting Ltd
Bury St Edmunds, Suffolk
Printed in Great Britain by
St Edmundsbury Press Ltd, Bury St Edmunds, Suffolk

Introduction

'A man's own observation, what he finds good of, and what he finds hurt of, is the best physic to preserve health.'

Francis Bacon: *Essays*, 30, *Of Regimen of Health*

In *The Alternative Dictionary of Symptoms and Cures*, I have described and defined both common— and some less common—disorders, together with their orthodox management and alternative forms of treatment. I have tried to take a 'whole' and unbiased view of both orthodox and alternative forms of medical treatment, thus making the book a logical extension—and a further application—of the holistic ideal.

In writing the *Alternative Dictionary*, I have had two main objectives. The first has been to provide a clear understanding of the underlying philosophy upon which alternative therapies are based, and of how alternative therapists work. Secondly, in doing so, I have tried to indicate the opportunities that exist in this country both for complementing traditional treatment with alternatives, or for choosing the 'natural' approach in preference to that of traditional medicine. Limitations of length, however, have precluded my including specific childhood complaints with the exception of childhood infections and obstetric problems.

At this point, however, I must add a cautionary word. It is vital, in the case of all serious acute or long-standing health problems, to obtain at least a definitive diagnosis from an orthodox doctor, and (except in rare instances) to undergo the recommended course of treatment, perhaps complemented by one or two appropriate alternative treatments.

In some conditions, for example, acute appendicitis, septicaemia, bronchopneumonia, accidents resulting in serious burn injuries or fractured bones—no substitute exists for orthodox treatment, and the majority of alternative practitioners are the first to acknowledge this.

Treatment for cancer requires special mention. Neither holistic nor orthodox medicine can yet claim to 'cure cancer', although many victories can be claimed by both. Because of the side effects of some types of orthodox treatment, many people are drawn instinctively to the gentler approach offered by natural medicine. However, because of the cures and remissions many patients experience as a result of orthodox medicine, one would have to be very brave—and perhaps foolhardy—

to counsel a cancer patient to forgo established treatment methods.

The choice is probably the most distressingly difficult that any individual has to make; and, sadly, for the time being, the choice must be made by the individual him or herself. Far from having to make it alone, however, a decision of this nature is best made after careful counselling both by orthodox specialists and alternative practitioners, preferably working in close co-operation with one another and with the patient.

My personal choice—were I ever asked to make it—would be to combine the best that orthodox medicine and the appropriate alternatives had to offer. I would also pursue every avenue of self-help at my disposal, such as specialised diet, meditation and positive visualisation.

At this point, a word about self-treatment seems appropriate. Many minor ailments can quite safely be treated with 'over the counter' remedies, of which thousands—both orthodox and alternative—exist. However, where the diagnosis is in doubt, or the problem troublesome and recurrent, it is vital to seek help and advice either from an arthodox doctor or from a qualified alternative therapist.

For insight into the usefulness of many of the alternative therapeutic methods mentioned in the *Alternative Dictionary*, I must thank the many authors to whose works I have turned time and again as sources of reference. In this context, my thanks are due particularly to Brian Inglis and Ruth West (*The Alternative Health Guide*, Michael Joseph, 1983); Andrew Stanway (*Alternative Medicine*, Penguin 1986); Stephen Fulder (*The Handbook of Complementary Medicine*, Coronet Books, 1984); Earl Mindell (*The Vitamin Bible*, Arlington Books, 1983); Roger Newman Turner (*Naturopathic Medicine*, Thorsons, 1984); Mark Bricklin (*The Practical Encyclopedia of Natural Healing*, Rodale Press, 1976); Maurice Messegué (*Health Secrets of Plants and Herbs*, Pan Books, 1981); and to the editors and contributors of *Here's Health*, *New Health* and the *Journal of Alternative Medicine*.

Appreciative thanks are also due to the therapists who have given their time so generously in discussing suitable applications of their respective disciplines; and to the numerous patients whom I have interviewed during the course of various types of treatment, for their invaluable opinions regarding the usefulness of the help they were receiving.

Finally, I should like to acknowledge the great debt owing to Caroline Ball and Paul Barnett who have worked so hard in editing the manuscript; and to Dr Chris Sinclair who has read the 'orthodox' parts and has made numerous constructive criticisms and suggestions.

Contents

vii

PART ONE

A–Z OF SYMPTOMS AND CONDITIONS

–A–

Abdominal pain PAIN arising in the abdomen due to disordered abdominal or pelvic organs. The stomach, bowel, digestive organs, kidneys, bladder and womb (uterus) are the most usual sources of discomfort, and generally the type of pain, its situation and the accompanying symptoms will suggest its origin.

Hollow organs initially give rise to a dull pain in the midline of the abdomen, and it is often accompanied by a feeling of NAUSEA. Examples are the stomach and upper small bowel, disorders of which often produce pain below the breastbone; and the appendix and lower small bowel, disorders of which can cause pain around the navel.

INFLAMMATION (e.g. gastritis [see I/13], appendicitis [see I/16]), muscle SPASM (e.g. COLIC), gut INFARCTION and an interrupted blood supply (e.g. strangulation of HERNIA) can all cause pain in the abdomen. In some cases, the pain gradually shifts from the midline to the particular area involved. The pain of an inflamed gall bladder, for example, will move after a few hours from the midline to the upper-right quarter of the abdomen. The pain of appendicitis (see I/16) also settles after some hours over the inflamed organ, which is in the lower-right quarter of the abdomen.

STRESS REACTIONS, emotional problems and anxiety (see XIV/4) often produce abdominal pain for which no physical cause can be found. They can also be partly responsible for several common stomach and bowel disorders, such as PEPTIC ULCER and diverticulitis (see I/32).

Occasionally, abdominal pain accompanies disorders affecting other parts of the body. Small children often complain of 'tummy ache' rather than a sore throat when they are suffering from tonsillitis (see II/6).

Abscess A collection of pus in a pocket of healthy tissue (the best known example is a boil). Abscesses are formed when the body's defence mechanism of INFLAMMATION traps germs (bacteria) and seals them off, but doesn't actually destroy them. The pus consists of the fluid and white cells which leak from the blood vessels in the infected area, together with bacteria (both dead and alive) and pieces of damaged tissue.

3

Orthodox treatment
An abscess is lanced, the pus is scraped out under a local anaesthetic, and a sterile gauze wick is inserted to drain off any further pus that may form. An antibiotic injection is usually given.

Homeopathic treatment
For abscesses that are slow to mature: *Hepar Sulphur*. For mouth abscesses: *Mercurius Solubilis*. When pus has formed and is slow to clear: *Silicea*. For an extremely painful boil, very sensitive to touch: *Hypericum* tincture.

Acid stomach   The return of digestive acid into the mouth, or the excessive production of acid by the stomach, associated with duodenal ulcer (see I/11). The acid, often mixed with partially digested food, can come from the stomach, where it is produced, or small bowel (duodenum). There is often a burning sensation (HEARTBURN) in the food-pipe (oesophagus), BELCHING and a feeling of food 'getting stuck' just after it is swallowed. (A persistent feeling of food 'getting stuck' should be investigated medically.) Symptoms are most likely to occur when bending over or lying down, or when a heavy weight is being lifted, and may be a sign of hiatus hernia (see I/7) or of peptic ulcer (see I/9).

Orthodox treatment
A commonly prescribed medicine for 'acid-stomach' symptoms is a suspension such as Polycrol, a gel or tablets containing activated dimethicone, magnesium hydroxide, and aluminium hydroxide gel.

Herbal treatment
A cup of camomile tea in which three or four fresh mint leaves, or a pinch of dried mint, have been steeped.

Acne   A collection of inflamed spots and blackheads caused by the overactivity of the grease (sebaceous) glands on the face, chest and back. See VII/1.

Addiction   See DRUG DEPENDENCE.

Addison's disease   A disorder of the adrenal glands, which fail to produce sufficient quantities of steroid hormones.

Adenitis   INFLAMMATION of a lymph gland (lymph node). See LYMPHADENITIS.

Adenoids When the condition 'adenoids' is diagnosed, enlarged adenoids are meant, as adenoids themselves are simply large clumps of lymphoid tissue comparable to tonsils and present in all normal children. Enlarged adenoids are discussed in II/7.

Adhesions Fibrous bands joining normally separate tissues. They are a consequence of the healing process following INFLAMMATION, which in turn usually follows INFECTION, injury or a surgical incision. Surgical scars can bind internal organs to one another because the fluid which is produced when healing starts contains the coagulation factor fibrinogen, which is able to form a clot. Into this, tendrils of connective tissue grow. This process can, for instance, 'stick' a fresh surgical scar on the large bowel (colon) to a neighbouring coil of small bowel (jejunum).

Adhesions following surgery cause pain because they interfere with normal processes, and frequently become inflamed themselves. They are, however, rarely dangerous.

Agoraphobia An unreasonable fear (phobia) of wide open spaces. See XIV/7.

AIDS (acquired immunodeficiency syndrome) A new viral illness, first described in the spring of 1981. See VIII/5.

Alcoholism See DRUG DEPENDENCE.

Alexia See DYSLEXIA.

Allergy The abnormal formation by the body of antidotes (antibodies) to substances with which it comes into contact. This is a misuse of its natural immune defence mechanism against infection. The substances (allergens)—such as metals, food or clothing—produce no unpleasant effects on first encounter. At second and subsequent meetings, though, the antibodies formed during the first meeting react and produce symptoms due to the release of the chemical histamine. This can produce skin RASHES, ECZEMA, ASTHMA, HAY FEVER and HIVES.

Occasionally, the body produces antibodies against some of its own tissues and an **autoimmune disease** results. Examples of this are rheumatoid arthritis (see VI/3) pernicious anaemia (see VIII/1) and, probably, ulcerative colitis (see I/29).

The significance of food allergies (or intolerances) is becoming more widely recognized, by both alternative therapists and orthodox doctors.

They are now thought possibly to be associated with a wide range of disorders, including migraine attacks (IX/2), asthma (II/15), colitis (I/29; I/30), schizophrenia (XIV/1), insatiable food cravings, CATARRH, feeding problems and poor growth in babies and children, and feeling 'generally unwell' in a way that is difficult to describe. There are two types of food allergy, some involving a straightforward allergic reaction and others having more in common with chemical dependence or addiction. See DRUG DEPENDENCE.

Orthodox treatment
Treatment may consist of advice to the patient to eliminate certain foods from his diet, or it may consist of gradual desensitization. Suspected food allergy can often be confirmed by an elimination diet in which the patient, generally under supervision, confines his foods and liquids to two or three basic 'hypoallergenic' items. A possible choice is lamb, rice and pears, with boiled tap water to drink. Suspect food items are reintroduced one by one, once the patient's reaction to exclusion has settled, the patient noting any recommencement of previous symptoms. In the United Kingdom there are NHS clinics at which food-allergy testing is carried out. Negative skin tests and blood tests are generally unreliable.

Alternative treatment
Applied kinesiology is often used both to diagnose and to treat food allergy. Alternatively, dietary desensitization may be employed.

Amnesia The loss of memory over a particular timespan. There are two main types. One, *anterograde amnesia*, results from an intolerable emotional shock. This *suppresses* the person's memory of his own identity and of familiar surroundings, and of the shock itself. It is a protective mechanism against emotional suffering. Various means (e.g. hypnotherapy) can be used to recall the memories. The other, *retrograde amnesia*, occurs following head injury. Loss of memory of the events immediately before the injury is complete and permanent. Other causes of amnesia include disease and abuse of drugs (e.g. of alcohol).

Anaemia A shortage of the oxygen-carrying pigment (haemoglobin) in red blood cells. This condition means either (a) that the body is losing too much haemoglobin or (b) that it is making it in insufficient amounts. See VIII/1.

Aneurysm An abnormal bulge in the wall of an artery, caused by the pressure of the blood within on a weakened area. This weakness can be present from birth, or caused by fatty deposits (ATHEROMA), injury or INFECTION later in life. If an aneurysm in a major artery bursts suddenly, it can be fatal.

Orthodox treatment
The only satisfactory method of dealing with an aneurysm is by surgery.

Alternative treatment
Little can be done about the mechanical problem of an arterial aneurysm, but hypertension (see **III/5**) poses a special risk in such cases, and its reduction by alternative forms of treatment can be very helpful.

Angina pectoris Chest pain due to oxygen shortage in the heart muscle. This means that the coronary arteries, which supply the heart with oxygen-rich blood, are failing to satisfy its demands. These demands are higher if the heart is beating more rapidly—for instance, during exercise or as a reaction to strong emotion. Other aggravating factors include obesity (see WEIGHT PROBLEMS), smoking, living at high altitudes where the air's oxygen content is low, and ANAEMIA.

An insufficient oxygen suppy from the blood means that the energy-generating chemical reactions inside the muscle cells are incomplete. Chemical substances (metabolites) are formed which cause PAIN (which can be agonizing) by irritating the nerve endings in the heart muscle. Angina is typically felt in the centre of the chest, sometimes spreading up into the neck and down either arm, usually the left.

The commonest disease process affecting the coronary arteries is ATHEROMA. Besides exercise, anything which causes the heart to beat more rapidly, such as excitement, fear, shock or an indigestible meal, can bring on an attack.

Orthodox treatment
Orthodox drugs for angina include glyceryl trinitrate (Suscard Buccal), timolol (Betim) and sotalol (Sotacor). A coronary artery bypass operation is offered to some patients with very severe coronary artery disease—see **III/4**.

Herbal treatment (to help prevent attacks)
An infusion of two pinches of sage and two pinches of lime flowers in a cup of water.

Ankylosing spondylitis (bamboo spine) See SPONDYLITIS (ankylosing).

7

Anorexia Loss of appetite. This is a common symptom found in a wide variety of disorders. Generally speaking, when poor appetite results from a minor disorder such as a common cold (II/2), a FEVER or following injury, it is better not to try to force food but to allow the appetite to return of its own accord.

Anorexia nervosa A nutritional illness of psychological origin, found most commonly in women in their teens and twenties and featuring severe weight-loss. See XIV/8.

Anus, bleeding from This can be due to a disorder of the digestive system, such as a peptic ulcer (see I/9) or a TUMOUR, giving the motions a black, tarry appearance due to altered blood. See MELAENA.
   Alternatively, the blood can be bright red and fresh, and most likely due to piles (I/34) or a FISSURE in the skin around the anus.
   As with bleeding elsewhere, the underlying cause should always be identified.

Anus, itching See PRURITUS ANI.

Anus, painful This can be due to piles (see I/34), bowel TUMOURS, or an anal FISSURE. See also PROCTALGIA.

Anxiety An unpleasant mood of tension and apprehension, arising for no concrete reason that is apparent to the patient. See XIV/4. Persistent anxiety, accompanied by symptoms, constitutes a neurotic illness.

Aphasia The inability to speak, due to a disorder of the brain. See DYSPHASIA.

Aphthous ulcer (mouth ulcer) See I/3.

Apoplexy (stroke) See IX/7.

Appendicitis Acute INFLAMMATION of the appendix. This is the commonest emergency in abdominal surgery, and needs to be dealt with before the appendix ruptures and causes PERITONITIS. See I/16.

Arrhythmia An abnormal, often irregular, heart rhythm. See HEART RHYTHM (irregular).

Arteries, hardening of (arteriosclerosis) Loss of elasticity and flexibility from the walls of arteries; one of the chief aspects of ageing. There is a loss of the normal expansion and recoil which occurs in the walls of healthy arteries as the heart pumps the blood rhythmically into the arterial system. After a time, the delivery of normal supplies of blood may be hampered to, for instance, the heart muscle, resulting in ANGINA.

Most hardening of the arteries is due to the deposition of fatty plagues within the lining of the arterial walls—see ATHEROMA. When the walls lose their smooth interiors and, in addition to losing their pliancy, become roughened, blood clots can form. See THROMBOSIS.

Arteriosclerosis   See ARTERIES (hardening of).

Arteritis, temporal   INFLAMMATION of the temporal artery or arteries of the scalp. A painful complaint, usually seen in elderly people, and treated with steroid drugs.

Arthritis   Pain and stiffness in a joint, due to INFLAMMATION or degenerative changes. Varieties include gout (see **VI/4**), osteoarthritis (see **VI/2**) and rheumatoid arthritis (see **VI/3**).

Asbestosis   See PNEUMOCONIOSIS.

Ascites   Collection of fluid in the abdominal cavity. The abdomen swells and becomes tense and uncomfortable. Causes include heart failure (**III/3**), cancer (**XIII**) within the abdomen or pelvis, and disorders of the kidneys and liver.

Asthma   A disorder typified by difficulty in breathing, especially in breathing out, due to muscular SPASM in the walls of the lungs' air tubes. See **II/15**.

Astigmatism   A common visual defect in which the front of the eyeball is not perfectly spherical. When the lines of an object are 'seen' clearly, those at right angles to them are distorted, resulting in a blurred image.

Orthodox treatment
Corrective spectacles.

Alternative treatment
Bates's eyesight training may be useful.

Ataxia   Lack of the muscular coordination required to perform a normal, voluntary movement (for instance, picking up a pencil or walking across a room). See also FRIEDRICH'S ATAXIA.

Atheroma   A fatty deposit, largely of cholesterol, in an arterial lining. The arterial walls become thick and stiff as a result, and this problem (known as atherosclerosis) is the commonest type of arteriosclerosis (see hardening of the ARTERIES). Besides hampering the free flow of blood within an artery, atheroma weakens the structure of its walls and makes it liable to bleed; it also encourages the formation of an ANEURYSM.
   Many factors are believed to encourage atheroma formation, the most important being excessive amounts of dietary saturated (animal) fats and refined sugar, a deficiency of fibre, overeating, insufficient exercise, obesity, tobacco smoking (very notably), a raised blood-pressure (see HYPERTENSION) and emotional stress.

Athlete's foot   INFECTION of the feet with ringworm fungus. See VII/6.

Attention deficit disorder   See HYPERACTIVITY.

Autism   A mental disorder, of unknown cause, appearing in children. It may possibly be related to schizophrenia in adults. See XIV/9.

Autoimmune diseases   See ALLERGY.

–B–

Backache   Pain in the back, arising either from the structures in this region or as a symptom of disorder elsewhere. The commonest cause is mechanical strain due to unaccustomed exercise or bad posture. Other causes include: a damaged vertebra; muscle SPASM; overweight (see WEIGHT PROBLEMS); tension (see STRESS REACTIONS); lack of exercise; and nerve compression. Conditions associated with backache include SCIATICA, slipped DISC, painful periods (see V/12) and SCOLIOSIS. See also FIBROSITIS, KYPHOSIS, LORDOSIS and LUMBAGO.
   Also known to aggravate back problems are remaining too long in

the same position (sitting or standing) and sleeping on either too soft or too hard a mattress. 'Emotional backache' is a form of PSYCHOSOMATIC DISORDER. The emotional disturbance involved is usually the result of constant stress (see STRESS REACTIONS); the back pain results from ligaments being weakened as a result of hormonal imbalance.

Orthodox treatment
For musculoskeletal backache, pain-killers such as paracetamol and aspirin and muscle-relaxant drugs such as diazepam (Valium) and chlormezanone (with paracetamol in Lobak) are generally prescribed.

Lumbar pain is sometimes dealt with by means of a fusion operation whereby two of the lower lumbar vertebrae are joined together. Traction and/or a corset are other alternatives. Hydrocortisone injections are sometimes given for back and shoulder pain to reduce local INFLAMMATION.

Alternative treatments
Osteopathy can be very useful in freeing strained joints and the accompanying restricted blood supply.
Chiropractic manipulation helps to correct posture and normalize joint movement.
The *Alexander technique* teaches the patient to correct his or her posture and to relinquish habits that stress and tense the body.
Applied kinesiology can help relieve back pain since its aim is to restore muscular balance and backache is very often due to muscular tension and imbalance.
Acupuncture is frequently used to relieve backache.
Relaxation has been found very helpful in the relief of 'emotional backache'. *Hypnotherapy* would also be useful in this context.

Bad breath (halitosis) See BREATH (bad).

Balanitis INFLAMMATION of the tip of the penis, usually caused by the foreskin being too tight to be pulled back properly (a condition known as 'phimosis'). In babies, ammonia from stale urine can irritate the penis tip. The condition needs investigation in older boys and men, as it may be a sign of diabetes mellitus ($X/2$) or of CANCER of the penis.

Orthodox treatment
Babies' balanitis is treated by changing the nappies more frequently, washing the area well, drying thoroughly, and applying antiseptic cream.

Herbal remedy
Bathe, dry, and apply *Aloe vera* gel.

Baldness (alopecia)   See VII/5.

Bedsores   Large, open sores arising at the body's pressure points in bedridden, debilitated or paralysed patients who cannot move about in bed. The commonest sites are the heels, ankles, hips and buttocks, where skin and flesh are pressed by the patients' weight against a bony surface. Often little PAIN is felt, as the pressure prevents the conduction of pain messages back to the brain.
   A badly fitting fracture plaster can also produce pressure sores.
   Preventive measures include efficient and regular skin cleansing, frequent changing of the patient's position, and cushioning of those parts likely to be affected. Treatment includes immediate relief from pressure as well as careful cleansing and dressing of the sores.

Herbal remedy
In addition to the above treatment, a lotion made up by decocting one handful each of fresh periwinkle leaves and of flowers in a litre of water can be used. Bathe the sore with this whenever dressings are changed.

Bed-wetting (enuresis)   By their third birthday the majority of children are dry at night, but those who continue to pass urine while they are asleep tend to do so for emotional rather than physical reasons. Anger with the child tends only to worsen the condition. Drugs can be prescribed, but a better method of treatment is the use of an electrical alarm system, which rings a bell and wakes the child up as soon as a special pad becomes damp.

Aromatherapy
Rub the child's lower abdomen before he/she goes to bed with olive oil and 10 per cent cypress essence (*Cupresses sempervirens*). Also, give child three drops of this essence three times daily between meals on a little brown sugar.

Bee sting   See STINGS.

Belching (burping)   The passage of gas from the stomach up through the foodpipe (oesophagus) and mouth, generally accompanied by a sound. It is often a sign of eating or drinking too rapidly, so that air is introduced with the food/drink into the digestive tract, or of drinking very gaseous liquids. Swallowing too much gas at once (for instance, by drinking straight from a can of beer or cola) can cause severe gastric pain which is relieved by the passage of the gas.

Traditional treatment
Sucking a strong peppermint has a 'carminative' effect—i.e. it causes stomach wind to be released.

Beriberi   See DEFICIENCY DISEASES.

Bile   The bitter fluid stored in the gall bladder and passed into the small bowel (duodenum) to help digest fats. It is sometimes returned to the mouth during a VOMITING attack or in the condition known as ACID STOMACH.

Bilious attack   The term really implies an attack 'affected by BILE', but it is often used simply to denote an attack of NAUSEA and VOMITING.

Birthmark (naevus)   A skin blemish present at birth, as displayed by many babies. Birthmarks can be due to a collection of pigment cells or to visible blood vessels. The latter (vascular) type—bright red and raised slightly—is known as a strawberry mark; it usually enlarges before shrinking and then finally disappearing altogether. At present the only known way of dealing with birthmarks is by surgical removal —although, of course, being generally harmless they are usually just left alone.

Blackout   Momentary loss of consciousness due to insufficient oxygen reaching the brain cells. Pilots occasionally 'black out' when they fly in excess of a certain speed because the blood is propelled away from the head. A sudden fall in blood-pressure on standing up suddenly can also cause a brief loss of consciousness (see HYPOTENSION). See also BREATH-HOLDING.

Bleeding disorders   A group of abnormalities in which bleeding either starts when it ought not to or fails to stop when it should. There are three ways in which the normal mechanisms which control bleeding can be disturbed.

- The tiny blood vessels (capillaries) can become very fragile (see SCURVY).
- There can be a fall in the number of platelets (small particles in the

blood, responsible for plugging damaged blood vessels to prevent bleeding). This can occur in normal people for no apparent reason, or result from diseases of the bone marrow, such as leukaemia (see VIII/3) and as a result of RADIATION SICKNESS.

- One of the blood chemicals or 'factors' responsible for clot formation may be missing (see HAEMOPHILIA).

Blister   A pocket in the outer layer(s) of skin, containing fluid. Causes include BURN injuries, rubbing garments or shoes, or certain disorders (for example, SHINGLES rashes appear at first as blisters). Friction blisters can safely be popped with a sterile needle after the area has been washed and patted dry. Large burn blisters should be dealt with by a qualified practitioner.

Blood, coughing up (haemoptysis)   A sign of disease (for example, TUBERCULOSIS [see **XII/8**] or CANCER [see **XIII**] or injury to part of the air passages or lungs. A qualified practitioner should always be consulted.

Blood, loss of   See HAEMORRHAGE.

Blood, vomiting of (haematemesis)   This is a sign of disease or injury to part of the upper digestive tract, such as the stomach or foodpipe (oesophagus). A qualified practitioner should always be consulted.

Blood poisoning   INFECTION of the blood. Often infection spreads from an original site (e.g. a wound) first into the surrounding tissues (CELLULITIS) and ultimately to other parts of the body by means of the bloodstream (SEPTICAEMIA).

Blood pressure   For raised blood pressure see HYPERTENSION; for low blood pressure see HYPOTENSION.

'Blue baby'   A newborn baby in which, due to a congenital heart defect, some of the blue (deoxygenated) blood is circulated around the body rather than passing to the lungs for reoxygenation. One of the commonest causes is HOLE IN THE HEART.

Body odour (BO)   Bacterial action on sweat, in the absence of sufficient oxygen, produces the characteristic 'coffee-grounds' or 'over-ripe-cheese' odour. Areas where this is most likely to occur are in the armpits, between the toes and in the genital area since, for most of the year in temperate climates, all of these regions are covered with one or more layers of clothing. The best way of combating the problem is to wash daily, dry the affected area(s) thoroughly, and use plenty of talcum powder between the toes and in the pubic region (without getting powder in the immediate area of the urethral opening or in or on the vaginal lips).

Antiperspirants and deodorants are usually recommended by chemists and doctors for underarm odour, but recently there has been some concern about products containing aluminium compounds since they might prove toxic. 'Intimate' deodorants (i.e. for use in the vaginal area) are effective but best avoided by anyone prone to cystitis (see **IV/5**).

It is also helpful to avoid nylon underwear. Cotton garments and loose-fitting clothes that allow air to reach the areas where sweat gathers are good choices.

Mineral-supplement treatment
20–30mg chelated zinc daily. Baking soda (sodium bicarbonate) between the toes and in the armpits is an alternative to commercial products.

Boil
A small ABSCESS inside a sweat gland or surrounding a hair root. Several boils grouped together comprise a carbuncle. A common place to find a boil is on the back of the neck.

Botulism   A highly dangerous, fortunately rare, form of FOOD POISONING.

Bradycardia   An abnormally slow pulse, at a rate of less than 60 beats/minute. Causes include pressure on the brain. A common type is sinus bradycardia, which is often found among healthy individuals.

Breath, bad (halitosis)   Common causes of halitosis are bad teeth and poor dental hygiene (see **I/4**). THRUSH infection of the digestive tract can be another cause of bad breath, which can also accompany chronic CONSTIPATION.

Herbal treatments
Common herbal remedies for bad breath include chewing parsley, drinking peppermint or fenugreek tea, and taking chlorophyll tablets. In all cases, however, the underlying cause(s) of the halitosis should be treated.

Breath-holding Holding the breath causes the waste carbon dioxide which we normally exhale to gather in the blood, which at the same time becomes increasingly short of oxygen. Ultimately, the respiratory centre in the brain is stimulated and a breath is drawn by reflex action. It is possible by holding the breath to BLACKOUT for a few seconds, something which some young children use as a means of attracting attention.

Breathlessness There are many causes, ranging from physical exertion to PANIC ATTACKS. Chronic shortage of breath may be due to a lung disorder, anaemia (see **VIII/1**), heart failure (see **III/3**) or chronic anxiety (**XIV/4**). A medical practitioner should always be consulted.

Bronchiectasis A chronic condition of one or more of the main air tubes (bronchi) of the lungs, which become stretched and fail to regain their normal shape and size. Mucus (PHLEGM) collects in the nearby area of lung and generally becomes infected. A typical symptom is an early morning COUGH. There are several causes of bronchiectasis, including the congenital disorder CYSTIC FIBROSIS, whooping cough (see **XII/4**) and pneumonia (see **II/14**). Orthodox doctors prescribe antibiotics and cough elixirs to reduce the stickiness of the mucus.

Traditional treatment
A tablespoonful each of fresh lemon juice and honey, taken up to eight times daily, for a bronchial cough. Honey also helps fight INFECTION.

Bronchitis INFLAMMATION of the air tubes in the lungs. See **II/11** and **II/12**.

Bronchopneumonia INFLAMMATION of the lung. See **II/14**.

Bruising Bleeding under the skin from damaged capillaries (minute blood vessels). This usually results from a fall or from a hard blow to the area, which injures the capillaries causing them to leak blood, but can also occur when the capillaries themselves are fragile (see SCURVY). Bruising also occurs spontaneously when the number of platelets in the blood falls below a certain level (see THROMBOCYTOPENIA and BLEEDING DISORDERS).

Orthodox treatment
This generally consists of bathing the area with cold water (also a form of hydrotherapy see page 94).

Herbal treatment
Swab with a solution of witch hazel, available from chemists' shops.

Homeopathic treatment
Arnica ointment.

Bulimia See **XIV/8**.

Bunion A swelling of the joint between the first metatarsal bone and
the base of the large toe, with an overlying tissue sac or bursa (see
BURSITIS) which becomes inflamed and painful due to shoe pressure.
Minor cases can be relieved by changing to soft, comfortable footwear
and sometimes by splinting the bones to correct their faulty position.
Severe bunion deformities can be corrected by surgery.

Burns Burn injuries can result as much from contact with corrosive or
boiling liquids, an electric current or radiation as from naked flames,
the common factor being the destruction or 'denaturation' of protein,
resulting in the death of tissues. The severity of a burn injury depends
upon the area of tissue destroyed and the volume of fluid (plasma) that
leaks from damaged capillaries. When a burn exceeds 15 per cent of an
adult's (10 per cent of a child's) skin area the blood circulation is likely
to be affected. SHOCK results unless the lost fluid is replaced by an
intravenous drip; this is one of the most important early aspects of
dealing with burn injuries.
  Local treatment of the burnt area depends upon its depth. *First-
degree burns* involve only the outer, non-vital (i.e. dead) layer of skin
cells and require little beyond the application of soothing antiseptic
ointment and perhaps treatment for shock. *Second-degree burns* involve living tissue but leave enough undamaged for new skin to develop.
Careful cleansing and wound-care under sterile conditions are important, as INFECTION must be avoided at all costs. *Third-degree burns*
destroy the whole skin thickness, and the area can best be protected by a
skin graft. This speeds recovery and reduces the risks of infection and
scar formation. When a large area of scar tissue is allowed to develop,
shrinkage inevitably occurs and deformity results.
  First aid for burn injuries normally includes immersion of the area in
cold water. This applies equally to corrosive burns, for attempting to
neutralize them with their chemical opposite (e.g. an acid with an alkali)
generates heat and worsens matters. BLISTERS should be punctured only
under sterile conditions. The best first-aid burns dressing is a piece of
sterile gauze or of freshly laundered household linen. Butter, cooking oil

and other non-sterile substances should under no conditions be applied to burns, as infection can easily result.

A good rule of thumb is to seek professional advice for all but the most trivial of burn injuries. In particular, burns from electric currents can be misleading as the damage occurs below the level of the skin and is generally worse than it appears to be.

Herbal/vitamin treatment
Aloe vera plant extract has been used under medically sterile conditions to treat burns[1], and can produce rapid healing in some patients. Rapid healing has also been claimed for the application of Vitamin E oil and for treatment with Vitamin C. This latter has been applied as a 1 per cent solution to the burned area, and also administered to patients by mouth or by injection four times every day, in doses of 200–500mg[2].

Bursitis The INFLAMMATION of a bursa, a small sac of fibrous tissue with a smooth, moist lining like that in the interior of a joint. Bursas are a part of our normal anatomy, and are found sandwiched between tendons or ligaments and underlying bone, where they help to reduce friction. Examples are found on the front of the kneecap or patella, around the shoulder joint and over the point of the elbow. Additionally, bursas may arise as a result of unusual pressure or friction.

Bursitis, too, generally develops in response to repeated friction or pressure. The sac becomes filled with fluid and the overlying skin becomes inflamed. Some types of bursitis are named after the trade with which they are most frequently associated, e.g. HOUSEMAID'S KNEE and dustman's shoulder. The most effective treatment is to remove the source of pressure or friction causing the trouble.

Byssinosis A lung disease caused by inhaling dust, bacteria, moulds and fungi present in flax, cotton and hemp. See PNEUMOCONIOSIS.

–C–

Cachexia Severe weight-loss and wasting of the body due to an underlying illness. The fact that muscular tissue is lost as well as body-fat helps to distinguish cachexia from the emaciation caused by starvation (as in ANOREXIA NERVOSA) where stored body-fat is used up before muscle. Cachexia is a frequent feature of cancer (see **XIII**).

Calcaneal spur   A small spur-shaped projection of bone growing out of the back of the heel bone or calcaneum. This can give rise to persistent pain on walking, and is diagnosed by X-ray. The best form of treatment is surgical removal of the spur of bone.

Calcium deficiency   The main diseases linked to a calcium deficiency are RICKETS, OSTEOMALACIA (due also to a deficiency of Vitamin D) and, most importantly, osteoporosis (see **VI/8**).

The recommended daily intake of calcium for an adult man or woman is 800–1,200mg[3]; in one study as much as 1,400mg daily was found necessary to keep calcium in neutral balance in post-menopausal women, 1,000mg in pre-menopausal women. Up to 2,500mg daily has been found necessary to produce a positive calcium balance in women with post-menopausal osteoporosis[4].

Best natural sources include milk and milk products, sardines, salmon and peanuts. Two reliable supplements are dolomite (five dolomite tablets supply 750mg of calcium) and chelated calcium. (See also IRON DEFICIENCY.)

Calculus   (1) A chalky deposit found around the base of the teeth. (2) See STONE.

Cancer   See **XIII**. For cancer of the foodpipe (oesophagus) see **I/8**; for cancer of the pancreas see **I/20**; for cancer of the gall bladder see **I/28**; for large-bowel cancer see **I/33**; for bladder cancer see **IV/6**; for breast cancer see **V/I**; for cancer of the cervix see **V/9**; for cancer of the blood see **VIII/3**; and for cancer of the brain see **IX/4**. See also CARCINOMA.

Candida infection   INFECTION with the yeast microbe *Candida* (*Monilia*) *albicans*. See THRUSH.

Carbohydrate intolerance   Often misinterpreted as an allergy, true carbohydrate intolerance is due to a lack of certain enzymes secreted by the small intestine. The function of these is to break down the large molecules of dietary sugars (disaccharides) into simpler molecules (monosaccharides) which can then be absorbed. The most usual enzyme to be missing is lactase, which breaks down lactose (milk sugar) into glucose and galactose. Lactose itself cannot be absorbed, and, when it remains in the bowel, acts as a purgative, attracting water to itself and causing DIARRHOEA; this is the characteristic symptom of carbohydrate intolerance. Other symptoms include a 'bubbly', unsettled sensation in the abdomen, gaseous distension and WIND. The large amounts of gas are a result of unabsorbed sugar in the large bowel.

When it is lactase which is absent, the symptoms arise after milk and milk products have been taken. Two other enzymes, sucrase and maltase, can also be absent, although this is much less common; symptoms then arise after foods containing sugar and starch have been eaten. Some patients diagnosed as having spastic colon (see I/30) in fact suffer from lactose intolerance.

Carcinoma   A cancer (see **XIII**) which develops in covering and lining membranes; for example, bronchogenic carcinoma is cancer arising from the cells lining the air-tube (bronchus). Carcinoma is the most usual form of cancer. See also SARCOMA. For carcinoma of the liver see I/25; for carcinoma of the ovary see V/2.

Caries   Dental decay. See I/4.

Carpal tunnel syndrome   Symptoms of pins-and-needles, pain and numbness in the thumb and first three fingers, often associated with weakness of the thumb muscles. The cause is compression of the median nerve, which enters the hand at the wrist joint by passing through an anatomical space called the 'carpal tunnel'. INFLAMMATION or injury can result in the compression of the median nerve within the carpal tunnel, but often there is no apparent cause. The condition is commonest in middle-aged or pregnant women.

Orthodox treatment
A usual form of treatment is to inject the area with hydrocortisone and/or splint the wrist at night. Persistent symptoms usually respond to a simple operation in which the fibrous band covering the wrist tendons is cut.

Vitamin treatment
It is now believed[5] that drug-induced pyridoxine (Vitamin B$_6$) deficiency—for example, by some monoamine oxidase inhibitor antidepressant drugs—can cause carpal-tunnel syndrome. Pyridoxine supplementation can correct both the deficiency and the syndrome, and it is certainly worth trying a course of organic pyridoxine before accepting the offer of surgical relief. The dose used was 300mg pyridoxine daily

over an eight-week period. Such treatment should form part of a normal supplementation programme (see page 436).

Cataract A disorder of the lens of the eye, most often found in elderly people but sometimes caused by injury and occasionally present at birth due to faulty development. The lens is opaque rather than transparent; vision is dim, and sometimes lost altogether.

Orthodox treatment
This consists of removing the lens, and is usually very effective. Poor focusing ability can be corrected with spectacles.

Catarrh For catarrh affecting chest, throat and nasal passages, see PHLEGM. For vaginal catarrh (leukorrhoea) see WHITES.

Catatonia A severe type of schizophrenic attack (see **XIV/1**) in which the patient is in a remote and trance-like state. He/she may remain in the same position, absolutely motionless, for hours on end.

Cellulitis INFLAMMATION of tissue cells. A common cause is INFECTION by streptococcal bacteria following a contaminated wound.

Orthodox treatment
Antibiotics are often necessary to prevent the condition from spreading further into adjacent tissues.

Herbal treatment
A compress of half a handful each of ivy and celandine to two litres of water; or bathe with the same ingredients. Also, an infusion of a pinch of each of the following in two cupfuls of water: mint, lavender, lime flowers, basil and vervain.

Cerebral haemorrhage Bleeding within the brain. See **IX/7**.

Cerebral palsy See SPASTICITY.

Cheloid See KELOID.

Chest pain PAIN in the chest due to a disorder therein, or in the diaphragm or chest wall. See ANGINA PECTORIS, HEARTBURN, PLEURISY and **II/11**. Like unexplained pain anywhere, chest pain should always be investigated.

Chickenpox (varicella).   A common infectious illness normally contracted during childhood. See **XII/1**.

Chilblain   An itchy, burning swelling arising typically on the toes and fingers in cold weather. In people who are highly sensitive to the cold, the blood vessels in the skin contract to such an extent that the extremities are deprived of blood and oxygen. Chilblains are the outcome.

Poor skin circulation, and hence chilblains, are aggravated by tobacco smoking (nicotine causes further constriction of the small blood vessels), and improved by alcohol. The best remedy is prevention, which means wearing adequate clothing in cold weather.

Orthodox treatment
Vasodilator drugs such as thymoxamine (Opilon), can be used to counteract the skin vessels' tendency to constrict at a low temperature. Doctors might also advise the use of an embrocation containing an aspirin derivative, menthol and camphor, such as Balmosa.

Traditional treatment
A single application of the following is said to relieve and generally cure bad chilblains. Take one tablespoonful each of honey and glycerine, and mix with an egg white and enough flour to make a fine paste. Spread over the chilblains, having made sure first that the inflamed areas are clean and dry. The chilblains should then be protected by a cloth as the paste is sticky. Leave for 24 hours.[6]

Chill   (1) An attack of shivering, or RIGOR, generally occurring during an infectious illness and due to a rapid rise in body temperature. (2) A popular expression for the effect of cold on the body—e.g. a 'chill on the bladder'. See **IV/5**.

Cholecystitis   Gall-bladder INFLAMMATION, usually associated with gallstones. See **I/26**.

Chondromalacia patellae   An early sign of degenerative change in the knee joint (between the kneecap—patella—and the lower end of the thigh bone, or femur). This condition produces PAIN and fluid inside the joint. It appears most often in young adults following an injury to the joint.

Orthodox treatment
Commonly, aspirin or non-steroidal anti-inflammatory drugs (NSAIDs) such as indomethacin (Indocid) and piroxicam (Feldene).

Manipulative therapy
Chiropractic manipulation may be helpful.

Chorea Uncoordinated movements of the body resulting from poor muscular control. *Huntington's chorea* is an inherited variety of this disorder, and is accompanied by progressive mental deterioration. Symptoms generally start when the patient is in his 30s or 40s, and life expectancy following diagnosis is between 5 and 20 years. *Sydenham's chorea* (St Vitus's dance) is now a rare disease of childhood. It is usually associated with RHEUMATIC FEVER, and is a complication of earlier INFECTION with a certain type of streptococcal bacteria.

Cirrhosis A disorder of the liver in which fibrous scar tissue gradually replaces healthy liver cells. See I/24.

Claudication (usually 'intermittent claudication') A limp caused by CRAMP in the calf muscles after walking a comparatively short distance. Like ANGINA PECTORIS in heart muscle, it is a result of diseased arteries bringing an inadequate supply of blood to the area (see ATHEROMA). The PAIN brings the sufferer to a halt after a certain distance, and disappears after resting.

Orthodox treatment
Surgery is sometimes possible, but the best treatment is regular, frequent exercise, which stimulates the growth of new, healthy blood vessels in the affected area.

Alternative treatment
Recovery can be greatly aided by combining walking with Vitamin E supplementation, (300–400iu daily). Trials conducted of this treatment show that improvement takes place over several months.[7]

Claustrophobia A terror of being confined in a small space. See XIV/7.

Cleft palate This and HARE LIP are developmental abnormalities present at birth, affecting one baby in 500. They are due to the various components of the lip and palate in the developing baby failing to grow towards one another and fuse. Surgery is the only realistic approach.

Climacteric   The menopause. See V/14.

Clubfoot (talipes)   A deformity of the foot, generally due to faulty development but sometimes due to bone INFECTION (see OSTEOMYELITIS), nerve injuries, polio (see XII/7), or an abnormality of the spine.

Orthodox treatment
Minor and moderate degrees of clubfoot often respond well to manual manipulation. In other cases, surgical correction of the deformity is required.

Manipulative therapy
Osteopathic manipulation may be helpful.

Coccydynia (coccygodynia)   INFLAMMATION of the coccyx ('tail' end of the spine), causing great discomfort when sitting on a hard surface, or driving a car.

Orthodox treatment
This includes warm sitz baths, massage, tranquillizers and local anaesthetic injections.

Manipulative therapy
Osteopathy is the most effective treatment. Sitting on a foam-rubber ring relieves the discomfort.

Coeliac disease   A disease most commonly found in small children, the chief symptoms being chronic DIARRHOEA and malnutrition. The small intestine of the sufferer is incapable of digesting and absorbing food properly, as a result of the intestinal lining being sensitive to gliadin, a protein found in gluten. Generally treatment is by keeping to a gluten-free diet for the rest of one's life. (See also GLUTEN INTOLERANCE and SPRUE.)
   The relationship between coeliac disease and gluten was discovered during the Second World War when Dutch children with the ailment were found to improve when bread was unavailable.

Cold   (1) The common cold. See II/1, II/2. (2) See CHILBLAIN, FROSTBITE, HYPOTHERMIA, and RAYNAUD'S DISEASE.

Cold abscess A slowly developing ABSCESS, generally tuberculous, with little apparent INFLAMMATION. See under tuberculosis (**XII/8**).

Cold sore A BLISTER on the lip due to an INFECTION by the *Herpes simplex* virus. See **XII/3**.

Colic Spasmodic PAIN arising from an internal organ, due to the powerful contraction of its muscular walls. It is usually a symptom either of INFLAMMATION (e.g. intestinal colic, as occurs in FOOD POISONING) or of obstruction (e.g. renal colic, which occurs when the kidney tube [ureter] is blocked by a STONE). WIND can often cause colic, especially in babies.

Colitis INFLAMMATION of the large bowel. The symptoms include mild abdominal discomfort (see ABDOMINAL PAIN), and CONSTIPATION or DIARRHOEA. These are followed by more severe abdominal pain, and sometimes by the passage of mucus and/or blood from the back passage (see ANUS [bleeding from]). See **I/29**, **I/30**.

Colour blindness The inability to distinguish between certain colours, most commonly between red and green. Women can pass on the defect to their sons; daughters will only be affected if they happen to have an affected father and a 'carrier' mother.

Coma A state of unconsciousness in which the activity of the brain is depressed and from which the sufferer cannot be aroused. Common causes include: HYPOGLYCAEMIA; POISONING (e.g. following a drug overdose, or too much alcohol); injury; and pressure on the brain due to a TUMOUR or ABSCESS.

Common cold See **II/1**, **II/2**.

Concussion Temporary disturbance of consciousness caused by the brain receiving a sharp jolt. The disturbance may be mild, or may consist of a deep COMA. See retrograde AMNESIA.
  Anyone who has been concussed—if only for a few seconds—should be carefully observed for the following 24 hours in case the brain is bleeding internally. The main symptoms are persistent drowsiness, NAUSEA and VOMITING.

Confusion Unclear, muddled thought processes, amounting to a definable symptom in certain disordering, e.g. DEMENTIA.

Congestion (1) Obstruction of the nasal passages, as occurs in the common cold (see II/1, II/2) and HAY FEVER.

(2) An accumulation of blood in one particular region of the body, due to increased supply (e.g. the pelvic organs during the premenstrual phase of the female cycle—see PREMENSTRUAL SYNDROME), or inefficient drainage (e.g. heart failure—see III/3).

Conjunctivitis See PINK EYE.

Constipation A reduction in the usual frequency with which a healthy person opens his/her bowels. Bowel habits are highly individual, and failure to open the bowels daily should not be regarded as a symptom requiring treatment. Symptoms of true constipation include lassitude, discomfort, abdominal distension, and hard, pellet-shaped motions. Possible causes include insufficient fibre in the diet, not enough exercise, the habitual use of drugs containing codeine or related compounds, and—unusually—a TUMOUR obstructing the large bowel.

Orthodox treatment
Laxatives (e.g. bisacodyl [Dulcolax], sterculia [Normacol]) in conjunction with dietary and exercise advice. Powerful purgative medicines should in the main be avoided.

Naturopathic treatment
Lifestyle advice regarding high-fibre diet and exercise.

Convulsion (fit, seizure) The uncoordinated jerking of muscles ordinarily under conscious control. Epilepsy (see IX/1) is one cause of convulsions; another very common one in childhood is high FEVER.

Corn A core of hardened, dead tissue in the outer layer of the skin, generally found on the foot. Common causes include badly fitting shoes and structural deformity.

Orthodox treatment
This usually consists of chiropody.

Herbal treatment
A trial carried out at the Marigold Clinic, St Pancras Hospital, London,[8] showed that 'mass' (material) from certain marigold (*Tagetes*) plants, used together with cavity pads, relieved the pain after one application, and the same results were obtained with callosities

(hard skin). Marigold products are manufactured by the Homoeo-pathic and Chiropody Laboratory Ltd under DHSS licence and patent number UK 2083356B.

Coronary thrombosis   The obstruction of a coronary artery by a clot of blood (thrombus), with consequent interruption of the blood supply to the relevant area of heart muscle. The irreversible damage normally suffered by the heart muscle as a result is called a myocardial INFARC-TION. It is this that is generally referred to when someone is said to have had a 'coronary', but in fact a THROMBOSIS or clot can occur in a coronary artery without damaging it, if the blood clot is small or if a good alternative arterial route exists.

Cough   Although a cough is often voluntary, the cough mechanism is basically a reflex action which expels irritants. It also arises as a symptom of many disorders of the windpipe (trachea), air tubes (bronchi) or lungs. Persistent dry coughs should always be investigated.

Orthodox treatment
This should be decided upon when the underlying cause has been determined. Relief of symptoms can be gained by use of 'anti-tussive' compounds which suppress the cough reflex (e.g. codeine linctus) and expectorants which help bring up PHLEGM (e.g. Actifed expectorant: triprolidine with pseudoephedrine and guaiphenesin).

Traditional treatment
For an obstinate cough, mix equal quantities of honey, linseed oil and whisky. Take a tablespoonful three or four times a day.[9]

Cramp   A painful, sustained contraction of a muscle or group of muscles. Examples are COLIC (although this has other causes); 'night cramp' in the muscles of the calf or foot; CLAUDICATION; and ANGINA PECTORIS.
   A sudden cramp in the calf can best be relieved by gently stretching the clenched muscles. Adding salt to the diet can help, should the cramp have been caused by excessive loss of sodium chloride in heavy perspiration.

Orthodox treatment
For 'night cramp', quinine sulphate tablets.

Dietary supplement treatment
For 'night cramp', Vitamin E (300–400iu daily) and/or dolomite or bonemeal tablets (4–6 tablets before retiring).

Crohn's disease ('regional ileitis', 'regional enteritis') This is an inflammatory disorder of the bowel, generally affecting the ileum (the last part of the small intestine). See I/15.

Croup A disorder of small children due to INFLAMMATION of the epiglottis, the chief symptoms being difficulty in breathing, and a harsh, croaky COUGH. See II/9.

Cyst An abnormal, benign swelling in the body, containing fluid or semisolid material. An example is the very common wen, or sebaceous cyst, which forms from a sebaceous gland in the skin when its opening becomes clogged.

Cysticercosis See WORMS.

Cystic fibrosis (mucoviscidosis) An inherited disorder chiefly affecting the function of the pancreas and lungs. The underlying problem is the production of thick, sticky mucus, which blocks the pancreatic duct and the small air passages in the lungs. The pancreatic digestive enzymes fail to reach the duodenum, and digestion of certain nutrients —particularly fat—is affected. The motions are bad-smelling, bulky and pale because of their high fat content, and malnutrition often results unless treatment is started early.

In the lungs, obstruction of small airway passages results in severe impairment in lung function, and in serious and frequent chest INFECTION.

The sweat test is usually used to confirm the diagnosis of cystic fibrosis. The sweat of someone suffering from the condition contains an abnormally large amount of sodium. The high fat content of the motions of the patient following a test meal also indicates the disorder, as does a history of lung complaints. Blood tests can also be used to confirm the diagnosis.

Orthodox treatment
This consists of a low-fat diet plus pancreatic enzymes and fat-soluble vitamins (A, D, E) taken orally. Antibiotics, inhalations and chest physiotherapy are also given.

Naturopathic/dietary treatment
Fresh vegetable juices, used to clear the body of mucus. Recommended for a six-month-old child with the illness is 30g of white radish juice and 150g of carrot juice, freshly juiced and strained through cheesecloth into a feeding bottle.[10] (As a substitute for the 30g of white radish juice, 30g of any of the following juices can be used: beetroot, cucumber, spinach.) Later the child should be weaned onto oatmeal, millet, lamb, white meat of turkey and chicken, and white fish (all with pancreatin added), plus fresh vegetables, blended in a liquidiser.

Cystitis   INFLAMMATION of the membranous lining of the bladder. See IV/5.

–D–

Dandruff (scurf)   A condition of the scalp in which dead skin cells are shed in greater numbers than normal; occasionally, it may take the form of thick, greasy scales. Sufferers are sometimes more prone than others to bacterial skin INFECTION, and their skin may be supersensitive to chemicals. Dandruff is commoner in people with greasy skin, and is often associated with acne (VII/1) and ROSACEA. Professor John Yudkin believes that dandruff may be associated with a high consumption of sugar, which contains no B vitamins but depletes the supplies already present.[11]

Orthodox treatment
Cetrimide or selenium sulphite shampoo. A mild, unmedicated shampoo designed for babies is often more effective if used daily.

Dietary/herbal treatment
Omitting sugar from the diet often helps. The Vitamin B complex in the recommended daily supplement should prove especially helpful.
   Scalp itchiness frequently responds dramatically to Vitamin E oil applied to the scalp every night for two or three weeks. Only a loose scarf should be worn if it is felt necessary to protect the pillow case.[11]
   Another remedy is daily application of a hair tonic made by infusing 30g each of rosemary and sage in half a litre of water for 24 hours.

Deafness Impairment or loss of hearing, generally due to a defect of the ear or of the auditory nerve. When the fault lies in the conduction of sound vibrations from the surrounding atmosphere to the internal ear, the deafness is called *conductive deafness*. When the problem lies between the internal ear and the brain, it is known as *nerve deafness*. *Mixed deafness* is a combination of these two. The fourth variety of deafness—*psychogenic deafness*—is the result of emotional upset.

Tuning forks are often used to test hearing. The selected fork is made to vibrate, and its base is then applied to the forehead of the patient. In this way, sound is conducted both by the bone of the skull and by the air. Deafness caused by poor air conduction can be differentiated from problems associated with abnormal bone conduction (and sometimes from nerve deafness). The difference is important in the choice of hearing aid: the type inserted into the ear amplifies air-conducted sound, and the type placed behind the ear amplifies bone conduction.

Deficiency diseases Diseases caused by dietary deficiency. Examples are kwashiorkor, a protein-deficiency disease which claims many lives in underdeveloped countries, and beriberi, also prevalent in underdeveloped countries, which is due to a shortage of Vitamin B_1 (thiamine). RICKETS, caused by lack of Vitamin D, iron-deficiency anaemia, and SCURVY, due to a shortage of Vitamin C, are other examples.

As more is becoming known about the importance in the diet of vitamins, minerals and trace elements, more modern deficiency conditions are being identified.

Degenerative diseases Disorders comparable to and often associated with the ageing process, but distinct from it in that they are prevalent in one particular body system. The factors common to most degenerative disorders are a loss of active tissue cells, the development of extra connective tissue, and a reduction in tissue flexibility. Examples include arteriosclerosis (see hardening of the ARTERIES and ATHEROMA), osteoarthritis (see **VI/2**) and senile DEMENTIA.

Dehydration Condition in which the total water content of the body is abnormally low, due either to the loss of a large amount of fluid from the body (as in DIARRHOEA or VOMITING) or to too little water being consumed—or to a combination of both. Excessive sweating in a hot atmosphere can also cause grave water depletion, as can untreated DIABETES and certain kidney disorders in which large volumes of urine are excreted. Water loss from the body invariably involves a depletion of the body's mineral salts—potassium, in particular, is lost during vomiting and diarrhoea, and may reach dangerously low levels which can impair the function of the heart.

Water deprivation can result either from an insufficient supply or from the patient's inability to swallow or to retain fluid in the stomach during a vomiting attack.

Symptoms of severe dehydration are thirst, loss of skin elasticity, exhaustion, muscular weakness and DELIRIUM. The correct treatment is the gradual replacement of the lost fluid, either by mouth or by intravenous drip. (See also DIARRHOEA).

Déjà vu Meaning literally 'already seen', this term refers to the feeling that people, places or situations encountered for the first time are in fact familiar. Normal individuals can experience déjà vu, especially when very tired. It also affects some epileptic patients (see EPILEPSY), in whom it can herald an attack, and people suffering from phobic anxiety neurosis (see XIV/4). See also JAMAIS VU.

Delirium A disturbance of the brain in which consciousness is affected, and confusion and disordered perception occur. The patient is extremely restless and anxious, and frequently suffers from HALLU-CINATIONS which increase his/her level of fear and excitement. The onset is usually sudden, and an attack may last for a few hours or for several days. Causes include: head injury; FEVER; some INFECTIONS; excessive amounts of certain drugs (e.g. amphetamine—'speed'—and some antidepressants); brain HAEMORRAGE; brain TUMOUR; and abrupt drug or alcohol withdrawal from a dependent person (see DRUG DEPENDENCE).

Skilful nursing of the delirious patient is essential, as are identification and treatment of the underlying cause. Sedatives are sometimes prescribed to combat extreme restlessness and the dangers of self-injury and physical exhaustion.

Delirium tremens ('DTs') The type of DELIRIUM caused by abrupt alcohol withdrawal after a lengthy bout of intoxication. One patient in four experiences a full-blown epileptic fit (see EPILEPSY) at the start of an attack, and the 'shakes' (uncontrollable trembling), restlessness and terrifying HALLUCINATIONS are usually prominent features.

Sedatives and anticonvulsants offer useful short-term control of an attack, but the only really effective management of 'DTs' comprises treating the underlying chronic alcoholism.

Delusion A firmly held belief which is clearly irrational (to a normal individual), and which cannot be explained in terms of the patient's educational, social and religious upbringing or environment. Examples of delusions are persecution fears, or the personal conviction of being, say, Napoleon, Julius Caesar, or a millionaire—or, conversely, of being a worthless 'nobody'. Delusions are symptomatic of certain mental illnesses such as manic-depressive psychosis (see **XIV/2**) and schizophrenia (see **XIV/1**).

Dementia Mental deterioration—in particular, poor memory for recent events—which results from physical changes in the brain. Degeneration, arterial disease, chronic POISONING, brain injury and INFECTION can all cause the condition.

The best known type, found among the elderly, is *senile dementia*, which arises as a result of degeneration of the brain cells, shrinkage of the brain and loss of the normal contours of the cerebral cortex. It can be distinguished from the usual mild loss of intellectual capacity common in old people by its progressive nature, the ultimate loss of all intellectual ability and emotional control, and the inevitable personality changes that occur.

A very similar type of dementia can occur in an elderly person as a result of atherosclerosis (see ATHEROMA) of the arteries of the brain. Occasionally, an identically progressive dementia occurs in a much younger person (Alzheimer's disease) and results in early death.

There is some evidence that nutritional deficiencies, of vitamins in particular, may be one of the causative factors in the development of senile dementia.[12] There has also been a suggestion that senile dementia and particularly Alzheimer's disease may be linked with aluminium toxicity.[13] A deficiency of choline (a B-complex vitamin) may also be a contributory factor.

Depression A common mental illness in which the chief symptom is intense misery, which either has arisen for no apparent reason or is disproportionate to the event that triggered it. See **XIV/3**.

Dermatitis Literally, INFLAMMATION of the skin. For all practical purposes, dermatitis can be taken to mean the same as eczema (see **VII/2**).

Diabetes The word 'diabetes' refers to the passage of abnormally large volumes of urine. *Diabetes insipidus* is a rare disease in which the large volumes of urine result from the deficiency of a hormone called ADH (antidiuretic hormone) secreted by the pituitary gland at the base of the brain. ADH is responsible for limiting the volume of urine formed by the kidneys. Lack of ADH secretion can result from INFLAMMATION, TUMOUR formation or injury to the pituitary gland, including surgery in that region.

For diabetes mellitus see X/2.

Diarrhoea The frequent passage of stools, or the passage of watery. The commonest cause is INFLAMMATION of the lining of the large bowel where the fluid part of our diet is normally absorbed. An inflamed bowel lining produces a watery mucus, and hampers the absorption of the fluid we ingest. The bowel contracts more frequently, so hastening the arrival of watery bowel contents at the rectum. The increased contractions of the inflamed bowel cause the COLIC pains we associate with an attack of diarrhoea, and the sudden arrival of fluid stools at the rectum causes the intense sense of urgency experienced during acute diarrhoea attack. The commonest cause of acute diarrhoea in a normally healthy person is INFECTION by a virus (as in GASTRO-ENTERITIS, especially in children) or by bacteria (e.g. bacterial FOOD POISONING).

If the diarrhoea is bloodstained, DYSENTERY may be the cause. *Salmonella* bacteria produce typical food poisoning within about 72 hours of the contaminated food being eaten. (See also TYPHOID FEVER.)

Holiday diarrhoea is due either to a harmful strain of *Escherichia coli* bacteria or simply to a change in the nature of the harmless bacteria normally present in the bowel. Holiday (or travellers') diarrhoea is usually self-limiting after a three-day period.

Other causes of acute diarrhoea include POISONING, drugs, food ALLERGY and poor tolerance of carbohydrates. Intense worry and ANXIETY can also be responsible, and these are best dealt with by learning effectively to deal with stress. The treatment of choice for most acute diarrhoea attacks is replacement of the lost salts and water. Half a litre of water added to a quarter-litre of fresh orange juice together with a teaspoonful of salt and a dessertspoonful of glucose is a reliable recipe. This should be drunk at the rate of half a litre per hour until the symptoms have subsided.

Chronic diarrhoea consists of increased frequency of bowel habit occurring over a period of time—the consistency and frequency of daily motions are less important. Possible causes include diverticulitis (see I/32), Crohn's disease (see I/15), spastic colon (see I/30), ulcerative colitis (see I/29), hyperthyroidism (see X/1), large-bowel TUMOURS, and certain types of MALABSORPTION.

33

Orthodox treatment

Diarrhoea is a symptom and its underlying cause should be established. However, the occasional attack may safely be treated symptomatically. Drugs used by orthodox doctors to control diarrhoea include loperamide (Imodium), diphenoxylate (Lomotil), and a suspension of kaolin together with codeine phosphate (Kaodene).

Homoeopathic treatment

For diarrhoea due to mild food poisoning: *Arsenicum Album*; for diarrhoea due to nervous excitement/anxiety about forthcoming events: *Argentum Nitricum*; for chronic, offensive, urgent stools, driving patient out of bed in the morning: *Sulphur*.

Diphtheria An acute INFECTION, almost invariably of the mucus membrane lining the throat. It was once a major cause of death in many countries, the two chief dangers being obstruction of the opening of the windpipe (trachea) and the poisonous effects of the toxin produced by the bacteria.

Disc, slipped A bulge in the tough casing of an intervertebral disc, resulting from severe strain. The gelatinous contents of the disc are squeezed into the bulge, and cause symptoms by pressing on nerve fibres. SCIATICA is a common outcome of a disc that has slipped in the lower lumbar region of the back.

Orthodox treatment

The PAIN can be excruciating, and patients are usually recommended by their doctors to lie flat on a hard surface (board beneath the mattress, mattress on floor, etc.) until it has eased a little. They are given muscle-relaxant drugs to ease the muscular SPASM (e.g. chlormezanone [Lobak], diazepam, [Valium]) and pain killers such as paracetamol or aspirin.

Manipulative therapy

Manipulation by either an osteopathic or a chiropractic practitioner can help a great deal with slipped discs.

Diverticulitis INFLAMMATION of small bulging pockets of large intestinal lining (diverticula) which protrude through the outer surrounding muscle at weak points. See I/32.

Dizzy spells There are several possible reasons for suddenly feeling dizzy. One of the commonest is low blood pressure (HYPOTENSION) of a postural type, which comes on as a result of getting up too quickly from the sitting or lying position. The small blood vessels are slow to respond to the change in posture, and dizziness is experienced for a few seconds until the blood supply to the brain is fully re-established.

Other causes are anaemia (see VIII/1), anxiety (see XIV/4), sudden blood-loss (see HAEMORRHAGE), PANIC ATTACKS, HYPOGLYCAEMIA and VERTIGO.

Down's syndrome   The old name for Down's syndrome was 'mongolism'. The condition affects about one child in every 600, and occurs most often in babies of mothers over the age of 40. Its characteristics are defective mental and physical development: adults with Down's syndrome have an intelligence equivalent to that of a child aged between 3 and 7 years. Physical characteristics include a flattish face, a round, small skull, slanting eyes which sometimes lack eyelashes, a large fat tongue, short stubby fingers and a characteristic skin crease across the palms of the hands.

Genetically, Down's-syndrome individuals have an extra chromosome, so that their total chromosome count is 47 instead of the usual 46. This has two possible causes. Either one of the smallest pairs of chromosomes in the mother fails to split when the egg (ovum) is formed. The resulting ovum then has 22 single chromosomes and one complete pair. (The correct configuration is 23 singles, which will pair up with the 23 single chromosomes in the sperm to form a normal embryo with the correct complement of 46, or 23 pairs.) If the ovum with a total of 24 chromosomes is then fertilized by a sperm, the resultant embryo will develop into a Down's-syndrome child with a total of 47 chromosomes.

The other possibility, which is far less common, is an abnormal chromosomal arrangement in one or other parent. The effect is confined to a tendency to form genetically abnormal sperm or ova, regardless of age.

Down's-syndrome children and adults are educable in only a limited way; but they are friendly, cheerful people, usually very gifted with animals and extremely fond of listening to music. They are nearly always very much loved by their families and relatives.

Down's-syndrome children have been found often to be zinc-deficient, and to have a lowered level in the blood of circulating thymic hormone, similar to that found in people over 50. It is believed that the decline in the activity of this hormone, both as people age normally and in the premature ageing noted in Down's-syndrome individuals, is more

35

likely to be due to a lack of zinc than to primary malfunction of the thymus gland.

Down's-syndrome children and adults have been found also to have low blood levels of selenium compared with normal people. Both of these findings emphasize the need for a full supplementation programme for Down's-syndrome subjects in order to allow them to function at their highest potential level. A test is available early in pregnancy which can reveal whether a developing baby will suffer from Down's syndrome.

Dropsy Swelling of the body due to fluid retention. See OEDEMA.

Drug dependence Traditional usage defines physical dependence on a drug as 'addiction' and psychological dependence as 'habituation', but the World Health Organisation prefers 'drug dependence' and 'drug abuse' as diagnostic terms.

Physical dependence implies that withdrawal symptoms occur if the drug is suddenly stopped or its dose radically reduced. This 'abstinence syndrome', as it is sometimes called, occurs because the body cells have become reliant upon regular amounts of the drug.

The *opiates* (morphine, heroin) invariably cause physical dependence, even when administered legally for the relief of severe PAIN, and ever-increasing doses are required by the body to achieve the same effect. Sudden withdrawal of the drug causes muscular CRAMPS, acute mental distress and profuse sweating.

Other potentially addictive drugs include *amphetamine compounds* ('speed'); amphetamine-like drugs used to curb the appetite, and which are abused because of the 'high' they induce (e.g. diethylpropion [Tenuate Dospan, Apisate]); *barbiturates* and other sleeping tablets (such as quinalbarbitone [Seconal] and nitrazepam—[Mogadon]); and *tranquillizers* such as diazepam (Valium), chlordiazepoxide (Librium), meprobamate (Equanil), and lorazepam (Atrian). When a person who has been taking Valium for months or years then tries to stop taking it, unpleasant symptoms are likely to develop, including sweating, NAUSEA, PANIC ATTACKS, unsteadiness, tearfulness, and PALPITATIONS, and perceptual changes; rarely, CONVULSIONS can occur. These symptoms prove very frightening, and the patient is likely to return to the drug as the lesser of the two evils.

Tobacco smoking is highly addictive; as is the use of *alcohol*, when it is heavy and regular.

Some of the *hallucinogens*, such as lysergic acid diethylamide (LSD, 'acid') and mescaline (from the peyote cactus), which alter perception, are very potent and can cause profound personality disorders, but are not physically addictive. *Cannabis* (marijuana, hemp, 'pot') is not addictive, but it is possible that it may cause harmful effects in other ways.

Cocaine ('Charlie', 'snow', 'crack') is rapidly broken down by the body and, when used infrequently in very small quantities, rarely produces physical dependence. It is capable of doing so if it is used chronically and in large quantities. Abrupt withdrawal produces strong cravings for the drug, prolonged sleep and intense fatigue. High doses can also result in cocaine psychosis, which has many features in common with classical schizophrenia. See **XIV/1**.

Glue sniffing (solvent abuse) has been recognized in the UK since 1970. The yearly death-toll rose from single figures during 1971–74 to 80 in 1983. The symptoms produced include intoxication, antisocial behaviour, HEADACHES and sometimes VOMITING. Telltale signs include glue-stains on the face or clothes, a RASH around the mouth, and a chemical smell on the breath. The habit does not appear to be addictive.[14]

Orthodox treatment

The best way to stop dependence upon a prescribed drug such as a tranquillizer (provided there is no special reason why the patient *has* to take it) is for the patient to work together with his/her general practitioner, coming off the drug little by little. It may take three to six months of hard effort, and supportive psychotherapy or hypnotherapy can be very helpful.

Patients on drugs with a short 'half-life', such as the benzodiazepines (lorazepam [Ativan], oxazepam [Serenid]. temazepam [Euhypnos]) generally have their dose cut by one-eighth every 2–4 weeks.[15] When a sufficiently low dose has been reached the patients are switched to the lowest suitable dose of a benzodiazepine with a long 'half-life', such as chlordiazepoxide (Librium) or diazepam (Valium).

Patients already on long-'half-life' benzodiazepine drugs (other examples are nitrazepam [Mogadon, Remnos], flurazepam [Dalmane] and chlorazepate [Tranxene]) likewise have their dose reduced by one-eighth every 2–4 weeks, until finally the drug is withdrawn. Unpleasant withdrawal symptoms are controlled using propranolol (Inderal), 60–120mg daily, or oxypertine (Integrin), 10–20mg daily.[15]

Tobacco smoking is sometimes treated with chewing-gum containing nicotine, to reduce the craving. A new treatment may soon prove efficient: it consists of one—or at the most two—injections of the steroid drug, Acthar gel.

Alcohol dependence (alcoholism) has been best researched by Alcoholics Anonymous, an excellent organization well worth recommending to anyone with a drinking problem, great or small.

Antabuse (disulphiram) is still prescribed by doctors as a deterrent to alcohol abuse: it induces severely unpleasant symptoms if alcohol is taken with it. Antabuse implants may soon be put into practice. Psychotherapy, including group therapy, is also used.

With respect to addiction to illegal drugs, heroin is available to registered addicts nowadays only through special centres and clinics. Addiction to heroin is a growing problem. Attempts to wean narcotics addicts off morphine, pethidine, etc., with methadone unfortunately created many methadone addicts. However, efforts are still made to ease patients off 'hard' drugs with less harmful drugs. Analysis and group therapy are also extensively employed. Such work is most effectively carried out in a drug-addiction centre specifically designed for the purpose and staffed by specialists in the field. Sympathetic support and encouragement from friends and family are enlisted wherever possible.

Alternative approaches

Naturopathy is applicable to all types of addiction. The needs of the addict as an individual are established with respect to the emotions, the diet, the exercise requirements, and the stress factors to be coped with.

The naturopathic approach usually involves the use of other forms of therapy, too. One of the best combinations is naturopathy with supplementary acupuncture and supportive hypnotherapy. Acupuncture, which has an excellent record with addiction cases, apparently works without the patient having to undergo withdrawal symptoms. Hypnotherapy, which is sometimes used with analysis, works by ego-strengthening and by aversion-planting.

There are a number of herbal treatments. Alcoholics can benefit from taking evening primrose oil (Efamol) as a source of gamma-linolenic acid (GLA), which many of them fail to manufacture in their bodies despite an adequate intake of linoleic acid. This occurs because alcohol blocks the chemical processes involved in the transformation of linoleic acid into GLA.

Taking Efamol (six capsules, with a multivitamin and mineral supplement) before a drinking session prevents a HANGOVER. In addition, it helps to prevent the mood-swing that results from a low GLA level (due to the consequent lowering of useful prostaglandins) and also helps to protect the liver from damage due to excessive intakes of alcohol.[16]

Chewing sunflower seeds is said to help relieve nicotine cravings.

Herbal medication can also be used to reduce the lengthy withdrawal regimens suggested by the description above of orthodox treatments. Herbs are prescribed not as substitute tranquillizers but to relax somatic (i.e. bodily) and psychological tensions, thus allowing the body and mind to regain a natural 'nervous tone'. This approach is based on the view that the innate healing mechanisms of the body will do what is necessary, given the chance: the herbs give that chance. Each patient has unique requirements, but both Skullcap and Valerian are likely to be prescribed. Supportive herbs might include Pasqueflower, Motherwort, Oats and Lavender.[15]

Dry-eye syndrome   Lack of sufficient tears. This can occur alone or as part of a disorder known as Sjogren's syndrome, in which there is accompanying dryness of the mouth and nose, and sometimes a form of arthritis (see VI/1).

When the dry eye occurs alone, it is believed to be due in part to a lack of an essential fatty acid which we make ourselves, called gamma-linolenic acid (GLA). This deficiency can be made good by supplying GLA direct as a dietary supplement. The dry eye of Sjogren's syndrome may also respond to this.

Herbal treatment
Evening primrose oil (Efamol), take three 500mg capsules twice daily together with daily nutritional programme.[17] (Evening primrose oil is a rich source of GLA.)

Duodenal ulcer   An erosion of the lining of the duodenum (small intestine) caused, like other varieties of peptic ulcer, by the corrosive action of acid and pepsin produced in the stomach. See I/11.

Dysarthria   Slurred speech, resulting from weakness of muscles involved in speech or from a disorder of the nervous pathways involved.

Dysentery   An INFECTION of the colon (large bowel) either by bacteria or by amoebae (tiny single-celled animals). The chief symptoms are DIARRHOEA, ABDOMINAL PAIN and blood and mucus in the stools. Both types of dysentery are spread by poor hygiene, in particular the failure to control flies around food and to wash and dry the hands after visiting the lavatory. See I/31.

Dyslexia   Great difficulty in comprehending the written or spoken word, coupled with inability to perceive the difference between left and right. Dyslexics, who are often of normal intelligence, may have any number of a wide range of language problems, all in general stemming from their failure to grasp the significance of letter, word and symbol sequences. A similar condition is *alexia*, but this is a result of disease of the brain's left hemisphere (right hemisphere in left-handed people). Alexics may only have difficulty in reading, while yet being able to write, speak and understand the spoken word perfectly capably; conversely, they may have trouble with all of these functions.

Different theories exist and sometimes conflict about the cause or causes of dyslexia. At one time it was attributed to 'brain lesions'. Since then it has been categorized as a type of 'organic brain dysfunction', a term applied to children who prove to be slow learners or who do not respond 'normally' to a particular stimulus. The underlying disorder here is thought to cause specific learning problems through the continued presence of certain central-nervous-system reflexes which in normal subjects become inhibited by a higher part of the brain during infancy, and through disturbance of the oculomotor cranial nerve which supplies some of the eye's muscles.[18]

It is also accepted that earlier educational traumatic experiences and other factors can hamper later learning.

Orthodox treatment
There are many orthodox approaches to the problem of dyslexia. They are mostly very time-consuming and take years of persevering application.

Applied kinesiology
The claim has been made that recent research using the simple muscle-testing and energy-balancing of basic applied kinesiology has uncovered ways to diagnose specific dyslexic patterns and to correct them, thus giving immediate help to sufferers. The new approach, developed in California, is called 'one-brain integration', and consists of balancing the right and left sides of the brain, and of overcoming 'blockages' between the front part of the brain (the area involved with present thought processes) and the back brain (involved in reasoning processes based upon past experiences).[19]

Dysmenorrhoea Abnormally painful periods. See V/12.

Dyspareunia Painful intercourse. This symptom is of two types. The first (primary dyspareunia) affects girls and women only, and is caused by the involuntary contraction of the pelvic muscles surrounding the vagina. This is a defence mechanism, known also as VAGINISMUS and often due to an association in the sufferer's mind between intercourse and pain, guilt or fear.

Secondary dyspareunia can be experienced by both sexes, and is 'secondary' to—i.e. a symptom of—some disorder such as a structural defect or INFLAMMATION. Examples are inflammation of the penis tip (see BALANITIS) in a man, and vaginal INFECTION in a girl or woman (see *vaginitis*, **V/8**).

Dysphagia Difficulty in swallowing. The commonest cause is a sore THROAT.

Dysphasia A speech difficulty, which may affect not only the spoken but also the written word. It is a result of a localized disorder of the speech pathways in the brain. Speech loss is termed *aphasia*. See SPEECH (disorders of).

–E–

Earache PAIN in the ear, commonly due to pressure, injury or INFLAMMATION. The eardrum is extremely sensitive, and pain due to unequal pressure on its inner and outer surfaces can be acute in sensitive people when swimming underwater or flying above a certain altitude. This problem can also arise when the Eustachian tube is blocked by catarrh, when EAR WAX accumulates or when a foreign body is introduced into the outer canal (small children often push beads, matchsticks, etc. into their ears). See **XI/2**.

Ear wax The accumulation of the yellow waxy secretion of the glands lining the outer ear canal. This can harden into solid brown lumps and severely impair hearing. It should first be softened with a special solvent or with warm olive oil. Later it can be removed by syringing the ear with warm water.

Herbal treatment
A little warm almond oil poured gently into the affected ear, and allowed to remain in place for as long as possible, helps to soften wax prior to syringing and may dissolve a small amount altogether. The oil should be introduced nightly for up to a week, depending upon results.

Eczema Non-infectious INFLAMMATION of the skin, arising in response to an irritant or as a result of ALLERGY. See VII/2.

Ejaculation, premature This is a very common problem, especially with young men, and can cause distress, embarrassment and tension early in marriage, especially if the man's partner is upset by it or unsympathetic. It consists of ejaculation occurring earlier in love-making than he or his partner would desire, and is usually due to incomplete control having been established over the ejaculatory impulse. Sexual counselling should be taken if the problem continues for too long.

One method that doctors sometimes recommend is for the woman to clasp her partner's penis firmly between thumb and finger just below the head of the penis. This should be done when the desire to ejaculate is starting to increase to orgasmic proportions. This sometimes enables control to be achieved by the man. No drugs are considered to be of any value.

Homoeopathic treatment
The most helpful remedy is *Lycopodium*. For the stressed, intolerant, angry person: *Nux vomica*.

Embolism Obstruction of a blood vessel by an embolus (clot of blood, air bubble, fat globule, or fragment of a TUMOUR carried in the blood stream). The effect depends upon the relative size of the vessel which becomes blocked, the importance of the part of the body deprived of blood, and whether blood can reach that part by any other route. A small embolus which obstructs the flow to one tiny section of leg muscle will pass unnoticed. An embolus big enough to block a large brain artery often results in a STROKE. A lung (pulmonary) embolism in which the pulmonary artery or a branch of it is obstructed results in death in 5 per cent of cases.

Clots of blood are a common variety of embolus. Usually, a clot will form on the wall or in the valves of the left side of the heart or inside a blood vessel (see THROMBOSIS). The leg and pelvic veins are common sites. The clot is then carried in the bloodstream and is likely to lodge in, and obstruct, a smaller vessel.

TUMOUR cells form an embolus when the tumour erodes a blood vessel and a piece breaks off. Fat globules can be released into the bloodstream when one of the long-limb bones is fractured and some of the bone-marrow fat dispersed. Air bubbles can enter the bloodstream if an intravenous injection is given incorrectly, and are a major hazard to 'main-lining' drug addicts. An air embolus in the heart can cause instant arrest of the heartbeat and death. Nitrogen bubbles in the bloodstream are responsible for the condition known as the 'bends' occurring in deep sea divers.

Emesis   See VOMITING.

Emphysema   Condition of the lungs in which the tiny air sacs (alveoli) become overdistended, resulting in the rupture of many of their thin dividing walls. See II/13.

Empyema (pyothorax)   A collection of pus in a cavity, generally inside the chest between the lung and the outer chest wall. See also ABSCESS and PLEURISY.

Encephalitis   INFLAMMATION of the brain, generally due to a virus. Encephalitic conditions are today largely unknown in the West, although on rare occasions they may arise as part of a mumps attack (see XII/6). Other ailments associated in one way or another with encephalitis include polio (see XII/7) and Parkinson's disease (see IX/3).

Endometriosis   The presence of fragments of the same type of tissue as that lining the womb (uterus) in abnormal sites in the pelvis (e.g. inside the ovary) or within the muscular wall of the womb itself. See V/11.

Endometritis   INFLAMMATION of the lining of the womb or uterus (endometrium), due in most cases to bacterial INFECTION. See V/6.

Enteritis   INFLAMMATION of the intestine, generally the small intestine. INFECTION by bacteria or viruses present in food (see FOOD POISONING) or water is the commonest cause. When the stomach lining is inflamed as well the condition is known as gastroenteritis (see I/14). Symptoms are HEADACHES, DIARRHOEA, VOMITING and FEVER. Other causes include food ALLERGY and excessive amounts of alcohol.
   Chronic enteritis is associated with MALABSORPTION. Regional enteritis is chronic inflammation of an isolated segment of small bowel (see Crohn's disease, I/15).

Enuresis   See BED-WETTING.

Epidemic parotitis   Mumps. See XII/6.

Epilepsy   Any of several different types of recurrent attack produced by disorganized electrical activity in the brain. See IX/1.

Epistaxis   See NOSEBLEED.

Ergot poisoning   POISONING due to items of food made from rye infected with the fungus *Claviceps purpurea* which contains ergot alkaloids. Death can occur. Other victims have developed gangrene in fingers and toes due to the constrictive effect of ergot on the walls of arteries.

Erysipelas   A dangerous, contagious skin INFECTION due to the bacterium *Streptococcus pyogenes* contaminating a surgical wound or minor abrasion. The inflamed area of skin is bright red and swollen, with a clearly demarcated edge, and it spreads diffusely unless successfully treated. The patient is likely to run a high FEVER and suffer from NAUSEA and VOMITING. The use of appropriate antibiotics is usually highly effective. In untreated patients, the infection can spread and lead to collapse and death.

Herbal treatment
Foot baths and hand baths of a handful of each of the following in two litres of water: artichoke leaves, fern leaves, nettle leaves.

Extrasystole (ectopic beat)   An extra systole (contraction) of the heat muscle, in which a 'flutter', 'missed beat' or additional beats are felt. Derived from an impulse which arises outside the normal controlling system, extrasystoles are usually harmless and do not, of themselves, indicate heart disease or require treatment. Stress, excitement, strong coffee, drugs and nicotine can all cause extrasystoles to occur. See irregular HEART RHYTHM.

Eyes, sore   The commonest causes are PINK EYE and EYE STRAIN.

Eye strain   Tiredness of the eyes caused by reading in poor light or by failing to wear appropriate spectacles to correct a visual defect. Although eye strain does not appear to cause physical damage, much discomfort results from holding intricate work or reading material too close to the eyes in order to focus on it. Optrex is a popular preparation easily available from the chemist's shop for bathing the eyes.

Herbal remedy
An eyebath of a decoction of five camomile flower heads in a litre of water.

–F–

Failure, heart   See III/3.

Fainting (syncope)   Temporary reflex loss of consciousness, either complete or partial, due to an inadequate supply of blood to the brain.

Standing still for long periods causes blood to pool in the lower legs and feet. Fainting sometimes results but can be avoided by contracting and relaxing the calf muscles every few minutes.

Fainting which occurs on standing up suddenly is due to the tardy reflex adjustment of blood vessels to the demands of a vertical position. This can be avoided by rising slowly.

Fainting due to an emotional shock, severe PAIN or terror is a result of overstimulation of the parasympathetic nervous system. This reduces the heartbeat and the output of blood by the heart, and relaxes the blood vessels in the abdomen, where the blood then pools. The blood supply to the brain is temporarily inadequate.

Recovery from fainting is always rapid once the head is lowered and the blood supply to the brain restored. Occasionally the patient may show small twitching movements, and the fainting attack can be mistaken for a CONVULSION.

Fallopian tubes, inflammation of   See salpingitis (V/4).

Farmer's lung (thresher's lung)   A lung disorder associated with the inhalation of dust from mouldy hay, grain and grass over long periods. See PNEUMOCONIOSIS.

Favism   A severe ALLERGY to a type of broad bean, *Vicia fava*, grown in Italy. The effects include profuse DIARRHOEA and the destruction of red blood cells, causing haemolytic anaemia (see VIII/1).

Fertility problems   See V/16.

Fever (pyrexia)   Raised body temperature, the normal range lying between 36°C and 37.2°C(97–99°F), taken in the mouth. ('Fever' is also the name for any disorder of which raised body temperature is a feature.)

A fever is one of the body's defence mechanisms against INFECTIONS. The setting of the 'thermostat', lying in the hypothalamic region of the mid-brain, is altered so that the body reaches a higher temperature before the alert is given to reduce it. Then the skin capillaries dilate and sweat is produced, lowering the temperature. The rise in body temperature during a fever helps to eliminate the bacteria or viruses responsible for the infection.

Babies and small children sometimes have CONVULSIONS when a fever comes on rapidly. Adults are liable to have RIGORS (uncontrollable attacks of violent shaking affecting the whole body) at this time.

There are a number of non-infective causes for raised body temperature. Overactivity of the thyroid gland (hyperthyroidism—see X/1), some forms of cancer (see XIII) and certain types of brain disease are among them. Orthodox practitioners treat high temperatures with aspirin, sponging with tepid water, ice-packs and fans.

Biochemic tissue salt treatment
Ferrum Phos. for early signs of fever; Kali Mur. for second stage, when fever has been present for a few hours and the tongue is white-coated. Dose: four tablets every half-hour, reducing dose as symptoms are relieved.

Fibrillation The rapid, disorganized contraction and relaxation of muscle fibres. The term is usually applied to heart muscle, and is denoted 'atrial' or 'ventricular' according to which chambers of the heart are affected.

Atrial fibrillation is a relatively common cardiac arrhythmia (see irregular HEART RHYTHM), and it can be diagnosed by an 'irregularly irregular' pulse—i.e. a pulse with no discernible pattern or rhythm to it. It is due to the muscle of the atrial (upper two) chambers of the heart contracting and relaxing irregularly and far more quickly than usual. The normal number of contractions is between 60 and 80 per minute, each being followed by a contraction of the ventricular (the lower two) chambers. When fibrillation occurs the atrial contractions speed up to a rate of around 500–600 per minute, and the ventricles cannot respond to all of them. Instead, some 100–150 waves of contraction do reach the ventricles, and this is felt at the pulse point as a fast, irregular beat, some beats being strong and others barely perceptible.

Fibrillation can be a symptom of heart disorder (e.g. rheumatic heart disease resulting from RHEUMATIC FEVER) or a feature of a disorder elsewhere (e.g. HYPERTENSION or hyperthyroidism, see X/1). Occasionally, a bout of atrial fibrillation lasting a few hours can arise for no apparent reason, although this has been related by some workers to an episode of unusually heavy alcohol consumption, an excess of strong coffee, and/or tobacco smoking.

The symptoms accompanying fibrillation are an 'odd' feeling in the chest and sometimes the throat, and breathlessness. Persistent atrial fibrillation can lead to heart failure (see III/3), and the sufferer runs an increased risk of clot (thrombus) formation inside the atria, leading to EMBOLISM.

Orthodox treatment for fibrillation aims at treating the underlying cause. It also uses digitalis compounds (e.g. digoxin [Lanoxin] and lanatoside C [Cedilanid]) to reduce the rate of the ventricular contractions, and sometimes a drug such as Kiditard, or Kinidin Durules (both are quinidine bisulphate) to correct the irregular rhythm.

Ventricular fibrillation, a type of cardiac arrest, is a great deal more serious than the atrial type—it is always fatal unless corrected immediately.

Alternative treatments
For atrial fibrillation any treatment should be carried out by a skilled practitioner, e.g. a homoeopathist or a herbal doctor.

Fibroid   Benign (i.e. non-cancerous) TUMOUR of the womb (uterus), consisting of muscle and fibrous connective tissue. See V/11.

Fibrositis   A poorly defined condition featuring PAIN and stiffness in varying areas, most frequently the neck, shoulder girdle and upper back. See VI/6.

Fissure   A split, or narrow ULCER, in skin or membrane tissue. An anal fissure lies at the point on the anus where skin and rectal lining meet; it can start as a tear due to straining to pass a hard motion. Its frequent contact with faeces (stools) makes it slow to heal, and the pain it causes encourages CONSTIPATION, which results in it being torn further. The best remedy other than surgery is to overcome constipation by using a natural, mild laxative until the fissure is healed, and to avoid constipation thereafter by the inclusion of more fibre in the diet.

Orthodox treatment
A compound soothing cream, suppository or ointment (e.g. Anusol, Anacal) is often prescribed. Surgery is sometimes used.

Herbal treatment
A hip bath of a decoction of one handful of chervil to a litre of milk.

Fistula   An abnormal connecting channel between two hollow structures, or between an organ and the exterior. For example, a knife wound in the bladder might cause a fistula between bladder and overlying skin, or an ulcer in the wall of the small intestine (ileum) affected by Crohn's disease (see I/15) might penetrate through and form an abnormal channel between the diseased ileum and another segment of bowel.

Fit   See CONVULSION.

Flash burn   A radiation burn to the front of the eye, an injury most frequently sustained by welders. *Aleo vera* gel has proved soothing, and the use of one or two direct installations speeds healing.

Flatulence   See WIND.

'Flu   See INFUENZA.

Flushes, hot   A symptom common during the menopause. See V/14.

Flutter, atrial   An irregularity of the heartbeat (see irregular HEART RHYTHM). It consists of the upper chambers of the heart (the atria) heating very rapidly, at around 300 beats per minute, while the lower chambers, or ventricles, cannot respond as quickly and so contract only to every second or third beat. Atrial flutter is found in a variety of heart disorders and sometimes in hyperthyroidism (disorder due to an overactive thyroid—see X/1). The treatment depends upon the underlying condition causing the flutter.

Food allergy   See ALLERGY.

Food poisoning   Intestinal disorder, usually sudden in onset, resulting from eating or drinking foods or liquids contaminated by bacteria or their poisons (toxins). *Staphylococcus* and *Salmonella* are two types of bacteria commonly responsible. The first of these (often found in dairy products or cooked meats and fish) releases a toxin which causes violent symptoms for a relatively short time. Staphylococcal food poisoning requires the relief of symptoms only.

Salmonella, found in many different types of food, produces an attack which takes longer to start and longer to wear off. *Salmonella* outbreaks can spread from animals to man—duck eggs are notorious for this. HEADACHES, shivering, prostration, VOMITING and DIARRHOEA can all occur with *Salmonella* poisoning, and the patient may require hospital treatment. Antibiotics are sometimes needed to combat the poisoning.

Botulism is a rare but very dangerous form of food poisoning. It is caused by the bacterium *Clostridium botulinum*, whose spores can withstand boiling and which has been the cause of a number of cases of botulism resulting from home canning. *C. botulinum* multiplies in preserved food and exudes a toxin which is absorbed by the intestinal lining and enters the central nervous system. Symptoms include double vision, difficulty in swallowing and dilated pupils. Emergency admission to hospital is vital, but even that may not prevent death from respiratory paralysis and cardiac arrest.

Meticulous hygiene when handling food is the best way of preventing food poisoning. No preserved food that is in the least bit suspect should be eaten, and no fruit or vegetables should be consumed fresh unless washed first. Tap water abroad, unless adequately treated, should be avoided.

Orthodox treatment
Solids are withheld and fluids are given to combat DEHYDRATION.

Alternative treatments
See DIARRHOEA and VOMITING.

Fracture A broken bone. A bone usually breaks completely—partial breaks (greenstick fractures—see below) occur only in children's bones. The commonest sites for fractures are the collarbone (clavicle), the radius bone at the wrist (Colles' fracture), the ankle (Pott's fracture), and, in elderly people, the hip (neck of the femur, or thighbone).

Signs and symptoms of a fracture include PAIN, swelling, loss of movement, shortening of the limb and deformity in shape. X-rays confirm the exact location, and the type, of the fracture.

Different types can be distinguished. In a *closed fracture* the overlying skin is not broken, while in an *open* or *compound fracture* the broken bone-ends pierce the skin, making infection a likely complication. A *greenstick fracture* is a bone broken on one side only. An *impacted fracture* has one fragment of bone driven into another and locked into position. In a *complicated fracture*, a nearby important structure such as an artery has been damaged; and a *pathological fracture* occurs due to bone disease, such as a bone TUMOUR or osteoporosis (see **VI/8**).

First aid is directed first at the patient as a whole to see that he/she is still breathing, and not bleeding heavily. Wounds should be covered over with the cleanest improvised dressing available, and the fracture and its nearest joint should be supported and immobilized. This is done by strapping the injured part as firmly as possible to the nearest secure, uninjured part of the patient.

Herbal treatment
To speed healing, Comfrey tablets, or Comfrey ointment at the site of the fracture.

Framboesia See YAWS.

Friedrich's ataxia A form of ATAXIA which begins in childhood and is inherited. The site of the disorder is within nervous pathways running between the spinal cord and the cerebellum. The chief sign is clumsy walking movements, but speech, arm and hand incoordination follow later. Patients may later go blind due to atrophy of the optic nerve. Some patients die of heart disorders that develop in early adult life. There is no known orthodox cure.

New holistic approach
Cell therapy, a holistic approach, has been pioneered in Germany and used in combination with a wholefood diet, enzyme substitution, spirulina (a food supplement) and Efamol (the evening primrose oil used in clinical trials and hospitals). Cell therapy consists of implanting cells from foetal organs into sufferers to aid regeneration of the organs and tissues destroyed by the disease. Although this does not cure sufferers from Friedrich's ataxia, considerable improvement has been noted. This work has yet to be carried out outside Germany.[21]

Frigidity Lack of sexual desire or responsiveness in a woman. Underlying causes include fear of pregnancy, painful or distasteful previous experience, poor communication of needs between sexual partners, and lack or unawareness of stimulating foreplay techniques. Poor general health is sometimes a cause, as is early indocrination that the sex act is 'dirty' or 'shameful'. TENSION, fatigue and stress (see STRESS REACTIONS) can rob a normally responsive woman of all desire for sex—just as it can rob a normal man, temporarily, of his potency (see IMPOTENCE). So many normal women feel an aversion towards sexual activity during the premenstrual phase of their cycles that loss of libido

then is regarded as one of the symptoms of the PREMENSTRUAL SYN-
DROME (PMS).

Many normal middle-aged women who have enjoyed sex all their
lives start to feel after a certain age that they should no longer be
interested in sexual love. When this supposed social taboo is coupled
with menopausal and post-menopausal vaginal dryness and soreness,
frigidity can gain a firm hold unless advice is sought (see V/14).

Reassurance, more information where necessary, and expert sexual
counselling can help individual women—or marital couples—
overcome frigidity in many instances. Sometimes particularly severe
cases require psychiatric help and psychotherapy. Greatest of all help is
that provided by an understanding, imaginative and gentle sexual
partner.

Homoeopathic treatment
For excessive anxiety and tension, of recent origin or associated with a
psychological trauma: *Natrum Muriaticum*. For a timid fair-haired girl,
tearful, passive, changeable, cannot tolerate heat: *Pulsatilla*. For phobic
personality, intolerant of heat, but more assertive than *Pulsatilla*
individual: *Argentum Nitricum*. When there is marked pain and SPASM:
Belladonna.

Frostbite   Injury inflicted on skin and sometimes deeper tissues by
exposure to very low temperatures. Prolonged exposure to severe cold,
without actual freezing, interferes with the circulation and causes skin
damage. True frostbite is more serious, and involves the formation of
ice crystals in the exposed tissues, besides impaired circulation and the
clotting of the blood. The extremities and the prominent areas of the
face are most likely to be affected, and, as the affected person may not
notice frostbite at first, companions in cold climates should observe one
another for the signs. These include, most notably, changes in skin
colour, first to pallor, then to reddish blue, and finally to black when the
tissue dies. Nails and skin often slough off but sometimes regrow.

Prevention by adequate clothing is the best approach to frostbite;
surgery must be resorted to once tissue death has occurred, but, in the
early stages, frostbitten areas can be revitalized by gradual rewarming
at body-heat. Frostbitten areas need to be bandaged carefully under
sterile conditions (or, at least, using the cleanest possible dressings) as
they are extremely susceptible to infection.

Funny attacks   See QUEER TURNS.

Furuncle   Another name for a BOIL.

–G–

Gall stones STONES in the gall bladder or bile ducts, often associated with chronic cholecystitis (see I/27).

Ganglion (1) Any structure consisting of a collection of nerve cells. (2) A tense, spherical CYST which develops from a tendon sheath or joint capsule. The commonest site to find a ganglion is on the back of the wrist joint. Usually painless and always benign, they can be removed surgically if they become a nuisance.

Gangrene Localized death and putrefaction of body tissue. Firstly the blood supply to a particular region fails, and this is soon followed by the destruction of the tissue by bacteria. Possible causes include: injury to a main artery in an area of the body where no adequate collateral (i.e. supplementary) blood vessel exist; obstruction through a blood clot in a diseased artery (see THROMBOSIS); or spasm of the artery walls due to ERGOT POISONING.

Antibiotics are powerless to control the bacteria, since they cannot reach the area of tissue concerned. Gangrenous tissue should always be removed surgically as the bacterial infection can spread from the dead tissue to surrounding healthy tissue (see CELLULITIS).

The reason why gangrene does not develop in all dead tissue—for instance, in the brain following a stroke (see IX/7)—is that in some areas of the body there are no bacteria to cause the necessary decay.

Gas gangrene can occur if badly damaged crush injuries are infected with clostridial bacteria which multiply and spread to healthy tissue, which they break down with the formation of gas.

Gastric ulcer An erosion in the stomach lining caused like other varieties of peptic ulcer by the corrosive action of the acid and pepsin produced in the stomach. See I/10.

Gastritis INFLAMMATION of the lining of the stomach. See I/13.

Gastroenteritis INFLAMMATION of the lining of the stomach and small intestine. The commonest cause is infection by bacteria or viruses present in water or food. See I/14.

German measles (rubella) A contagious viral infection common in childhood. See XII/2.

Gingivitis INFLAMMATION of the gums caused by bacterial infection. See I/5.

Glandular fever (infectious mononucleosis) An acute, viral infection in which the lymph glands become enlarged and tender, and the throat inflamed. See VIII/2.

Glaucoma Abnormally high fluid pressure inside the eye. See XI/5.

Glioma A TUMOUR found in the brain or spinal cord. See IX/4 (cancer of the brain).

Glomerulonephritis INFLAMMATION of the glomeruli, the minute filtration units of the kidney responsible for forming urine. It is the commonest cause of chronic kidney (renal) failure (see IV/2).

Glossitis INFLAMMATION of the surface of the tongue. It is extremely rare in healthy individuals, but is found in a number of conditions including anaemia (see VIII/1) and VITAMIN DEFICIENCY.

Gluten intolerance The inability to tolerate gluten, a protein found in wheat, rye and other grains. The effects of gluten sensitivity are chronic DIARRHOEA and malabsorption of fat, vitamins and other nutrients. Two forms of the disease exist (see COELIAC DISEASE and non-tropical SPRUE).

Goitre Enlargement of the thyroid gland in the neck. Simple goitre is due to a lack of dietary iodine, a mineral usually obtained from seafood (seaweeds are especially rich), vegetables or drinking water. Simple goitre is endemic in areas where the soil is iodine-poor, usually in mountainous regions close to the hearts of continents. In England, where the condition is still sometimes referred to as 'Derbyshire neck', goitre is especially prevalent in a belt extending from Derbyshire to Somerset. Adding iodine to table-salt is a measure aimed at reducing the number of simple goitre cases.

Toxic goitre (thyrotoxicosis or Graves's disease) is over production of thyroid hormone due to a functional abnormality. See X/1.

Gonorrhoea   One of the commonest venereal diseases. It is caused by INFECTION of the genital organs and urinary outlet (urethra) by the bacterium *Neisseria gonorrhoeae*, also called the gonococcus. About three days pass between contracting the infection and the appearance of symptoms. A woman may develop no symptoms but nevertheless be capable of transmitting the infection—on the other hand, she may suffer from a discharge of pus, and pain at the entrance of the urethra and the vagina. A man develops an infected urethral discharge and also experiences pain.

Since urinary obstruction and sterility can develop in either sex if gonorrhoea is left untreated, early treatment is essential. Unborn babies are not affected by the mother having this condition, but during birth they frequently contract an eye infection which can lead to blindness if not treated effectively.

Orthodox treatment
Antibiotics, in particular penicillin, are the mainstay of treatment.

In the UK it is an offence for anyone other than a registered medical practitioner to treat or prescribe remedies for any venereal disease.

Gout   a very painful, recurrent form of arthritis (see **VI/1**) due to the deposition of crystals of uric acid in and around joints. See **VI/4**.

Gynaecomastia   Abnormal development of breast tissue in a boy or man. Temporary breast enlargement is normal in baby boys, the swelling being a response to their mother's hormone levels. It may recur in adolescence for a short time; and very obese children and adolescents often appear to have gynaecomastia on account of their heavy fat distribution. Real gynaecomastia, however, is related to hormonal imbalance, and does not disappear when excess weight is lost. One cause is a rare chromosomal abnormality called Klinefelter's syndrome. Others include overactivity of the pituitary or thyroid glands (see **X/1**), TUMOURS in the kidneys or lungs, and certain drugs—such as oestrogen, given to control acne (see **VII/1**); digitalis, given in certain heart conditions; and cimetidine (Tagamet).

–H–

Habitual spasm   See TIC.

Haematemesis   The vomiting of BLOOD.

Haematoma   A swelling due to bleeding into the tissues.

Haematuria   Blood in the urine; see URINE (discoloured).

Haemolytic anaemia   Anaemia arising from the excessive destruction of red blood cells. See VIII/1.

Haemophilia   A BLEEDING DISORDER due to the inherited lack in the blood of a vital clotting factor known as Factor VIII or antihaemophilic globulin. This disease affects between two and three people in 100,000 and, because of the manner in which it is passed on genetically, men are generally affected more severely than women (in whom the condition is extremely rare). Women who have inherited the tendency are unlikely to develop symptoms themselves, but they 'carry' the disease, and there is a 50/50 chance that they will transmit it to their children, the girls again being the carriers and the boys the sufferers. A haemophiliac man, by contrast, cannot transmit the disease to his sons but is bound to transmit the ability to 'carry' haemophilia to his daughters.

There are mild and severe forms of haemophilia. Easy BRUISING is characteristic, and the bruise tends to affect the deep tissues below the skin rather than the skin region itself. Small wounds bleed excessively, and a minor blow or fall can cause joints to bleed inside. Diagnosis rests upon the history of abnormal bruising and bleeding, and on blood tests which show Factor VIII to be missing.

Orthodox treatment is carried out initially specialized hospital units. The basic approach consists of replacing the missing Factor VIII. Home treatment is arranged wherever possible.

Haemoptysis   The coughing up of BLOOD.

Haemorrhage   Bleeding, blood loss. Loss of blood can follow a disease process or injury which may be obvious and external, when an outer part of the body is involved, or unsuspected at first if the blood loss is internal. Examples of the latter situation are damage to the spleen or liver as a result of a violent blow or a penetrating wound to the upper abdomen; perforation of a peptic ulcer (see I/9); and cerebral haemorrhage, when a blood vessel in the brain ruptures (see STROKE IX/7).

Further examples of haemorrhage include a bleeding tooth socket; bleeding from varicose veins (see III/6); and bleeding from a peptic ulcer (see I/9) site, which might produce haematemesis (vomiting of BLOOD) or dark, tarry stools (see MELAENA). Sometimes a disorder of the blood-clotting mechanism is responsible for blood loss (see BLEEDING DISORDERS); this can result in blood being lost from any site, even after a very slight injury or knock.

The frequent loss of small amounts of blood, such as occurs with piles (see I/34) or a peptic ulcer can eventually lead to iron-deficiency anaemia (see VIII/1) once the body's stores of residual iron are depleted. Women are more prone to this condition than men, because their iron stores are likely to be lower in the first place on account of monthly menstrual blood loss. The signs of developing anaemia are exhaustion, DIZZY SPELLS, facial pallor and pale nail beds and mucous membranes.

The signs of the sudden loss of a litre or more of blood are FAINTING, dizziness, a fast 'thready' pulse, and maybe collapse and SHOCK. The patient is cold, sweaty and pale, his/her blood pressure falls dramatically (see HYPOTENSION), and death may ensue if expert treatment is not given.

The immediate need of an acutely haemorrhaging patient is to have the flow of blood staunched. This can best be done by compressing the edges of the wound, or by direct pressure over the artery. Tourniquets should be avoided wherever possible, as cutting off the blood (and oxygen) supply completely for more than 30 minutes can result in loss of the affected limb through tissue damage. However, if a tourniquet is applied, it should be as broad as possible (a long piece of cloth several centimetres wide, not a piece of string). It should be tied no tighter than necessary to stop the bleeding, and *always* released at 25-minute intervals. It should be reapplied only if the haemorrhage continues and after checking that the blood return to the limb is satisfactory.

Once in hospital, the bleeding can be stopped surgically by tying off the bleeding vessels or by heat-sealing them with electrocoagulation. Shock is treated by correcting the blood loss, with, as an emergency measure, a 'drip' of specially designed salt solution administered through a needle into an arm- or leg-vein. A small sample of the patient's blood is taken to determine his blood group, and, after cross-matching, a volume of blood equal to the patient's estimated loss is taken from the blood-transfusion bank. This can then be used to replace the patient's blood loss.

Haemorrhoids   Piles. See I/34.

Hair, loss of (baldness, alopecia)   See VII/5.

Halitosis   See bad BREATH.

Hallucination   Perception of sounds, sights, smells, etc., without physical origin, such as when a person 'hears voices' or 'sees things', and is convinced of their reality. Hallucinations can be caused by DELIRIUM, stress (see STRESS REACTIONS), extreme fatigue, epilepsy (see IX/1), hysteria (see XIV/6), liver failure, and injury or TUMOUR of the brain. However, persistent hallucinatory experiences strongly suggest mental derangement such as DEMENTIA, schizophrenia (see XIV/1) or manic-depressive psychosis (see XIV/2). The best way to get rid of hallucinations is to identify and treat their underlying cause.

A number of drugs cause hallucinations. These include the narcotics (e.g. morphine, heroin), mescaline (from peyote, a Mexican cactus) and LSD (lysergic acid diethylamide).

Hangover   The unpleasant symptoms that follow the drinking of too much alcohol. These include NAUSEA, VOMITING, intense HEADACHE, DIARRHOEA, stomach pain and PHOTOPHOBIA. The symptoms are caused by irritation of the stomach lining and by a degree of alcoholic POISONING by the breakdown products of alcohol.

Vitamin/herbal treatment
An extra Vitamin B complex supplement (100mg strength) plus six evening primrose oil (Efamol) capsules with a glass of water and a small piece of dry wholemeal bread is an excellent remedy. This combination is also, taken one hour before a drinking session, very good at preventing hangovers. (For further details see DRUG DEPENDENCE.)

Hare lip   Part of the same congenital abnormality as CLEFT PALATE, in which tissues forming the upper lip and palate in the developing embryo failed to meet together in the midline and fuse as they normally do. The only remedy is surgical repair.

Both conditions (in particular hare lip) were once regarded by country folk as a witch's curse, and the unfortunate mother who produced the child was referred to as 'hare shotten'. This was because it was believed that a witch worked the spell on her victim by shape-changing into a hare and running across the pregnant women's path, thus affecting the child in her womb by sympathetic magic.

Hay fever A very common allergic condition of the lining membranes of the nose, the main symptoms of which are a stuffy nose, sneezing attacks and watering eyes. See II/4.

Headache Pain experienced 'within' the head, but which can arise from three distinct sources:

- from structures outside the skull
- from the skull itself
- from the membranes (meninges) covering the brain

External structures are the commonest source. 'Tension' headaches are due to SPASM in the muscles of the scalp and at the back of the neck. Migraine attacks (see IX/2) are largely due to constriction of the scalp, temple and facial arteries, followed by dilation.

INFLAMMATION of the nasal sinuses (sinusitis—see II/8) of the skull, and raised fluid pressure inside the eye (glaucoma) [see XI/5], eye infection and eye inflammation can all produce headaches. So, too, can disorders of the teeth, ears, facial nerves (see trigeminal NEURALGIA), facial arteries (as in temporal ARTHRITIS), neck and jaw bone. Raised blood pressure (HYPERTENSION) produces tension-type headaches in some people; and head injuries are often followed by periods of severe headache, generally caused by tenderness at the injury site or muscular spasm around it.

Headaches originating inside the cranium are usually more serious in nature. Inflammation of the meninges, as occurs in MENINGITIS, produces severe head pain, and brain TUMOURS can cause pain by pressing upon sensitive nerve fibres. Headaches which accompany infectious illnesses and FEVERS are due to dilation of the arteries of the brain. The headache of HANGOVER is famous—or notorious.

Simple headaches usually respond well to a mild analgesic such as aspirin or paracetamol. The underlying causes of persistent headaches should be investigated rigorously.

Homoeopathic treatment
With painful, watering eyes and unable to bear bright light: *Euphrasia*.

Pain lessened by bending head backwards: *Hypericum*. With humming in the ears: *Kali Phosphoricum*. For a hammering headache preceded by misty vision or zigzag lights: *Natrum Muriaticum*.

Head injury   When a head injury results in bleeding within the skull, the greatest problem is compression of the brain since there is no room within the skull's fairly rigid framework for expansion. The only viable treatment is surgery, for it is vital to stop the blood flow and to relieve pressure on the delicate brain tissues.

Most deaths following head injuries are due to airway obstruction by the patient's tongue, or by vomited stomach contents. First aid for an unconscious person consists of laying him/her on his/her side, removing false teeth if present, and checking that the air passage at the back of the throat is unobstructed.

Medical help should be sought urgently. A description of the fall or injury sustained by the patient, the length of time he/she has been unconscious, the time of the accident and the amount of blood lost—all of these data are extremely helpful to the patient's management. See CONCUSSION.

Hearing, loss of   See DEAFNESS.

Heart attack   Damage to an area of heart muscle (see myocardial INFARCTION) due to the obstruction of blood flow in a coronary artery, either by a clot of blood (CORONARY THROMBOSIS) or by extreme narrowing of the artery's walls (see ATHEROMA). The chief symptom is severe chest pain which, unlike ANGINA PECTORIS, is not relieved by rest, and this is often accompanied by signs of SHOCK and by a slow pulse (see BRADYCARDIA).

When a very large area of heart muscle is damaged in this way, immediate death can occur. However, the vast majority of heart-attack sufferers survive.

Heart block   A block in the normal conducting pathways of the heart. See introduction to III (page 226).

Heartburn (pyrosis)   A burning pain in the midline of the chest, sometimes extending into the throat or the back. It is caused by INFLAMMATION of the lower part of the foodpipe (oesophagus), generally due to a reflux of the acid contents of the stomach. It can also follow a very large meal, or be due to a hiatus hernia (see I/7).

Orthodox treatment
Antacids (e.g. aluminium hydroxide gel [Aludrox]) are usually pre-scribed for heartburn. Heavy, overspiced meals should be avoided. The cause of recurrent heartburn should be investigated.

Herbal treatment
The very occasional bout of heartburn can safely be treated without recourse to a medical or herbal practitioner. Try 2–3 cupfuls of the following infusion per day: 5–10 pinches of aniseed to a litre of water, with perhaps a pinch each of mint and lavender.

Heart failure   In heart failure the heart does not, as the term might suggest, stop beating; instead, it fails to perform its work of maintaining the circulation through the lungs and around the body as efficiently as it should. See III/3.

Heart murmur   The normal heart produces two basic sounds detect-able with the stethoscope. The first is due to the closure of the mitral and tricuspid valves, and is referred to as 'lubb'. The second is due to the closure of the aortic and pulmonary valves, and is referred to as 'dupp'.
  Heart murmurs are sounds produced by the heart in addition to these normal sounds. They are due to a turbulent blood-flow, and are referred to as 'functional' when caused by the flow of blood through the chambers of a normal heart, and 'organic' when caused by valvular defects. Murmurs present in children can be due to a hole, or defect, in the walls separating the chambers of the heart (SEE HOLE IN THE HEART).

Heart rhythm, irregular   An abnormality in the rhythm of the heart-beat, termed an 'arrhythmia', can occur both in the presence and in the absence of heart disease. Occasional irregularities occur in normal people as a result of stress (see STRESS REACTIONS), too many cigarettes or too much coffee. No treatment is required, although removal of the causative factor is advisable. Some irregular heartbeats occur after a CORONARY THROMBOSIS. See also BRADYCARDIA, TACHYCARDIA, PAL-PITATIONS, EXTRASYSTOLE, FIBRILLATION and FLUTTER (atrial).

Heat rash (miliaria)   See PRICKLY HEAT.

Heatstroke   Illness due to exposing the body to excessive heat. The symptoms are caused by the heavy loss of both salt and water as a result of profuse sweating, and start with lethargy, HEADACHE and confusion. The body temperature remains near normal, but the blood pressure falls and the patient is pale, sweaty and usually nauseous. Visual disturbances and profuse VOMITING follow if no treatment is given, and COMA and death can result.

The best way to manage this condition is to remove the patient into a cool, dimly lit room, put him/her to bed and restore his/her salt and fluid balance—either in the form of a palatable drink or by intravenous infusion.

Hemiplegia   Paralysis of one side of the body as a result of injury or disease to the brain. Right-sided paralysis is due to interference with the movement (motor) area in the left half of the brain, and vice versa. Birth injuries and accidents later in life can produce hemiplegia; the commonest cause is disease of the cerebral arteries which supply the brain (see **IX/7**).

Hepatitis   INFLAMMATION of the liver, generally due to a virus INFECTION. See **I/23**.

Hernia ('rupture')   Protrusion of an organ from its normal position in the body into another area—e.g. of the upper part of the stomach through the diaphragm into the chest, to form a hiatus hernia (see **I/7**). Other examples include: a *groin (inguinal) hernia*, much commoner in men, in which a loop of bowel pushes through the weakened abdominal wall (direct type) or down the passage of the sperm cord on its way to the testicle (indirect type); a *femoral hernia*, commoner in women, which consists of a loop of bowel pushing out of the abdomen into the top of the thigh; and an *umbilical (navel) hernia*, seen in babies at birth. *Incisional hernias* can occur following an abdominal operation when the surgical scar is weak or incompletely healed.

Many hernias require no treatment. Large hernias, or hernias in danger of becoming trapped (i.e. not returnable to their proper place by finger pressure), require surgery.

Hernia, strangulation of   Sometimes, when a patient has a HERNIA, the tissue through which the herniating organ has passed tightens around it and nips it sufficiently hard to cut off its blood supply. This condition is a strangulated hernia, and an emergency. The urgency is due to the fact that any living tissue deprived of its blood supply—and therefore of oxygen and nutrients—quickly dies and becomes gangrenous (see GANGRENE). Early surgical repair is vital.

Heroin (diamorphine), addiction to   See DRUG DEPENDENCE.

Herpes simplex   A patch of sore, inflamed, crusted BLISTERS commonly found around the mouth and lips—cold sores—and the genitals —genital herpes. See **XII/3**.

Herpes zoster (shingles)   See **IX/6**.

Hiatus hernia   See **I/7**.

Hiccup (hiccough)   An involuntary spasm of the diaphragm, which draws air down the windpipe (trachea) in a sudden rush. This is cut short by the rapid closure of the sound-producing folds at the top of the windpipe, producing the jerky movement and the characteristic noise.

Hiccup attacks normally resolve themselves without much trouble. They are thought to be caused by eating or drinking too rapidly, with consequent irritation of the phrenic nerve which supplies the diaphragm. Normally they are of no clinical significance. Occasionally, long persistent attacks can result from a disorder of the stomach, diaphragm or chest.

Ways of stopping an attack of hiccups include eating a spoonful of sugar (possibly a spoonful of dry muesli would do just as well), holding your breath very determinedly, and drinking water out of the side of a glass furthest away from you.

Herbal treatment
A cup of sage tea, sipped slowly (one teaspoonful of sage to a cup of water). Or: aniseed tea, one cupful, sipped slowly.

Hirschsprung's disease (megacolon)   A condition some babies are born with in which a section of their large bowel (colon) lacks a network of nerve fibres. This prevents the colon muscles in the affected area from squeezing the food residue further along the length of the bowel towards the rectum. The result is a build-up in bowel contents and an enormous distension of the bowel. The only treatment is surgical removal of the affected segment of colon, the ends of which are then rejoined.

Hirsutism   The abnormal growth of body hair, particularly in women. The most likely areas for unusual hairiness are around the nipples, on the face and on the lower part of the abdomen. Disordered hormones are thought to account for only one per cent of cases, and in rare instances a genetic or metabolic disorder may be responsible. Usually, though, no cause can be found and hormone treatment is inapplicable. The problem then becomes a cosmetic one.

Hives (urticaria, nettlerash) An allergic reaction (see ALLERGY) to certain protein foods (especially fish and shellfish), insect bites and STINGS, and certain drugs, such as penicillin; it can also be triggered by ANXIETY and emotional stress (see STRESS REACTIONS). It is an intensely itchy (see ITCHING) rash similar in appearance to a batch of nettle stings, consisting of raised white blotches surrounded by reddened skin. Susceptibility to the condition tends to run in families.

Breathing can become difficult if the hives are accompanied by swelling of the throat, a fortunately rare condition known as 'angioneurotic oedema'.

Orthodox treatment for hives consists of antihistamine drugs and lotions.

Herbal treatment
Gentle dabbing of the rash with the following infusion, which is also recommended for foot- and handbaths (two daily): to two litres of water, add a handful of each of these ingredients: celandine, poppy, mallow, violet, sage and nettle.

Hodgkin's disease Cancer (see **XIII**) of the lymphatic system (see LYMPHOMA). Affected lymphatic tissue in the lymph nodes, bone marrow, spleen, and sometimes the liver and other organs, enlarges and can eventually press on other structures. Of greater concern is the effect of the disease on the lymphatic tissue's role in fighting infection and maintaining immunity. The cause of Hodgkin's disease is not yet known, but it is suspected that a virus is responsible.

Enlarged lymph glands in the neck, groin and armpits are often the first sign of the condition, as they are easy to feel and the patient notices that they fail to reduce in size in the normal way after an infection. There is no pain in the first few months of the illness, but early symptoms include FEVER, weight-loss, fatigue, itchy skin, and pallor due to ANAEMIA.

Orthodox treatment combines chemotherapy with radiation. It achieves sufficient success for life expectancy to be expressed in years rather than months, and there are many long-term survivors.

Hole in the heart Congenital heart defect in which a hole exists in the wall or septum separating either the two upper heart chambers (atria) or the two lower heart chambers (ventricles). The hole, wherever it is situated, is due to incomplete closure of the developing wall in the unborn baby. It permits the blood to pass from one side of the heart to the other, with the result that some deoxygenated blood gets passed around the body instead of being delivered to the lungs for reoxygenation. Deoxygenated blood is bluish in colour, and babies with this type of problem are sometimes referred to as blue babies.

About one baby in 1,000 is born with a hole in the heart. Those that require surgery can usually be operated on successfully. The hole, if a large one, is closed up with a patch of artificial fibre or a piece of tissue taken from another area of the patient's body.

Hordeolum See STYE.

Housemaid's knee (prepatellar bursitis) INFLAMMATION of the bursa, or small pocket of connective tissue (see BURSITIS), situated over the patella or kneecap. The bursa becomes filled with clear fluid, and the kneecap red and very painful. It is caused by prolonged kneeling on a hard surface. Treatment consists of withdrawing the fluid with a hypodermic syringe, giving anti-inflammatory drugs, and advising the patient not to kneel.

Hyaline membrane disease A lung disorder found in new born babies. See RESPIRATORY DISTRESS SYNDROME.

Hydrocephalus Enlargement of a baby's head due to the abnormal accumulation of fluid around the brain or inside the brain cavities. Sometimes found associated with SPINA BIFIDA, it is caused by a blockage of the normal circulation of the cerebrospinal fluid. Because the newborn baby's head is still distensible for a time after birth (the bony 'plates' forming the skull have not yet knitted together), the increased pressure causes the head to enlarge and the forehead to bulge.

A drainage operation is the usual form of treatment. One end of a small tube is inserted into a brain cavity and the other is connected with the jugular vein in the neck, allowing the excess brain fluid to escape into the bloodstream. Untreated hydrocephalus causes serious brain damage and can prove fatal.

Hydrocoele An accumulation of fluid around the testis. This can occur when the testis is diseased or injured, but generally no cause is found. The usual treatment is to remove the tissue sac containing the fluid. Sometimes, in elderly patients, the fluid is tapped (aspirated), but in this case it may reform.

Hyperactivity (hyperkinesis; attention deficit disorder) This is a disorder nowadays found with increasing frequency in infants and small children. Its chief feature is abnormally restless behaviour, with affected children appearing to be 'on the go' nearly 24 hours a day.

Hyperactive babies are restless and fidgety, cry nearly incessantly and sleep for only about 3–4 hours in the 24. Typically they are poor feeders, whether breast- or bottle-fed, and often suffer from eczema (see VII/2) or asthma (see II/15). They are not easy to comfort, even when picked up and cuddled.

Hyperactive children, after babyhood, are generally extremely difficult to manage—they are frequently cot-rockers and head-bangers, and tend to be hyperexcitable and often tearful. They seem to be unable to sit still for more than a minute or two at a time. Their coordination is poor and they are very accident-prone.

Despite a possibly high IQ, many hyperactive children have learning problems. They have very poor powers of concentration and are usually slow to learn to speak. There is a high incidence among such children of catarrh (see PHLEGM), HEADACHES, hay fever (see II/4), asthma and other respiratory disorders. Abnormal thirst is also common. Boys are more often affected than girls.

Orthodox treatment
The standard method of treatment has for a long time been the use of amphetamine compounds, for example, dexamphetamine sulphate (Dexedrine) or a mixture of equal parts of amphetamine and dexamphetamine (Durophet). Psychotherapy is also used in some children.

Naturopathic treatment
The findings of the Hyperactive Children's Support Group (HCSG) show that there is evidence that hyperactivity may be due to a deficiency of essential fatty acids (EFAs), either because these children cannot absorb them from their diet, or because they have a greater need than other children, or because they fail to metabolize the EFAs they do absorb (or possibly all three). Affected children are generally made a great deal worse by eating food containing artificial additives, and improve noticeably when such foods are withdrawn. They are often zinc-deficient (see ZINC DEFICIENCY).

A strictly wholefood diet is recommended (diet sheet provided by the HCSG), together with a multivitamin and mineral supplement. This regime is combined with a herbal remedy (used also by orthodox physicians and tested in hospital trials) of evening primrose oil. Six 500mg capsules of evening primrose oil (Efamol is the clinically tested brand) are prescribed, three taken at night and three in the morning. These supply an EFA the children have difficulty in making called GLA (gamma-linolenic acid). The capsules can either be taken orally or opened and the contents rubbed into the skin of the inner forearms or thighs.

Hyperglycaemia An abnormally raised blood-sugar level. Hormones, in particular insulin, usually keep the level of the blood sugar within normal limits, but this function is adversely affected in diabetes mellitus (see **X/2**) and the level of sugar in the blood is elevated. When it reaches a certain threshold level, the sugar spills over into the urine, where its presence can be detected with a simple test.

Hyperkinesis See HYPERACTIVITY.

Hypertension The normal blood-pressure reading of a healthy young adult is in the region of 120/80 millimetres of mercury (mm Hg). The first of these readings, the *systolic blood pressure*, is an approximation to the pressure inside the arteries during systole (pronounced 'sis-to-lee'). This occurs when the ventricle chambers of the heart contract and pump the blood out into the arterial circulation.
  The second reading, and the more clinically significant of the two, is named the *diastolic blood pressure*, and is a reflection of a factor known as 'peripheral resistance' during the diastolic phase of the heartbeat. The phase of diastole (pronounced 'di-as-to-lee') occurs as the heart relaxes between beats or contractions, and receives more blood from the veins which feed into it. This peripheral resistance is the resistance to the flow of blood in the small blood vessels distributed throughout the body. These vessels are responsible for delivering oxygen and nutrients to the tissues and organs, and for collecting waste material, including carbon dioxide.
  The 'give' in the arterial walls helps to even out the blood pressure —otherwise it would drop to nothing between heart beats! However, an excessive amount of pressure—i.e. much in excess of 80mm Hg indicates constriction of the walls of these small peripheral vessels, and requires treatment (see VASOCONSTRICTION). See **III/5**.

Hyperthyroidism See **X/1**.

Hyperventilation Overbreathing—i.e. breathing in and out rapidly, with the result that more carbon dioxide than normal is lost from the blood. The pH (or acidity) of the blood therefore alters, becoming less acidic and more alkaline. This can sometimes trigger an emotional release of pent up fear, anger or emotional pain, and for this reason controlled hyperventilation is used therapeutically in a technique known as rebirthing. Hyperventilation can also feature as a symptom in PANIC ATTACKS.

Hypocalcaemia   An abnormally low level of calcium in the blood (the normal level for an adult is between 0.84–1.02mg/ml of serum). The most important symptom is TETANY (cramp-like muscular spasms). Hypocalcaemia can have a number of possible causes, including under-activity of the parathyroid glands, OSTEOMALACIA, kidney disorders and severe malnutrition.

Hypochondria   A personality disorder in which an individual is un-duly preoccupied with his/her state of health. The cause of the person's complaint may be real or imaginary. Whatever the case, concern over a particular set of symptoms or the function of an organ takes on an obsessive nature, and the hypochondriac never loses an opportunity to describe his ailments in graphic terms to anyone willing to listen. Psychotherapy—including hypnotherapy—may prove helpful.

Hypoglycaemia   An abnormally and potentially fatally low level of sugar in the blood. This typically occurs in diabetics, either when they have received too high a dose of insulin or when, as a result of an unplanned burst of energetic activity, too much sugar has been used up (see $X/2$).

Hypoglycaemia can occur also in non-diabetics as a result of over-stimulation of the insulin-producing cells of the pancreas with heavily sugared snacks. The blood-sugar level soars until the insulin effect is felt, and then drops just as dramatically, often leaving the person with symptoms of hypoglycaemia. A deficiency of Vitamin B_5 (calcium pantothenate) may also be a contributory factor.

Symptoms include shakiness, weakness, a fast pulse, irritability, and confusion; and occasionally COMA in diabetics. The first five symptoms can be relieved rapidly by taking a spoonful of sugar, but hypogly-caemic coma requires immediate hospital admission.

Naturopathic treatment
Non-diabetic hypoglycaemia can be avoided by excluding sugar from the diet, and eating whole foods with a high proportion of unrefined, high-fibre carbohydrates.

Hypotension   Low blood pressure. Postural hypotension occurs in some people, especially the elderly, when they get suddenly to their feet after sitting or lying down. It is due to a slower-than-normal response in the mechanism which alters the blood pressure according to the body's position, raising it when the person is vertical. During the few seconds before the blood pressure has adjusted itself the room can swim and the person feel giddy. The answer is to change position as gradually as possible.

Hypothermia   A body temperature abnormally below the usual value of about 98.4°F (37°C). Seriously lowered body temperature can occur either through insufficient heat being produced by the body or through excessive loss of heat. Circumstances in which hypothermia typically arises include: immersion in cold water; hiking and camping in very cold, damp weather; states of exhaustion or illness where the victim is unable to move around; and, among elderly people living alone, poorly heated accommodation.

Symptoms begin when the body temperature falls to 95°F (35°C) and consist of confusion and listlessness. When the body temperature has dropped to 86°F (30°C), the respiration and pulse start to slow down, and the blood pressure starts to fall.

Treatment is the gradual restoration of body heat—sudden immersion in hot water can cause death.

Hypothyroidism   Underactivity of the thyroid gland. See **X/1**.

Hysteria   A variety of mental disorder in which the patient subconsciously develops symptoms which protect him from a difficult life situation. The symptoms can take many different forms, both psychological and physical, and CONVULSIONS can occur. See **XIV/6**.

–I–

Iatrogenic disorder   A physical or psychological illness resulting from treatment received for another disease. This definition does not refer to occasional, transitory side-effects of drug treatment, but refers instead to an illness, frequently unrelated to the original medical condition or the expected effects of treatment, due to the treatment and sometimes continuing after the treatment has ended.

Ichthyosis simplex A congenital disorder in which the skin is dry, scaly and rough as a result of the sufferer having too few sebaceous glands and sometimes too few sweat glands.

Illusion A false sense impression of something actually present. An illusion differs from an HALLUCINATION, in which the person imagines he sees something that is not actually there. An illuded person may see what is in fact a spouse or friend coming into the room, for example, and believe the individual concerned to be a police officer, the Pope or some other well known figure. Illusions, like hallucinations and DELUSIONS, are features of psychotic illness (see **XIV**).

Impetigo A highly contagious skin INFECTION, most commonly found in newborn babies and small children. See **VII/4**.

Impotence The inability to achieve or sustain an erection of the penis during sexual intercourse. Occasionally it is a physical disorder which causes this problem (see, for example, IRON POISONING) but in the vast majority of cases anxiety (see **XIV/4**) and a reaction to stress are the underlying cause. An understanding, patient partner can be very helpful, as can sex therapy. See **V/16**.

Incontinence Inability to control the passage of urine and bowel motions. Most children are 'dry' and 'clean' by the age of three or four, but a few normal children do not gain complete control over their bowels and bladder until they are five or six. After this age, a full investigation is needed to discover whether bladder infections or emotional problems are the cause. See BED-WETTING.

In adults, pelvic injuries, operations to the bladder outlet (urethra) or prostate gland, and multiple pregnancies can all predispose to urinary incontinence. Damage to the nerves supplying the bladder and rectum, or the spinal cord, can result in loss of bladder and rectum control—this is the cause of incontinence in children with SPINA BIFIDA. Elderly people are often incontinent due to poor sensation, inability to hurry to the bathroom, or simply through CONFUSION.

Occasionally, severe CONSTIPATION can produce in the large bowel a hard mass of impacted faeces which cannot be passed unaided and causes intense irritation of the bowel lining, resulting ultimately in uncontrollable DIARRHOEA.

Orthodox management of cases of incontinence may utilize drugs or surgery, or provide incontinence bags for patients who cannot be cured.

Herbal remedy
For urine incontinence, twice-daily hipbaths using a handful of hawthorn flowers and a head of crushed garlic to two litres of water.

Indigestion (dyspepsia) An imprecise term, referring to a range of symptoms associated with the stomach. These include HEARTBURN, distension, fullness, pain (see ABDOMINAL PAIN), BELCHING, WIND and NAUSEA. All of these symptoms can be associated with recognizable disease, and should be investigated if they are very troublesome or persistent. More often, however, they are due to bad habits, such as hurried meals, going for too long without food, overeating, inappropriate diet, smoking, swallowing air with food, or eating when the appetite has been reduced by anger, fear or drugs. The best treatment for indigestion for which no medical cause can be found is, then, to avoid these habits and to exclude from the diet any items of food and drink that seem to worsen the condition. Fatty foods can aggravate indigestion by retaining gas in the stomach for longer than is usual with non-fatty meals.

Orthodox treatment
This is aimed at relieving the symptoms of indigestion, and consists of antacids which neutralize the hydrochloric acid produced by the stomach, and drugs which counteract the irritability of the bowel. Examples of such substances are aluminium hydroxide gel (Aludrox), for excess acidity, and propantheline bromide (Pro-Banthine), for relaxing stomach spasm.

Homoeopathic treatment
For indigestion accompanied by much wind: *Carbo Vegetabilis*. For indigestion due to nervous causes: *Kali Phosphoricum*. For indigestion due to overeating: *Nux Vomica*.

Infarction The death, due to a blockage in its blood supply, of a portion of the tissue from which a whole body area or organ is made up. This can happen when the arteries supplying the area become narrowed due to ATHEROMA, or when the main artery is suddenly blocked by a blood clot (see THROMBOSIS) or some other material (see EMBOLISM). A *myocardial infarction* is the damage suffered by heart muscle (myocardium) during a HEART ATTACK or CORONARY THROMBOSIS.

Infection Invasion of body tissues by viruses, bacteria or fungi. Infections illnesses are discussed in **XII**.

Infertility   The inability to conceive or to fertilize. See **V/15**.

Inflammation   A defence mechanism of the body, enabling it to cope with tissue damage. Physical injury, chemical irritation, exposure to radiation and, most notably, infection all arouse the inflammatory response, which consists of the blood vessels in the affected area dilating, a process which helps to make their walls penetrable. This releases the white blood cells, which migrate out into the 'danger zone' and either ingest the harmful bacteria or release chemicals which break down damaged tissue cells. The white cells, dead bacteria and tissue debris mix with fluid from the blood to produce a usually whitish semi-liquid called pus.

The characteristic features of an acutely inflamed area of the body —for example, a scratch on the finger sufficiently deep to draw blood—are PAIN, some swelling, redness and heat. Function of the inflamed part is affected until healing is complete.

Influenza ('flu)   A virus infection spread by moisture droplets expelled during speech, coughing or sneezing. The incubation period is from one to four days, and symptoms tend to appear suddenly. They include FEVER, sore throat, HEADACHES, weakness, muscular aches and pains, DEPRESSION, loss of appetite and a dry COUGH.

Influenza reduces the body's resistance to bacterial infection, and bronchitis (see **II/11** and **II/12**), sinusitis (see **II/8**) and ear infections (see EARACHE) can result. The bronchitis, if left untreated, can progress to pneumonia (see **II/14**), and consequently influenza represents a particular risk to the very elderly, young children, invalids and convalescents, and patients with heart and lung disorders.

Orthodox treatment
This consists of bed rest, plenty of fluids, and perhaps aspirin to reduce the temperature and treat the muscular aches. The doctor should be consulted if green or yellow PHLEGM is coughed up, if chest pain is felt, or if the fever has not subsided within five days.

Traditional treatment
A honey and yarrow drink, consisting of a tablespoonful of honey added to an infusion of yarrow (four or five flowerheads to a half-litre of hot water). It should be drunk hot at bedtime and first thing in the morning.

Ingrowing toenail   Growth of the sides of a toenail, usually of the big toe, into the flesh of the nail groove. This is a painful condition, largely caused by cutting the nails too short at the sides, and by wearing ill-fitting shoes. The toenails should be cut straight across at the top, or cut with a slight dip so that the sides are slightly longer than the middle yet smoothly rounded off.

The PAIN can be relieved by gently inserting the tip of a pair of scissors under the embedded edges for a few minutes every day. This gradually encourages the nail to grow up out of the deep groove. As soon as it is long enough, the nail can then be cut correctly. Nails that discharge PUS and become brown and flaky should be seen by a doctor.

Occasionally, chronically infected toenails have to be removed under anaesthetic. They take just under a year to regrow.

Insomnia   Inability to fall asleep, or to remain asleep for long. This can exist for no apparent reason, or be caused by an underlying condition such as anxiety (see **XIV/4**), PAIN, mental disturbance or an overactive thyroid gland (see **X/1**).

Orthodox treatment
This is aimed at identifying and treating an underlying disorder, if one exists, and at relieving the symptoms with a mild hypnotic (sleeping tablet) if no cause can be found. Because even mild sleeping tablets are habit-forming (see DRUG DEPENDENCE), and lose their effectiveness if taken for too long, doctors usually prefer to prescribe them for a few nights only, in the hope that this will re-establish the normal sleeping pattern. Common sleeping tablets include nitrazepam (Mogadon) and temazepam (Euhypnos).

Herbal treatment
A number of proprietary brands of herbal compounds are available, Quiet Life being one the author has tried with success. If you wish to prepare your own, try this: an infusion of a pinch of lime flowers, a pinch of vervain and a pinch of marjoram to a cupful of hot water. Drink one cup before retiring.

Intermittent claudication   See CLAUDICATION.

Intertrigo   An area of soreness where two skin surfaces chafe against one another and sweat collects. It is found most frequently in elderly, obese people, and in babies who do not notice it in its early stages. The groin, the armpits, below heavy, pendulous breasts, and between the folds of the buttocks are common sites for intertrigo, and it is also found in the fold of skin behind the ear and between the scrotum and the thigh.

Orthodox treatment
The best remedy is to wash the area with super-fatted soap and dust it with talcum powder. Losing weight is helpful (if applicable). If the reddened area becomes infected a doctor should be consulted.

Herbal treatment
Bathe the inflamed areas with a decoction of burdock leaves.

Iritis INFLAMMATION of the iris, the coloured part of the eye. The symptoms are PAIN, a discoloured iris, contraction of the pupil, and often impaired vision. This condition should be treated by an eye specialist.

Iron deficiency The chief disorder that results from insufficient dietary iron is iron-deficiency anaemia (see VIII/1). Iron deficiency and CALCIUM DEFICIENCY are the two major mineral deficiencies in women, iron being lost in the blood shed monthly at menstruation.

A reasonable daily iron intake is 50mg for a man, 100mg for a woman; any excess should simply be excreted (although, in its ferric forms, iron destroys Vitamin E—see also IRON POISONING). Chelated iron is the form most easily assimilated. Foods rich in iron include pork liver, beef kidneys, heart, eggs (the yolks) and nuts.

Iron poisoning An excess of dietary iron is rare. In an uncommon condition known as *haemosiderosis* (iron-storage disease), excessive amounts of iron are stored in the body in one of three possible ways. Excessive amounts may be absorbed by the small bowel due to an inherited abnormality or in certain forms of anaemia (see VIII/1); or an excessive amount of iron may be taken in over a long period and large quantities absorbed as a result. In developed countries, this is mainly due to the regular consumption of red wine or iron-containing supplements and tonics. The third way in which iron poisoning may occur is when patients are receiving regular blood transfusions: iron can then accumulate in large quantities.

The most usual symptoms of excessive amounts of iron in the body result from the effects of the iron upon the areas where it is stored. The skin takes on a bronze appearance, and diabetes mellitus (see X/2), heart disorders, sexual IMPOTENCE, shrivelling of the testicles and joint pains can also occur.

Irritable-bowel syndrome Alternative term for spastic colon. See I/30.

Itching (pruritus) A sensation within the skin of irritation, provoking the need to scratch. The effect upon the individual depends upon the area involved, and upon the severity. A mildly itchy sensation can be pleasant, but intractable itching can drive a person to desperation.

Causes include external factors such as woolly clothing, foreign bodies, parasites, skin disorders such as eczema (see VII/2), psoriasis (see VII/3) or LICHEN PLANUS, and CHILBLAINS. Underlying disorders such as JAUNDICE, kidney disease, MYXOEDEMA, LYMPHOMA or other types of cancer can cause severe skin irritation. ALLERGY, emotional problems and hormonal changes are also often responsible. (See also PRURITUS ANI and PRURITUS VULVAE.)

Orthodox treatment
This includes detection of the underlying cause, which should be removed or treated if possible. Antihistamine drugs can be helpful, and steroid creams often control the symptoms. Tranquillizers and sedatives are sometimes prescribed.

Herbal treatment
A compress and foot and hand baths made using a handful of each of the following ingredients to two litres of water: elecampane, burdock, marsh-mallow roots, dandelion roots and rose petals.

–J–

Jamais vu (French, meaning 'never seen') A feeling of unfamiliarity with familiar things, people or places (contrast DEJA VU); also, a feeling that real objects are unreal, or far away. This condition can happen as a result of great fatigue, and can also be a symptom of EPILEPSY.

Jaundice Yellow discoloration of the skin and mucous membranes caused by the deposition of bilirubin, a yellow-orange bile pigment formed as a breakdown product of haemoglobin. (Haemoglobin is the iron-containing pigment in the red blood cells responsible for transporting oxygen around the body. It is broken down into its simpler chemical parts when the red cells some to the end of their natural lifespan of approximately 120 days.) Normally excreted in the bile, bilirubin is always present in small amounts in the blood, but it appears in the skin and tissues only when it is released into the bloodstream in abnormally large amounts. There are three important ways in which this can come about.

In *hepatic jaundice*, due to damaged liver cells, the formation of bile salts from bilirubin is adversely affected, and the level of bilirubin in the blood rises. Eventually the urine darkens, and the stools gradually become lighter in colour.

In *obstructive jaundice* the bile cannot reach the intestine due to blockage of the bile ducts by STONES or TUMOURS, and is reabsorbed into the bloodstream. In this type of jaundice the urine is very dark brown, and the motions are clay-coloured.

Haemolytic jaundice involves the abnormal destruction of the red blood cells and the consequent release of excessive amounts of haemoglobin into the blood: the level of bilirubin therefore rises. The motions are dark, the urine coloured as normal.

Orthodox management of jaundice is to detect the underlying cause, and to treat it.

Herbal treatment
Foot baths and hand baths of the following ingredients: one handful each of celandine leaves, artichoke leaves and dog's tooth roots, and a half handful each of chickory leaves and dandelion flowers, infused in two litres of water. Two baths daily.

Jet lag   Disordered bodily functions experienced when a person has crossed a number of time zones in the course of an international flight: the symptoms result from the physiological functions getting out of step with the time system, and can include feelings of intense fatigue coupled with INSOMNIA, an artificial 'high' which causes a brief spell of hyperactivity, a racing pulse, loss of appetite, disorientation and a dry mouth. Dehydration worsens the condition, and is very common due to the extremely low moisture content of the atmosphere in pressurized cabins and to the consumption of alcoholic drinks. The best way to avoid jet lag (as far as possible) is to eat light salad meals during the flight, drink mineral water and freshly squeezed fruit or vegetable juices in preference to alcohol, and sleep as much as possible both during the flight and during the first day abroad.

Vitamin therapy
In addition to your normal supplemental programme, take: extra stress

B complex, starting while on the 'plane (50–100mg strength, one morning and evening); a gram of Vitamin C with bioflavonoids (morning and evening); Vitamin E, (400iu, also morning and evening).

–K–

Keloid (cheloid)   Thickened, lumpy connective tissue at the site of an old wound. Keloids are disfiguring but essentially harmless, and may recur in the new scar area after surgical removal.

Keratitis   INFLAMMATION of the cornea, the transparent membrane covering the front of the eye. It can result from infection, overexposure to sunlight or ultraviolet light, or chemical irritation, but the commonest cause is Vitamin-A deficiency. Keratitis can be cured if it has not been allowed to progress for too long. The treatment consists of large doses of Vitamin A, given under professional supervision.

Ketosis   The presence of excess ketones in the blood; and the toxic effects upon the body of ketones (acetone and similar substances) formed when the breakdown of fats is disturbed. Normally ketones are rendered harmless and disposed of, but they collect in the blood of diabetics and of people on starvation diets, or in other people after persistent vomiting. Ketosis is apparent from the smell of acetone on the breath. A doctor should be consulted if a person has this symptom.

Knee joint   For pain and/or stiffness of this joint, see CHONDRO-MALACIA PATELLAE and the discussion of arthritis (**VI/1**).

Koilonychia   The development of thin, spoon-shaped fingernails due to a deficiency of iron (see **VIII/1**).

Koplik's spots   Small red spots with blue-white centres found on the inner lining of the cheeks in the early stages of measles (see **XII/5**).

Kraurosis vulvae   A condition affecting the vulva, the main symptoms being dryness, soreness and INFLAMMATION. See discussion of vaginitis (**V/8**).

Kwashiorkor   See DEFICIENCY DISEASES.

Kyphosis   Overemphasized curvature of the thoracic spine (i.e. in the region of the chest), producing an arched back in the upper trunk region (i.e. 'hunchback') and muscular strain.

–L–

Labyrinthitis   Inflammation of the inner ear (labyrinth); known also as OTITIS INTERNA. See XI/4.

Lacrimation   Production and discharge of tears. This can be excessive due to a foreign substance in the eye, emotional upset and blockage of the drainage apparatus. In the latter case, a small operation is usually performed.

Lactose intolerance   The inability to digest milk sugar, or lactose. This can occur in COELIAC DISEASE, Crohn's disease (see I/15), and other disorders of the bowel, and is due to the absence of activity of the enzyme lactase, which is responsible for breaking lactose down into its constituent simple sugars, glucose and galactose. Lactose intolerance is also a racial characteristic of Orientals and many African peoples.

Lactase deficiency is the underlying problem in at least some of the patients diagnosed as suffering from spastic colon (see I/30).

Yoghurt is a well tolerated source of milk for affected people since the bacteria present in it release lactase, thereby aiding the digestion of the lactose present.

Laryngitis   INFLAMMATION of the 'voice box' or larynx. See II/9.

Lassa fever   A highly contagious, serious viral INFECTION, first described in Lassa, Nigeria, in 1969, and confined to central West Africa. It is transmitted from rats or through close personal contact with an infected patient; it can also be airborne. The symptoms include FEVER, BACKACHE, NAUSEA and VOMITING, COUGH, sore THROAT, ABDOMINAL PAIN and DIARRHOEA. There is also an increased tendency to bleed. Most untreated patients die, and the best hope of survival is treatment

77

with a specific antiserum available in limited supply from laboratories around the world.

Lead poisoning Chronic lead poisoning results from the gradual accumulation of lead in the body. This can result from contaminated water supplies, excessive contact with (or, among children, the actual consumption of) lead-containing paint, the use of lead-glazed pottery for the storage of acidic drinks, industrial pollution, pollution from motor-vehicle exhausts, etc. The effects of lead poisoning in children can include mental irritation, mental retardation, CONVULSIONS and death. Minimal degrees of lead poisoning are believed to stunt intellectual development. Adults react to slight lead poisoning by becoming anaemic (see VIII/1), and to more pronounced poisoning by developing lead COLIC, discoloration of the gums, and muscular weakness due to interference with nerve function. This weakness is typically found in the muscles of the forearm. Lead poisoning is diagnosed by blood tests.

Uncombined lead is not easily excreted in either the urine or the faeces. Large supplements of calcium in the diet help to displace lead from the bones, and the chelating agent EDTA (calcium sodium edetate) is useful since it binds chemically with the lead to form compounds which are readily excreted in the urine.

Legionnaires' disease An acute infectious disease with a high mortality rate, usually producing a type of pneumonia. It derives its name from the large outbreak of the illness at an American Legion convention in Philadelphia in 1976, in which 29 legionnaires died and many others were affected. It is caused by a bacterium known as 'legionnaires' agent' (technical name *Legionella pneumophila*), first identified in the USA in the stagnant water in cooling towers and commercial air-conditioning systems.

Symptoms initially resemble those of INFLUENZA, and appear after an incubation period of between two and ten days (usually about seven). They include high FEVER, malaise, muscular pain, DIARRHOEA and HEADACHE. A severe pneumonia (see II/14), sometimes accompanied by PLEURISY, generally develops within a week. The most effective antibiotic so far is erythromycin.

Leukaemia Cancer of the white blood cells in both the blood and the blood-forming tissues (e.g. bone marrow). See VIII/3.

Leukoplakia Small white patches of thickened lining membrane on the tongue, the inside of the mouth or lips, or in the mucous membrane of the genitals. The condition is believed to be due to chronic irritation, such as a prolonged discharge in the genital area, or tobacco, ill fitting dentures, jagged teeth or excessive heat within the cavity of the mouth. Possible predisposing factors include deficiencies of sex hormones or Vitamin A, and coexisting SYPHILIS. The condition is more common in men.

Early, thin patches of leukoplakia can sometimes be cured simply by removing them or by treating the source of irritation. Unresponsive or advanced leukoplakia should be biopsied (i.e. a small portion of the lesion should be taken and the cells examined under the microscope) and then, together with a margin of surrounding healthy tissue, removed surgically. The reason for this radical treatment is that leukoplakia is sometimes precancerous.

Leukorrhoea (vaginal catarrh)   See WHITES.

Lichen planus   An inflammatory condition of the skin and the lining of the mouth. Small blotches appear on the skin, typically on the wrists, arms, legs and trunk, and can run together to form scaly patches. The raised areas are itchy and have a pink or violet sheen. The cause is unknown (it may be emotional upset) but the condition usually responds to a soothing lotion.

Aromatherapeutic treatment
To a lukewarm bath add 300g of pure bicarbonate of soda (Vichy salts) enriched with essence of common chamomile (50 drops). Stir well and climb in.

Lipoma   A benign swelling of fat cells, usually in the dermis (lower skin layer) or subcutaneous tissue (the layer below the skin), surrounded by a tough capsule of fibrous tissue. Most lipomata arise for no apparent reason, but occasionally they can result from disordered fat metabolism in patients with neurological or endocrine problems. Most appear on the back, neck, shoulders and abdominal wall. They are usually easy to remove surgically, and rarely recur.

Lockjaw (tetanus)   The disorder resulting from infection with the tetanus bacterium, *Clostridium tetani*, which lives without causing disease in the bowels of certain animals, especially horses and occasionally humans. Its spores are found in the soil and live bacteria can emerge after years of existence in this form. The conditions have to be exactly right for the bacteria to thrive—they need to do so away from a source of air (i.e. they are anaerobic)—and they often gain entry to the body through skin scratches without causing damage. Sometimes, however, they impregnate a wound in which the tissue has been killed—as a result of burn injury, chemical damage, previous bacterial infection, etc. This type of location lacks oxygen and is therefore favourable to the bacteria's needs, and they multiply there, producing an extremely dangerous toxin as they do so. This substance travels along the nearest nerve to the spinal cord, where it acts in a similar way to strychnine: the movement ('motor') nerves are affected in such a way that they function uninhibitedly, sending unrestricted movement impulses to the skeletal muscles which either twitch or go into SPASM in a completely uncoordinated fashion. The jaw muscles contract (see TRISMUS) and the patient's face is contorted into a ghastly, mirthless grin. His/her whole body convulses and he/she becomes physically exhausted—breathing movements, too, are often badly affected.

Orthodox treatment
Tetanus is not seen very often in the UK these days, chiefly because vaccination against tetanus infection is available. This has to be repeated every five years—and straightaway after an injury which has introduced particles of dirt and soil into a scratch or wound. The same antitoxin is used to treat cases of tetanus, although this can only combat the bacterial toxin which has not yet reached the central nervous system: it cannot affect the action of toxin already causing muscular spasm. Sometimes a muscle-paralysing drug such as curare has to be given to counteract extremely severe muscular spasm, especially if breathing difficulties are present. (Curare paralyses the muscles of respiration as well as skeletal muscles, so the patient has to be placed on an automatic respirator until the effects wear off.)

Skilful nursing and extremely quiet conditions are essential. Sedative drugs are also likely to be given (e.g. intravenous diazepam [Valium]).

Longsightedness (hypermetropia)   This is due to the lens of the eye focusing the rays of light from objects in the visual field behind the retina instead of upon it. By orthodox practitioners this is corrected by suitable spectacles or contact lenses.

Bates' eye-training technique
This is sometimes successful in improving the sight by natural means, including eye exercises and hydrotherapy.

Lordosis   Curvature of the spine in a concave direction towards the back. There is a natural lordosis, which produces the 'hollow' of the back in the lumbar region, but in some people with bad postures the lordosis is overemphasized; this can put considerable strain on the small joints of the spine and their attached muscles. The Alexander technique (see page 473) is helpful in correcting postural defects.

Lumbago Severe PAIN in the lower back. The possible causes include a slipped DISC and strain upon other structures in that area through faulty posture. See BACKACHE.

Lump See TUMOUR.

Lymphadenitis INFLAMMATION of the lymph glands (lymph nodes) due to INFECTION nearby. When the condition is acute, the glands can swell to twice their normal size and become very painful. When lymphadenitis is chronic, and caused by repeated infection of, for example, the tonsils or a tooth, then the glands which receive lymph from the infected area become enlarged but not necessarily tender. Treatment is directed at removing the underlying infection.

Lymphadenoma See HODGKIN'S DISEASE and LYMPHOMA.

Lymphangiitis INFLAMMATION of lymph vessels (as opposed to nodes —see LYMPHADENITIS) due to the spread of INFECTION, usually from a septic wound. The inflamed vessels can be seen as red lines in the skin travelling from the infected area to the lymph nodes which drain that area. They can throb painfully and the infection can spread rapidly, resulting in SEPTICAEMIA (blood poisoning).

Lymphoedema Swelling of a limb or limbs due to a blockage in their lymph flow. When finger pressure is applied, the tissues feel hard due to thickening of the skin and underlying tissues. Causes include congenital abnormalities of the lymph vessels; removal of lymphatic structures as part of cancer treatment; and thickened, inflamed nodes or vessels. Bandaging and elevating the limb can bring relief, but the only ortho-dox cure is surgical removal of the thickened tissue under the skin.

Lymphoma Cancer of lymphoid tissue. The different types vary in their overall malignancy, and can be identified by a biopsy (microscopic examination of cells from the area). Treatment depends upon the type, but surgery (where possible), radiotherapy and chemotherapy are the usual measures—see XIII. Two common lymphomata are HODGKIN'S DISEASE and LYMPHOSARCOMA.

81

Lymphosarcoma   A variety of LYMPHOMA with symptoms similar to those of chronic leukaemia (see **VIII/3**) and arising chiefly in middle-aged people. The malignant changes can start in any lymph node and the condition usually spreads rapidly, casting malignant cells into the blood stream at a later stage, so that the blood picture is similar to chronic lymphatic leukaemia. Patients experience abdominal discomfort due to a large spleen and liver, and fatigue and weakness due to anaemia (see **VIII/1**). With orthodox treatment, remissions gained by chemotherapy and radiotherapy can last for several years. See **XIII**.

–M–

Magnesium deficiency   There is no specific DEFICIENCY DISEASE due to dietary deprivation of magnesium, but chronic alcoholics tend to develop a low blood level of this metal. Symptoms include irritability, TETANY and CONVULSIONS; the condition can also lead to a low blood level of calcium (see CALCIUM DECIENCY). Recommended daily intake of magnesium is 300–400mg. The best natural sources include figs, lemons, grapefruit, yellow corn and almonds.[24]

Malabsorption   Impairment of the normal absorption of nutrients from the digestive tract, resulting in symptoms of malnutrition. The symptoms include weakness, DIARRHOEA and often anaemia (see **VIII/1**); and babies and children fail to thrive—they may even lose weight. See COELIAC DISEASE, CROHN'S DISEASE (see **I/15**) and pernicious anaemia in **VIII/1**.

Malaria   A parasitic INFECTION of the blood, found chiefly in the tropics and subtropics. See **VIII/4**.

Mania   A form of mental disturbance typified by aimless, uncontrollable euphoria and elation. See **XIV/2**.

Manic-depressive psychosis   One of the two main varieties of psychotic illness; see **XIV/2**. The other is schizophrenia (**XIV/1**).

Marihuana abuse   See DRUG DEPENDENCE.

Mastitis Literally, INFLAMMATION of the breast. Acute mastitis affects breast-feeding women, and exists in two forms. In the first, the breasts are swollen and painful in response to hormonal change and the patient's temperature is raised; in the second, *acute suppurative mastitis*, the inflammation is due to bacterial infection following contamination of a cracked nipple or milk duct, and pus forms. Antibiotics are invariably prescribed by orthodox doctors.

Mastoiditis Infection of the mastoid air cells, small spaces in the mastoid bone which projects as a rounded swelling immediately behind the ear. See EARACHE.

Masturbation Stimulation of one's own sexual organs by gentle or firm rubbing and stroking in order to gain sexual pleasure. Many parents worry about toddlers and children playing with their genitals, but masturbation is neither harmful nor dangerous. It is regarded as a normal part of psychosexual development, and excessive masturbation in children is a 'nervous' habit akin to thumb-sucking, denoting emotional insecurity rather than morbid preoccupation with sexual sensations. Masturbation is also a very common practice in adult men and women, and affords pleasure, comfort and relief from TENSION. Indulgence in masturbation to the exclusion of any other type of sexual activity can suggest the presence of emotional problems; a psychotherapist should be consulted only when the habit disturbs the patient him/herself or the marital partner.

Measles (rubeola, morbilli) An extremely infectious viral illness, most common in childhood. See **XII/5**.

Megacolon See HIRSCHSPRUNG'S DISEASE.

Melaena The production of black tarry stools containing chemically altered blood from somewhere in the upper end of the digestive tract—e.g. from a peptic ulcer (see **I/9**), VARICOSE VEINS around the foodpipe (oesophagus), or gastritis (inflamed stomach lining—see **I/13**). Other causes for melaena are blood swallowed during a NOSEBLEED or dental extraction, OESOPHAGITIS, and cancer of the stomach or foodpipe. Black tarry stools can also be due to taking iron supplements, charcoal or bismuth.

Melancholia Severe DEPRESSION.

Melanoma *Juvenile melanoma* is a benign pigmented skin condition seen in children, and does not predispose to *malignant melanoma*. This latter, by contrast, is a cancerous tumour of pigment cells (melanocytes) arising either in a previously harmless mole (this occurs only once in every one million moles) or elsewhere for no apparent reason. Increased pigmentation, itching, increased hair growth, bleeding, ulceration or changes in shape or size of a mole should be examined by a medical practitioner. Early diagnosis and treatment, usually by surgery, are vital since malignant melanoma spreads cancer cells rapidly to other body areas. Predisposing factors are believed to include sunlight on fair skin, X-rays, and contact with tar.

Ménière's disease   A disturbance of the inner ear; see **XI/3**.

Meningitis   INFLAMMATION of the membranes (meninges) enclosing the brain and spinal cord. This is a very serious INFECTION, and best dealt with in a hospital.

Menopause ('change of life', 'climacteric').   For menopausal symptoms see **V/14**.

Menorrhagia   Excessive menstrual bleeding—either just excessively heavy periods or these in association with abnormally frequent periods. During a normal period, approximately 50ml of blood are lost; menorrhagia can produce a loss of three times this amount per month, and so easily leads to anaemia (see **VIII/1**).

Common causes for menorrhagia include womb POLYPS and FIBROIDS, but in many women with menorrhagia no cause can be found. Orthodox treatment comprises dilatation and curettage (a 'D and C'), or womb scrape, in which the neck of the womb is dilated and its lining gently scraped out with a 'curette' (a specially designed surgical instrument rather like a small spoon on a long handle). A 'D and C' gives diagnostic information, and is sometimes curative in itself. When no cause can be found for menorrhagia, hormone therapy is sometimes successful. Hysterectomy is occasionally performed for severe and intractable menorrhagia.

Aromatherapeutic treatment
Three drops of essence of cypress (*Cupressus sempervirens*) on a little brown sugar three times daily.

Mercury poisoning   The possibility of mercury-amalgam dental fillings being responsible for a wide range of health problems has been a highly controversial topic for some time. Mercury has been used in this form for over 150 years but, if its use were proposed for the first time today, it is doubtful that it would be approved. The *Journal of the American Dental Association* deplores the rumours about amalgam toxicity and says that there is no scientific proof that it causes any harm. However, an article in the *American Journal of Forensic Medicine and Pathology* pointed to a possible link between multiple sclerosis and amalgam, and in 1952 demonstrations showed that amalgam generates electromotive forces which propel ionized mercury particles into the body. These trigger destructive electrolytic processes and can produce adverse electrochemical effects. A number of instruments are now available for the assessment of mercury release into the system.[25] Toxins and metallic ions from teeth have been shown to travel along nerve pathways from the mouth.

The range of possible symptoms in which mercury toxicity can result, include: the formation of POLYPS; oozing eczema (see VII/2); stomatitis (see I/1); HIVES; numbness of the extremities and of patches of skin around the mouth; gastrointestinal upsets; INSOMNIA; ULCER formation; a TREMOR; arthritis (see VI/1); NAUSEA; and DIARRHOEA.

Suggested treatment for the problem is the removal of mercury-amalgam fillings and their replacement by either plastic ceramic resin (known as 'composite') or gold ones. Other suggestions include detoxification by means of a cleansing diet, and the use of chelation therapy, either oral or intravenous or both. (Chelation therapy is discussed in some detail in the treatment of coronary artery disease; see III/4.)

Metastases See SECONDARIES.

Migraine Recurrent HEADACHE which usually occurs on one side of the head only, and is often associated with visual disturbance and VOMITING. See IX/2.

Miliaria (heat rash) See PRICKLY HEAT.

Mongolism The old name for DOWN'S SYNDROME.

Monilia Infection with *Candida albicans*. See THRUSH.

Motion sickness (travel sickness) NAUSEA and/or VOMITING associated with travelling by sea, rail, car, air, etc. It is due to the movement of the vehicle disturbing the balance organ in the inner ear, aggravated in many cases by the conditioned reflex of expecting to feel sick, plus a variety of psychological and emotional factors.

Orthodox treatment
This consists of drugs such as dimenhydrinate (Dramamine), or cinnarizine (Stugeron) taken half an hour to an hour before travelling.

Herbal treatment
Powdered ginger is excellent at preventing motion sickness. It is available in capsules: the dose is one to two capsules half an hour to an hour before travelling.

Mouth ulcers (aphthous ulcers)   See I/3.

Mucoviscidosis   See CYSTIC FIBROSIS.

Multiple sclerosis (MS, disseminated sclerosis)   A disorder in which small patches of the central nervous system and nerves are destroyed, and the healthy tissue replaced by plaques. See IX/5.

Mumps (epidemic parotitis)   A contagious viral illness involving INFLAMMATION of the salivary glands. See XII/6.

Muscular rheumatism   See VI/5.

Myopia   See SHORTSIGHTEDNESS.

Myxoedema   The disorder due to a deficiency of thyroxine (the thyroid hormone), resulting from a state of untreated hypothyroidism (underactive thyroid). See X/1.

–N–

Naevus   See BIRTHMARK.

Nailbiting   A very common habit, probably due to TENSION and insecurity. A common form of treatment is to paint the nails with an unpleasant-tasting yet harmless substance such as bitter aloes, which should act as a deterrent.

Hypnotherapy
Painting the fingernails does not eradicate the underlying tension problem. A form of psychotherapy is advisable to help discover the reason for the insecurity if the habit is persistent and troublesome. Hypnotherapy is the treatment of choice since hypnoanalysis can be used if necessary to discover the underlying problem, and hypnosis can then be utilized to suggest to the patient that he/she no longer needs to bite his/her nails.

Nails, flaking of   Like dry skin and coarse hair this can sometimes be due to a deficiency of prostaglandins of the E1 group, due in turn to a failure to manufacture GLA (gamma-linolenic acid).

Herbal treatment
Evening primrose oil is a source of GLA. The dose is three Efamol capsules twice daily for two months.

Nappy rash   See RASH.

Narcolepsy   See SLEEP DISORDERS.

Nasal polyp   See POLYP.

Nausea (feeling sick)   Sensation of wanting to vomit (see VOMITING). There is a very large number of possible causes for nausea. The two primary ones are that either the vagus nerves in the stomach become irritated and vomiting occurs as a reflex action, or that a revolting sight or a nasty smell produces sickness, the brain in this case generating impulses that stimulate the same nervous pathways. Whichever mechanism is called into play, the normal activity of the stomach contracting to squeeze its contents into the small bowel (duodenum) is interrupted, the duodenum tightens up and prevents the stomach emptying, and nausea is experienced.

Orthodox treatment
Either no treatment; or a drug such as metochlopromide (Maxolon).

Homoeopathic treatment
Ipecacuanha.

Neoplasm   An abnormal growth of new cells from previously normal tissue (see TUMOUR). A neoplasm can be benign (non-life-threatening) or malignant—i.e. a cancer (see XIII).

Nephritis   Inflammation of the kidneys. There are two basic varieties —GLOMERULONEPHRITIS and PYELONEPHRITIS.

Nephrotic syndrome (nephrosis)   The coexistence of protein in the urine, a low blood-level of albumen (a blood protein), and tissue swelling (OEDEMA).

Nettlerash (urticaria)   See HIVES.

Neuralgia   Pain originating in a peripheral nerve—i.e. a nerve which radiates from the central nervous system (brain and spinal cord) and conducts impulses to and/or from all parts of the body. Examples of neuralgic disorders are SCIATICA, which is pain felt in the buttock and down the leg, along the course of the sciatic nerve; and *trigeminal neuralgia* where the pain is felt in the face along the branches of the trigeminal nerve. Neuralgic pain can be mild or severe, a dull ache or a stabbing sensation. Mild pain killers are usually given.

Herbal treatment
An infusion of two pinches of vervain to a cup of water. See also PAIN (alternative treatment for).

Neurasthenia   An old fashioned term meaning literally 'nerve weakness'. The term was, and sometimes still is, used to describe a neurotic condition featuring fatigue, physical and mental irritability, and lassitude. There is no specific orthodox treatment for neurasthenia.

Aromatherapeutic treatment
Four drops of lavender essence on a little brown sugar half an hour before each meal.

Neuritis   Literally meaning 'inflammation of a nerve', this is a general term used to denote disorders of the peripheral nerves. Neuritis can involve one nerve or many simultaneously, and the affected nerve tissue may undergo degeneration with subsequent loss of feeling, poor muscular action, and severe pain or a tingling sensation when the relevant body area is moved.
   Many underlying causes exist, ranging from nerve compression to nutritional or vascular problems. Nerve compression and a temporary neuritis can be experienced by, for example, a person who has gone to sleep with an arm hanging over the hard back of a chair, with pressure being applied to the armpit. This compresses the radial nerve, and the

88

consequent pain, weakness and 'pins and needles' running down the arm are familiar to most people.

Alcoholics often suffer from *nutritional neuritis*; and diabetics are prone to a *vascular polyneuritis*, in which the peripheral nerves are generally affected.

Treatment of neuritis is aimed at its cause, wherever possible. Rest, physiotherapy and painkilling drugs are also used. See PAIN (alternative treatment for).

Neurosis   A general term embracing a large group of mental disorders, with a spectrum of complexity ranging from the nearly normal to the severely disturbed. Examples include depression, anxiety and phobia. See **XIV/3, XIV/4** and **XIV/7**.

Nicotine addiction   See DRUG DEPENDENCE.

Nonspecific urethritis (NSU)   See URETHRITIS.

Nosebleed (epistaxis)   A nosebleed can be caused either by a fall or blow on the nose or by sudden slight pressure on a blood vessel which has been weakened by a bout of INFLAMMATION. Orthodox medical treatment (if required) is generally to pack the nose with lengthy wicks of gauze to staunch the bleeding. Nosebleeds that continue despite this can be made to stop by use of a special balloon device which is inserted into the nose in a deflated state and then inflated, so that pressure is applied from within to the bleeding vessels.

Herbal treatment/first aid
Cotton wool moistened with a decoction or infusion of yarrow and then stuffed up the nose. For all nosebleed treatment, the patient should be sitting down, in a cool room, with his or her head tipped forwards.

–O–

Obesity   An excessive amount of body fat. See WEIGHT PROBLEMS.

Occult blood   Traces of blood in, for example, the stools (faeces), undetectable to the naked eye. These traces would be tested for in a hospital laboratory if episodes of bleeding in the digestive tract were suspected. Several samples of the motions would be taken, as a single negative test is insufficient to prove the total absence of unseen bleeding —for instance, from a PEPTIC ULCER. It is necessary to avoid eating meat for four days prior to an occult blood test, as the blood content of the meat can produce a false positive result. Occult blood can occur elsewhere—for instance, in the urine.

Oedema Swelling due to the accumulation of excess tissue fluid. This can affect the whole body (a condition commonly called dropsy) or can be confined to an area such as the lower limbs. Oedema occurs in people suffering from VARICOSE VEINS or from heart and kidney disorders (see III and IV); also, healthy people who stand for long periods of time often get swollen feet and ankles. Oedema of the peritoneal cavity (abdominal cavity) is called ASCITES.

Oedema of the legs and feet is a very common effect of air travel, when passengers go for several hours without moving from their seats or exercising their ankles or calf muscles. It occurs also in cases of malnutrition where protein or the B vitamins are severely lacking.

Orthodox treatment
This is properly directed towards the underlying cause. Diuretic drugs in injection or tablet form ('water pills') are used to rid the body of the excess fluid by stimulating the kidneys to excrete more water. A low-sodium diet is helpful in some cases, and cardiac stimulants help to relieve oedema caused wholly or partly by heart failure (see III/3).

Herbal treatment
Foot and hand baths twice daily of the following in 2 litres of water: a handful of celandine leaves, a bunch of cress, a grated onion, a bunch of parsley and a handful of meadowsweet.

Oesophageal varices Small VARICOSE VEINS in the lining of the oesophagus, often associated with cirrhosis of the liver (see I/24) and alcoholism (see DRUG DEPENDENCE).

Oesophagitis Inflammation of the oesophagus. The cause may be a virus or fungus (notably *Candida*), the ingestion of caustic acid or alkali, or frequent regurgitation of juices from the stomach (reflux oesophagitis); this last condition may be associated with a hiatus hernia (see I/7).

Onychomycosis Fungal infection of fingernails or toenails. Orthodox doctors treat this condition with fungicidal ointments, such as tolnaltate nystatin (Tinaderm-M) and miconazole (Dermonistat).

Orchitis INFLAMMATION of the testis. This painful condition can occur as a complication of mumps (see **XII/6**) or of GONORRHOEA.

Osteitis INFLAMMATION of bone. True inflammation of bone tissue is most likely to be found together with inflammation of the bone marrow (OSTEOMYELITIS). The term 'osteitis' is now more commonly used for other bone disorders such as osteitis deformans (PAGET'S DISEASE) and osteitis fibrosa cystica, a disease due to overactive parathyroid glands.

Osteoarthritis A degenerative disease of the joints, especially of the weight-bearing joints of the spine and the lower limbs. See **VI/2**.

Osteoma A benign TUMOUR of bone, occurring most frequently on the bones of the skull and the lower jaw as a hard, painless swelling. No treatment is needed unless the tumour causes pressure symptoms or looks unsightly, in which case surgical removal is the easiest method.

Osteomalacia Softening of the bones due to Vitamin-D deficiency and poor calcium deposition. It is comparable to the childhood deficiency disease of RICKETS, and is unknown in sunny climates. It is cured by supplementary Vitamin D.

Osteomyelitis Inflammation of the bone marrow and the bone as a result of INFECTION. This condition is most likely to be dealt with in hospital, possibly by surgery. Osteomyelitis can follow a compound FRACTURE or an infection elsewhere in the body (such as a streptococcal sore throat).

Osteoporosis Thinning, due to loss of minerals, of the bone substance, with consequent loss of structural strength. See **VI/8**.

Osteosarcoma Bone cancer. See **XIII**.

Otitis externa INFLAMMATION of the skin covering the ear and of the lining of the canal leading to the eardrum. See **XI/1**.

Otitis interna Another name for labyrinthitis. See **XI/4**.

Otitis media INFLAMMATION of the middle ear. See **XI/2**.

Otosclerosis   A hereditary cause of deafness due to the formation of spongy bone in the inner ear. It has been suggested that adequate intake of vitamin A throughout life help to prevent otosclerosis in old age.

Ovarian cyst   Fluid-filled swelling of the ovary (see CYST).

–P–

Paget's disease (osteitis deformans)   A bone disorder in which, in the early stage, calcium is lost from the bone substance and certain bones become deformed due to a loss of strength and rigidity. This is followed by an excessive amount of calcium being laid down in the affected bone(s), with consequent thickening and coarsening of the bone structure. Bone PAIN is often only mild, but patients with severe discomfort and incipient deformity can be treated with X-rays or the hormone calcitonin.

Pain   A sensation of extreme discomfort, due to injury, disease or psychological factors. It is a purely subjective experience, and an examining doctor or therapist cannot elicit it by physical examination. What he/she elicits on moving or palpating (pressing upon) a painful part is tenderness, which is pain's objective equivalent. Thus, for example, pressure on the lower right side of the abdomen over an inflamed appendix causes the patient to flinch with pain. Examiners assess the degree of tenderness they observe by comparison with their own experience of pain, and of tenderness in other patients. Since tenderness cannot be quantified, therapists express it in degree—i.e. 'mildly', 'moderately' or 'severely' tender. Also of great importance to the ultimate diagnosis are the answers to a series of questions about the pain, such as its localization, nature (sharp or dull), duration, accompanying symptoms and the existence of any factors which relieve or aggravate it.

The mechanism by which pain is felt is complex. Stimuli that produce it are carried by specific 'pain' nerve fibres which follow two pathways. One, equipped with fast conduction, carries a sensation which is interpreted as sharp pain; and the other, with slower conduction, transmits impulses interpreted as dull pain.

Pain itself is experienced not in the injured or disordered body area but in the area of the brain responsible for interpreting it as a conscious sensation. Besides the nature and severity of the injury or disease, the experience of pain is also influenced by the frame of mind of the patient. For example, if a person awaits an injection tensely and fearfully, the experience is very likely to be 'painful'. If, however, that same person badly grazes a knee in climbing out of a bedroom window to escape a fire, the chances are very high that he or she will be unaware of the injury, as his or her conscious awareness will be completely distracted by the stress of the moment.

Referred pain is experienced from a body area other than that in which the underlying cause is located. For example, the early pain of APPENDICITIS is referred to, and experienced, in the centre of the abdomen, around the navel. Only later does it settle in the lower right-hand quarter of the abdomen, immediately over the inflamed organ.

The ideal treatment of pain is never simply symptomatic—i.e. aimed only at relieving the pain itself. The real objective is to identify the underlying problem, and to treat that, thereby eradicating the pain at the same time. Sometimes, however, an immediate cause cannot be found; and sometimes pain needs to be alleviated long before its cause can be determined and treated effectively. An aspirin or herbal remedy for a headache whose underlying cause has not been discovered can be justly criticized as 'symptomatic' only, but in practice occasional minor pains are often treated in this way. However, there are no grounds for treating severe or recurrent pain purely symptomatically, and the practice of prescribing repeat medication for an unidentified pain that has not been investigated is iniquitous.

Orthodox methods of combating pain include analgesic (pain-killing) and other types of drugs; locally acting anaesthetics which are sprayed or smeared on—e.g. anaesthetic eyedrops for a corneal abrasion (scratch on the front of the eye)—or injected, as in the use of a 'ring block' to deaden a finger before its diseased nail is removed; the application of heated pads or of ice packs prior to painful manipulation, which also is aimed at pain relief; and neurosurgery, in which relevant nerves or areas of the brain or spinal cord are severed.

Many of the alternative methods of pain relief discussed below are used by orthodox doctors as well as alternative therapists. You can use them yourself, but make sure that you consult a qualified practitioner about any pain that continues despite treatment, or the cause of which is not known to you. Regard self-help treatment as a first-aid measure only.

Trigger points

These are small areas within muscles which, when pressed, feel extremely tender and also produce a painful reaction in a consistent spot elsewhere. Leon Chaitow's book *Instant Pain Control* illustrates 40 of these points. Having located a trigger point by pressing and squeezing the muscle you think is involved, carry out the following three stages of treatment.

- Press upon the trigger point with the tip of a finger for five seconds at a time, alternating pressure intervals with rest intervals of the same length. When there is a slight reduction in the referred pain (normally after about a minute), go to the next stage.
- Chill the area with ice or a vapocoolant spray, working from the trigger point to the referred pain area in a series of sweeping movements along the surface of the muscle.
- Place the muscle in the position of maximum stretch for a few seconds (do not strain or hurt it—the position should be the furthest comfortable position).

Avoid lumps, warts, moles, swellings, inflamed areas, the female breasts, varicose veins, and scars. Pregnant women should not be treated, and cancer patients and patients with rheumatoid arthritis should ask professional advice before treating themselves.

Hydrotherapy

Cold compresses applied to a painful joint will reduce pain, swelling and inflammation, but should be covered with flannel or wool so that the body-heat eventually warms the whole application. Cold compresses are useful for acute inflammatory conditions, such as a sprained wrist or ankle.

Alternate hot and cold applications are useful for chronic conditions (e.g. an arthritic joint), since they relieve pain and stimulate a sluggish local circulation. Dunking a suitable body area in hot and cold water alternately is one method. The temperatures should be as hot and cold as possible, without going to excess. The timings are roughly 10 seconds' hot application, followed by 5 seconds, cold. Alternate 10 to 15 times, always finishing with the cold. Gently move and stretch the painful area during and after hydrotherapy. Perform twice daily.

Nutrients

We manufacture our own natural pain-killing chemicals, but also 'degrade' them—i.e. break them down again chemically. The amino acid d-phenylalanine slows down the destruction of these useful substances, which are called endorphin and enkephalin; it is available together with l-phenylalanine (the form in which we meet it in proteins we eat), and the whole compound is known as DLPA.

Take two 375mg tablets of DLPA three times daily, half an hour before eating, for three weeks. If no improvement is noted, double the dose for a further three weeks. If this still does not work, you are one of the few people unable to respond. Once you get relief from pain, stop treatment until you need it again. DLPA should not be taken if you are taking MAOIs (monoamine oxidase inhibitor antidepressants, requiring that you avoid such foodstuffs as red wine, cheese, marmite and broad beans).

The essential fatty acid EIPA (eicosapentaenoic acid), available in oily fish and in Max EPA capsules, has helped the pain of rheumatoid arthritic joints. It should be taken with a diet very low in red meat at a dose of 10 capsules daily.

Vitamin B_3 (niacin), at a dose of a gram daily, can help relieve pain.

TENS therapy

Transcutaneous electrical nerve stimulation relieves pain essentially because one sensation reduces the access to the brain of another, painful one. You can buy TENS machines, but it is best to receive therapy from a practitioner.

Homoeopathic treatment

The following remedies aid pain relief—ask for details from your pharmacist or healthfood-shop proprietor.

- *Arnica*: mental or physical shock, dental extractions, sprains, concussion, bruises, fractures. Available as a cream and in tablet form. Take the latter hourly at first, then every four hours until symptoms cease.
- *Ledum*: for accidents from sharp pointed instruments, thorns, bites, stings, splinters. Use every half hour, hour or two hours, depending on severity. Helpful for black eyes.
- *Comfrey*: for slow-healing wounds, ulcers, fractures. Take three times daily.
- *Puta*: ideal for torn painful ligaments or tendons, and for SYNOVITIS. Use internally every two to four hours, or externally as an ointment.[26]

Palpitation   Sudden awareness of the beating of the heart, due either (a) to a forceful heartbeat being waited for and expected by a nervous subject or (b) to the heart actually beating more strongly than usual. Two conditions which cause patients to complain of palpitations are EXTRASYSTOLES and paroxysmal atrial TACHYCARDIA.

Palsy, cerebral   see SPASTICITY.

Panic attack   Classic symptom of anxiety (see **XIV/4**), characterized by a rapid pulse, a dry mouth and a feeling of immense fear without the sufferer being aware of the cause.

Papilloedema   Swelling and congestion of the optic nerve 'head' at the back of the eye. This can be seen with an ophthalmoscope (an illuminated instrument used for observing the interior of the eye, especially the retina), and is symptomatic of raised fluid pressure within the brain. The commonest causes of papilloedema are severe HYPERTENSION and brain tumours, blood clots and brain ABSCESSES. While unlikely to produce symptoms in itself (apart from poor eyesight if it is very severe), papilloedema is a sign that something may be seriously wrong and its cause should be investigated without delay.

Papilloma   A benign TUMOUR growing on skin or on lining membrane. Papillomata include WARTS and POLYPS. They can be removed by use of a cautery or by snipping the stalk by which they are attached. The commonest areas to find papillomata are the skin, the lining of the large bowel, and the lining of the bladder.

Paralysis   The loss of movement in a muscle or group of muscles normally under the individual's control. It can be caused by damage to the muscle tissue itself or to part of the nervous system. Paralysis can occur as a symptom of almost any nervous-system disorder; see discussions of multiple sclerosis (**IX/5**), Parkinson's disease (**IX/3**), polio (**XII/7**) and STROKE.

Paranoia   A chronic mental disorder in which the patient develops DELUSIONS of persecution and self-importance. Some psychiatrists deny that paranoia exists as a separate entity, and recognize only paranoid schizophrenia (see **XIV/1**), in which delusions of the above type play a significant role.

Paraplegia   PARALYSIS of the lower part of the body, usually due to a spinal-cord injury.

Parkinson's disease   A disease especially prevalent in old age, characterized by a TREMOR and rigid muscles. See IX/3.

Paronychia   See WHITLOW.

Pellagra   A disorder caused by a deficiency of niacin (nicotinic acid or nicotinamide—Vitamin B_3). The symptoms are poor appetite, headaches, irritability, digestive upsets and red discoloration of areas of skin exposed to sunlight. Pellagra is still seen in the corn-eating populations of several Middle-Eastern and African countries, notably in Egypt and Lesotho, and in some areas of central India.

Pelvic inflammatory disease   See V/3.

Peptic ulcer   See I/9.

Pericarditis   Inflammation of the pericardial membrane surrounding the heart. Causes include infection (such as tuberculosis—see XII/8) and an underactive thyroid gland.

Period pains   See V/12.

Peritonitis   INFLAMMATION of the peritoneum, the membranous lining of the abdominal cavity. This can be acute or chronic.
   The usual causes of the former are perforation of a hollow abdominal organ (e.g. the appendix) and infection spreading from an inflamed organ. Acute peritonitis either remains localized—for example, when the cause is an inflamed organ such as the appendix or gall bladder—or becomes generalized (i.e., involving the whole of the peritoneum) when an inflamed organ ruptures, spilling its contents into the abdominal cavity. A classic example of this is the peritonitis following a ruptured peptic ulcer (see I/9). At first the peritonitis is chemical in nature, reacting to the stimulus of the gastric or duodenal contents with which it has been brought into contact, but it soon becomes infective, and pus can fill much of the peritoneal cavity.
   The chief symptoms of peritonitis are severe PAIN, and tenderness of the abdominal wall when palpated (examined manually). The peristaltic, rhythmic, squeezing movement of the bowel ceases, and the abdomen becomes distended. As clinical SHOCK develops, the pulse races and the blood pressure falls. Peritonitis is a serious, potentially life threatening condition, and urgent medical attention is required.
   Generally, it is necessary to stabilize the patient's condition, with an

intravenous drip and possibly antibiotic therapy, before operating to drain the pus from the peritoneal cavity and attend to the underlying cause.

ADHESIONS are liable to form as peritonitis resolves, and sometimes cause obstruction of the intestine.

Chronic peritonitis sometimes results from TUBERCULOSIS of the peritoneum, which is now a rare disorder in the UK.

Pernicious anaemia   Defective formation of the red blood cells due to a deficiency of Vitamin B$_{12}$. See **VIII/1**.

Personality disorder   Defect in the structure of the personality with respect to lifestyle or behaviour. See **XIV/3**.

Pertussis (whooping cough)   See **XII/4**.

Phantom limb   The feeling that a recently amputated limb is 'still there', and perhaps even still painful. Someone who has lost a foot, for instance, may retain the sensations of touch, temperature and position in that foot, and complain that it continues to hurt. This ILLUSION comes about when nerves serving the remaining part of the limb, and containing fibres which used to serve the recently lost area, are stimulated. The sensation continues to be referred (see PAIN) to the lost region. Modern orthodox medicine treats persistent phantom-limb pain with drug therapy, heat application and sometimes vibration.

Pharyngitis   INFLAMMATION of the pharynx, the commonest cause of a sore throat. See **II/5**.

Phenylketonuria (PKU)   A rare cause of mental deficiency, inherited as a recessive character. This means that both parents (neither of whom has the disease) have to carry the trait, or tendency, for a one in four chance to exist, in every pregnancy the woman undergoes, of the disorder being passed on. An excess of the amino acid phenylalanine, a constituent of protein, accumulates due to the absence of the enzyme which usually deals with it, and this in some undefined way affects the nervous system.

Early symptoms of phenylketonuria include unusual irritability, VOMITING and progressive mental retardation. Sufferers are usually fairer in complexion than unaffected brothers and sisters, and are likely to suffer from dermatitis at six months. If they remain untreated or undetected, they can become so retarded that institutional care is necessary; and they often develop epilepsy (see **IX/1**).

The incidence of PKU in southeast England is one in 30,000; in Scotland it is one in 8,000. Nowadays newborn babies throughout the UK are tested routinely for PKU within a few days of birth. Treatment consists of early identification followed by strict adherence to a diet low in phenylalanine. Besides being found in many protein foods, phenylalanine is also one of the two constituent amino acids present in the sweetener aspartame. Foods and drinks which have been sweetened using aspartame ought therefore to be avoided by phenylketonuria sufferers.[27]

Phlebitis INFLAMMATION of a vein wall, often associated with THROMBOSIS inside the vein.

Phlebothrombosis THROMBOSIS inside a vein which is not inflamed. Compare THROMBOPHLEBITIS.

Phlegm (catarrh) A thick, moist secretion produced by the nose and frequently swallowed and coughed up. Uninfected phlegm is white and semitranslucent; infected phlegm is yellow or green.

Photophobia Abnormal sensitivity of the eyes to light. This is a common feature of migraine attacks (see IX/2), HEADACHE, MENINGITIS, measles, (see XII/5), PINK EYE, IRITIS, KERATITIS and HANGOVER.

Piles (haemorrhoids) Swollen VARICOSE VEINS within the rectum. See I/34.

Pink eye (conjunctivitis) INFLAMMATION of the white of the eye (conjunctiva) due to an allergy or an INFECTION by bacteria or viruses. The symptoms include intense ITCHING, a yellow secretion, and reddened conjunctivae. Antihistamine or antibiotic eyedrops are the mainstay of orthodox treatment.

Herbal treatment
A cornflower or marigold eyebath. This could perhaps alternate with antibiotic eyedrops or take over from them as soon as the symptoms show sign of abating.

Pinworms (thread worms) See WORMS.

Plantar wart (verruca plantaris) A WART on the sole of the foot.

Pleurisy INFLAMMATION of the pleural membranes which line the interior of the chest cavity and cover the outer surfaces of the lungs. Pleurisy occurs both in a dry form and in association with a (pleural) effusion—i.e. with a collection of fluid in the space between the pleura's layers. The commonest cause of pleurisy is bacterial or viral infection. Dry pleurisy produces a typical, sharp, stabbing chest pain, made worse by coughing or by taking deep breaths. Pleurisy with pleural effusion is painless because the fluid prevents the inflamed membranes from rubbing against one another, but the patient may be very breathless. Empyema is the name of an infected pleural effusion.

PMS See PREMENSTRUAL SYNDROME.

PMT See PREMENSTRUAL SYNDROME.

Pneumoconiosis Irreversible disorder of lung tissue resulting from the inhalation of certain types of dust; it is a common industrial hazard. Three main forms are distinguishable.

Simple pneumoconiosis causes little trouble and consists of the deposition of inert particles in the lungs—e.g. carbon from city air (anthracosis) and iron dust (siderosis).

Silicosis and asbestosis are due, respectively, to the inhalation of particles of silica and asbestos, both of which are extremely irritant and cause longstanding, debilitating illness. Patients with *irritant dust pneumoconiosis* are breathless, and suffer from a chronic COUGH and wheezing attacks. Lung tissue becomes thickened and scarred, and loses much of its elasticity—which accounts for its impaired function.

In the third type of pneumoconiosis, the main feature is ALLERGY to dusts such as moulds (FARMER'S LUNG), or cotton (BYSSINOSIS). These conditions produce symptoms of asthma (see II/15) and bronchitis (see II/11).

Pneumonia INFLAMMATION of the lungs due either to INFECTION by bacteria, viruses or fungi, or to chemical irritation. See II/14.

Poisoning There is a yearly increase in the number of people in our society who poison themselves, but despite this the death rate is lower than it was, due largely to improved medical techniques for dealing with cases of poisoning. Regardless of the nature of the substance taken, any unconscious person suspected of being poisoned should first be checked for clear airways—i.e. whether his or her nose, mouth and throat are free from vomit—and then placed in the classic recovery position: this consists of turning the person so that he or she is lying prone, with the head resting on an arm and the mouth and face directed sideways and downwards. Immediate transfer to hospital is the next priority; should breathing cease before this can be effected, mouth-to-mouth resuscitation should be applied.

The admitting doctor at the hospital can be greatly helped in the treatment of the patient if a friend or relative can answer questions on the patient's behalf. Any empty or half-empty containers that might be related to the poisoning or overdose should be taken along, or at least sent with the patient in the ambulance, in the care of the attendant. A specimen of vomit in a secure container can also be of great use.

In some cases, poisons have a specific antidote, but often the stomach or bowel ejects some of the irritant before it has been absorbed into the system. In many cases of poisoning, especially those of medicinal overdose, the stomach is washed out by means of an emetic (substance producing vomiting) or a stomach tube. Corrosive poisons cannot be treated this way, however, as vomiting worsens the degree of tissue damage already suffered. White of egg can be used instead to minimize the degree of internal burning. Other general antidotes include milk, charcoal and tannic acid in the form of strong cool tea.

All but the most trivial cases of poisoning are better off in hospital. Some poisons take several hours to produce symptoms, and artificial respiration, intravenous therapy to combat SHOCK, and even renal dialysis (removal of the poison from the blood by means of an artificial kidney machine) may become essential.

Poliomyelitis (infantile paralysis)   A viral infection of the digestive tract that can attack the central nervous system to produce paralysis of voluntary muscles. See XII/7.

Polyp   A benign (i.e. non-cancerous) TUMOUR growing from mucous membrane, to which it is attached by a stalk; the whole structure is rather like a berry. Common locations for polyps are the nose, the neck of the womb (cervix) and the womb itself (uterus); in none of these places are they likely to be malignant. They are more likely to develop in areas of longstanding superficial infection, and are uncommon in children.

Nasal polyps tend to occur in hay-fever sufferers, and can cause difficulty in breathing through the nose, NOSEBLEEDS, and a diminished sense of smell. Cervical or uterine polyps sometimes cause bleeding between periods. Polyps also occur in large numbers in the colon and rectum of individuals with a rare inherited disorder called familial adenomatous polyposis, in which malignant change sometimes occurs.

Potassium deficiency The balance of potassium in the body is critical, and diets that include little fresh food (especially fresh vegetables and fruit) can lead to a potassium-deficient state. A tendency to DIARRHOEA, frequent use of laxatives that produce a liquid bowel motion, and/or a course of diuretic drugs ('water pills') which are not of the potassium-conserving variety can create a state of clinical potassium deficiency which needs to be corrected.

A mild to moderate degree of potassium deficiency produces apathy, muscular weakness, mental confusion and abdominal distension; the passing of large quantities of urine (and consequent thirst) is also likely to occur. Severe potassium depletion lowers the output of the heart, often producing OEDEMA, and if untreated can cause death.

Potassium deficiency can be corrected in the first instance with supplements of potassium chloride; but further deficiency must be prevented by improving the diet, seeking professional advice about recurrent diarrhoea, ceasing to use laxative drugs, and taking potassium supplements when on a course of diuretics which deplete the body's resources.

Premenstrual syndrome (PMS) Known also by its old name of premenstrual tension (PMT), the premenstrual syndrome is a group of physical and mental symptoms affecting many women in the days before their periods start. These symptoms include tension HEADACHE, weight gain, bloating, tender breasts, spots on the face, sleep disturbances, food cravings or loss of appetite, intense irritability, poor emotional control, an increased tendency to violent behaviour (if the tendency already exists), loss of interest in sex and feelings of depression (see **XIV/3**).

Most of these symptoms are common ones in other circumstances, and, in order to be certain that they—or a selection of them—do indeed constitute the premenstrual syndrome, the best idea is to record in a diary both the day in the menstrual cycle on which they occur and the day on which they disappear. True PMS symptoms begin anything from two days to two weeks before 'day one' (i.e. the first day of the next period) and usually at the same point in each month for the particular sufferer. In addition, PMS symptoms *always* disappear shortly after menstrual bleeding starts—often within a few hours, but invariably during the first two to three days of the period. A complex of symptoms that continues throughout the period into the next cycle may resemble PMS but cannot be defined as this disorder.

Orthodox treatment
This includes tranquillizers to combat tension, sometimes antidepress-

ants, water pills (diuretics) to combat fluid retention, and either supplementary progestogens or bromocriptine (Parlodel) to reduce the secretion of prolactin hormone from the pituitary gland.

Naturopathic/herbal treatment
A wholefood diet with full supplements of vitamins and minerals, taken daily. Regular exercise is recommended. In addition, oil of the evening primrose flower taken as Efamol (the brand used in hospital trials), in the form of 500mg capsules. Minimum dose, two capsules twice daily, beginning in each cycle two days before the symptoms can be expected to commence. Maximum dose, 10–12 capsules daily, half in the morning and half in the evening, taken throughout the menstrual cycle; this quantity can gradually be reduced over the months as symptoms lessen.

Pressure sore   An area of dead tissue resulting from pressure obstructing the local blood supply. See BED SORES.

Prickly heat (heat rash; miliaria)   An irritating RASH caused by the sweat glands becoming blocked. This causes tiny blisters to appear. Prickly heat mostly affects people from temperate climates when they first visit the tropics. Keeping the body cool and wearing loose cotton clothing are essential.

Orthodox/alternative treatment
Cold compresses, cool showers, and cooling skin lotions.

Homoeopathic treatment
Aconitum Napellus.

Proctalgia (proctodynia)   In simplest terms, PAIN in the anus or rectum. *Proctalgia fugax*, which is probably due to muscle spasm, involves a severe PAIN suddenly affecting the rectum; it may persist for only a short time or for hours, and usually passes after a hot bath or a bowel motion—alternatively, the insertion of a finger into the rectum should ease it. See also PRURITUS ANI.

Prolapse   The unnatural descent of any organ from its normal anatomical position. The most usual organs to prolapse are the womb (uterus) and the bladder.

Orthodox treatment
The encouragement of weight-loss; the insertion of a rubber support

ring around the neck of the womb, changed six monthly; and surgical repair.

Alternative treatment
Weight reduction through swimming as a form of exercise; yoga, with special attention to the postures which strengthen the muscles of the pelvic floor.

Prostate gland, enlargement of See V/13.

Proteinuria The presence of protein in the urine, often as a result of a serious kidney or heart disorder.

Pruritus See ITCHING.

Pruritus ani Persistent ITCHING (pruritus) of the area from which stools are ejected (anus). Commoner in men, the usual causes are lack of adequate hygiene, the accumulation of sweat, added irritation from tight nylon or wool pants, sitting for long periods, and sometimes parasites. Likely culprits are pinworms, which lay eggs around the anus (see WORMS), and THRUSH. PILES also cause anal irritation, as does any form of discharge or RASH in that region.

Orthodox treatment
This seeks to identify and eliminate the underlying cause of the itching. Advice may be needed on hygiene, on clothing and on alternating long periods of sitting with regular exercise.

Aromatherapeutic treatment
To a lukewarm bath add 300g bicarbonate of soda enriched with 50 drops of essence of common chamomile.

Pruritus vulvae Itching of the vulva. The causes are similar to those of PRURITUS ANI, and are aggravated by the wearing of tight jeans and closed crotch pantyhose in addition to nylon panties. Abnormal VAGINAL DISCHARGE and THRUSH are other common causes. Orthodox treatment is aimed at the underlying problem.

Herbal treatment
As for PRURITUS ANI.

Psoriasis A skin disease affecting 1–2 per cent of the population and thought to be due to an enzyme disturbance in the skin itself. See VII/3.

Psychosis   Severe type of mental disorder characterized by a loss of touch with reality. A psychosis is termed either 'organic', if it results from damage to the brain, or 'functional', if no physical cause can be found for the mental disturbance.

Psychosomatic disorder   Any disorder in which mental disturbance causes physical changes to occur in the body. Emotions stored in the subconscious mind stimulate the autonomic nervous system. This works throughout the body, regulating activities such as breathing and hormonal release and the processes of digestion. The pituitary gland is likewise affected by emotion, and it in turn regulates the other endocrine glands throughout the body.

If an emotion and its bodily responses are brought into play often enough, physical change will ultimately take place. For example, frequent or perhaps almost continual stimulation of the tiny blood vessels to constrict will ultimately produce a high blood pressure; overactive stimulation of the digestive processes can lead in the end to peptic-ulcer formation. Migraine, asthma, spastic colon and circulatory disorders are further examples of disorders that sometimes have a psychosomatic cause.

Orthodox treatment
Psychotherapy, as well as symptomatic treatment for whatever disorder has been psychosomatically produced.

Alternative treatment
Psychotherapy, including hypnotherapy and positive visualization.

Pulse, irregular   See HEART RHYTHM, IRREGULAR.

Pulse, rapid   See TACHYCARDIA.

Pulse, slow   See BRADYCARDIA.

Purpura   Spontaneous bleeding of the skin, mucous membranes and elsewhere. There are two basic causes of purpura: (a) abnormally fragile capillaries (the smallest of the blood vessels, connecting the tiny ramifications of the arteries—arterioles—with those of the veins); or THROMBOCYTOPENIA, a shortage of blood platelets (tiny cell-like bodies), which normally act as a sealant when a capillary wall is damaged. The various disorders which can produce purpura include infections, wasting diseases, toxic reactions to drugs, malnutrition and certain allergic reactions.

Pus See INFLAMMATION.

Pyelitis INFLAMMATION of the hollow space (renal pelvis) within the kidney where the urine collects. In nearly all cases, the rest of the kidney tissue is also inflamed. See PYELONEPHRITIS.

Pyelonephritis Inflammation of the renal pelvis (see PYELITIS) and the main substance of the kidney (parenchyma), due to bacterial INFECTION.

Pyorrhoea Literally, a discharge of pus. The term as generally used refers to a gum condition, the full name of which is *pyorrhoea alveolaris*. It involves INFLAMMATION or degeneration of the gums, the bone around the tooth sockets, the ligaments around the bones and the connective tissue covering the root of the teeth. Pyorrhoea usually begins as gum inflammation (gingivitis – see I/5) and this develops into the more extensive periodontitis (see I/6).

Pyothorax See EMPYEMA.

Pyrexia Raised body temperature. See FEVER.

–Q–

Q fever An infectious illness similar to viral pneumonia (see II/14) and caused by the bacterium *Coxiella burneti*, which is carried by sheep and cattle and excreted in their stools and milk. Man contracts the infection either from drinking milk from a carrier animal or from inhaling dust particles containing some of the bacteria. The symptoms start after an incubation period of 14–28 days, and include FEVER, weakness, HEADACHE and persistent COUGH. The inflamed lungs usually respond to treatment with tetracycline, but occasionally damage to the heart may be apparent months after the original infection. Q fever is very rarely fatal, but can become chronic and relapsing despite treatment.

Queer turns Also known as the COQIW ('come over queer in Woolworths') syndrome, and as funny attacks. Patients generally find it very hard to be specific about the symptoms they have experienced. Sometimes, consciousness is lost for a few seconds or longer. In other varieties of queer turn, DIZZY SPELLS are experienced but consciousness is retained. Possible causes include simple FAINTING spells, postural HYPOTENSION, and HYPOGLYCAEMIA. Queer turns should always be reported to a doctor and their cause investigated. Sometimes the underlying problem is a disorder of the heart or of the nervous system, but frequently the cause is simple and easily remedied. Quite often, despite thorough investigations, no cause whatever can be found.

Quinsy (peritonsillar abscess) This condition, an ABSCESS in the region of the tonsils, is an occasional and very painful complication of acute tonsillitis (see II/6). Swallowing becomes progressively more difficult, and muscular SPASM occurs around the jaw. Treatment consists of bed rest and a fluid diet until the abscess either bursts and releases its pus or is incised and drained by an ear, nose and throat specialist.

–R–

Radiation sickness Illness caused by exposure to undue radioactivity, usually a side-effect of radiation treatment. Symptoms normally include temporary hair loss (see VII/5), mouth ulcers (see I/3), VOMITING and DIARRHOEA; anaemia (see VIII/1) is common. INFLAMMATION occurs around the irradiated site, and, depending upon where this is situated, can cause trouble at a later date by becoming chronic. Recurrent ABDOMINAL PAIN, for example, can result from the laying down of fibrous tissue following radiotherapy to an abdominal area. Sometimes the bone marrow is affected, giving rise to disorders of the blood such as THROMBOCYTOPENIA. This can result in excessive blood loss following injury.

Rash A skin eruption, often bright pink or red. A rash can be confined to one or several areas, or cover the entire body, and may or may not be itchy. The source of the problem can be an actual skin disorder, such as eczema (see VII/2) or psoriasis (see VII/3), or it may lie elsewhere in the body, as for example in measles (see XII/5) or SCARLET FEVER. Alternatively, the rash can result from the action of an external agent, such as mosquitoes or parasites (see SCABIES). See also HIVES and PRICKLY HEAT.

Nappy rash is a type of dermatitis resulting from irritation by dirty or wet nappies.

Orthodox treatment
The inflammation is treated with a soothing, antiseptic cream, and the nappy area is kept dry by leaving the nappies off for long periods. Changing those nappies that are worn as soon as they become soiled helps to prevent recurrence of the rash. Superimposed fungal infection (such as by *Candida albicans*—see THRUSH) is treated with antifungal creams.

Herbal treatment
After thorough, gentle bathing and drying of the sore area, spread pure *Aloe vera* gel on all inflamed parts.

Raynaud's disease Sudden episodes of coldness and pallor of the fingers or toes, which may last for an hour or longer. The condition is due to a disorder of the small arteries, whereby their walls periodically go into SPASM, greatly reducing the blood supply to the affected area. The spasm is brought on by trivial factors which do not produce that effect in normal arteries—examples are slight cold, vibration, anger and fear. The phenomenon is an exaggeration of the normal response, since healthy vessels also contract in this way but only when there is a physiological need for them to do so—e.g. in conditions of extreme, not slight, cold.

Orthodox treatment
This uses vasodilator drugs—i.e. drugs that dilate the small arteries and prevent them from going into spasm. Examples are nicofuranose (Bradilan) and isoxsuprine (Duvadilan).

Acupuncture
This may be successful in improving Raynaud's disease.

Reiter's syndrome A male disorder with three main distinguishing features: (a) urethritis (INFLAMMATION of the bladder outlet, or urethra —see IV/5) which does not arise from infection with the gonococcus (bacterium responsible for GONORRHOEA); (b) arthritis (see VI/1) and (c) PINK EYE.

Respiratory distress syndrome (RDS; hyaline-membrane disease) This disorder is most frequently found in premature babies (sometimes full-term babies), within the first four hours of their lives. Its main symptoms are breathing problems and a bluish tinge to the skin (cyanosis) as a result of insufficient oxygen in the blood. The underlying cause is stickiness of the tiny air sacs (alveoli) of the lungs, due to the absence of a surface agent that normally prevents the stickiness from occurring. This agent is almost always present in the lungs of babies born at full term, but does not appear until a relatively late stage of embryonic development has been reached. Thus RDS is a possible complication of all premature births. Tests can now be performed, before a pregnancy is induced, to make sure that the respiratory agent has been produced.

When babies develop RDS they are treated with a special type of artificial respiration to minimize the chance of the delicate lung sacs collapsing.

Restless legs syndrome An aching, burning irritation of the lower limbs coupled with the need to move the legs restlessly. This typically comes on while at rest, most frequently after getting into bed at night. The skin over the legs sometimes burns and itches, and attacks of cramp can occur in the leg muscles. The cause of this syndrome is inefficient return of blood from the veins of the lower limbs upwards towards the heart. The result is partial stasis of the bloodflow and the development of back pressure in the tiny vessels (capillaries) of the lower limbs. Fluid seeps out of the capillaries and into the spaces between the tissues. This condition, known as *chronic venous insufficiency*, predisposes the patient to VARICOSE VEINS.

Orthodox treatment
This consists of weight reduction (where appropriate), elastic stockings, exercise advice and the drug oxerutins (Paroven).

Vitamin treatment
Vitamin C/bioflavonoids complex, 1g twice daily.

Retinopathy Damage to the light-sensitive membrane at the back of the eye (retina) resulting from diseased blood vessels. The age-related degenerative disorder arteriosclerosis (hardening of the ARTERIES) affects the blood vessels supplying the retina (in common with blood vessels throughout the rest of the body). If undue strain is placed upon the fragile vessels, for instance by high blood pressure, then small HAEMORRHAGES occur into the retina and affect the vision.

Malignant HYPERTENSION—i.e. a blood pressure reaching or exceeding a reading of 250mm over 150mm Hg—can damage the retina of younger people in this way. Similarly, nine out of ten patients who have had DIABETES for more than 25 years have a degree of retinopathy. This can lead to complete blindness at an early age, but can be treated if diagnosed sufficiently early.

Rheumatic fever   An acute illness, commonest in children and young adults, which occurs as a delayed complication of a haemolytic strepto-coccal throat INFECTION. In its mildest form the illness may involve a slight degree of FEVER and only fleeting aches and pains in the arms and legs; alternatively, the fever may be more prolonged, with PAIN and INFLAMMATION appearing in one large joint after another. The under-lying process is the inflammation of connective tissue, occurring at various points in the body but most often in the heart valves and the large joints (e.g. elbows and knees).

Some children develop a condition known as Sydenham's CHOREA, which consists of strange, involuntary, restless, fidgeting movements in the muscles normally under conscious control. Both this and the inflamed joints recover, but the heart may remain permanently dam-aged. See III/1.

Rheumatism   A collective term for painful disorders of muscles and associated tissues which are not directly due to injury or infection. See VI/5.

Rheumatoid arthritis   A chronic inflammatory disorder of the connec-tive tissue of the joints. See VI/3.

Rhinitis   INFLAMMATION of the lining of the nose, as occurs in the common cold (see II/2) and in hay fever (see II/4).

Rickets   A childhood disorder, resulting from Vitamin-D deficiency. The typical symptom is bone softness and irregular bone growth, resulting in skeletal deformities, swollen joints and misshapen limbs. Rickets is far less common than it once was in developed countries, but it can still be seen occasionally. The most likely cause is insufficient exposure to sunlight. Treatment is by Vitamin-D supplementation and, where possible, a change in lifestyle to permit greater contact with sunlight. See also OSTEOMALACIA.

Rigor   Violent attack of shivering at the start of a FEVER, as a result of a rapid rise in body temperature.

Ringworm (tinea)   A very common skin disorder, resulting from a fungal infection of the outer skin layers. See **VII/6**.

Rodent ulcer   A malignant skin ULCER of the face, most commonly found above an imaginary line joining the tip of the earlobe to the lowest point of the nostril on a particular side of the face. Rodent ulcers can be treated by surgical excision or by radiotherapy, and, although cancerous (see **XIII**), do not form secondary deposits elsewhere in the body.

Rosacea (acne rosacea)   A chronic skin condition which colours the skin of the forehead, nose, cheeks and chin a bright red or pink, as a result of dilated skin capillaries (minute blood vessels); lumpy and pus-filled spots are often found as well. Some authorities attribute rosacea to the consumption of coffee, tea and alcohol, others to hormonal imbalance. Typical orthodox treatment consists of a course of tetracycline, and cortisone ointment. The drug metronidazole can be helpful.

Rotator cuff syndrome   See TENDINITIS.

Roundworms   See WORMS.

Rubella   German measles. See **XII/2**.

Rupture   See HERNIA.

–S–

St Vitus's dance   See CHOREA.

Salpingitis   INFLAMMATION of one or both fallopian tubes. See **V/4**.

Sarcoma   Malignant growth of muscle, bone or connective tissue. It is one of the two major varieties of malignant TUMOUR, the other being CARCINOMA; sarcoma is by far the less common of the two. The commonest variety occurs in bone tissue. See **VI/9**.

Scabies   A skin disorder causing a great degree of ITCHING. It is due to the itch mite, a very small parasite formally named *Sarcoptes scabiei*, generally picked up from infested bed linen. Orthodox treatment is to paint the area with gamma benzene hexachloride solution (Quellada).

Herbal treatment
Soak a handful of ivy leaves in a litre of wine vinegar for 24 hours, strain, and apply to skin twice daily.

Scarlet fever (scarletina)   An infectious illness usually encountered in children, resulting from a THROAT infection caused by a certain strain of streptococcal bacteria (see **XII/9**).

Schizoid personality   People with this type of personality tend not to form close relationships with others, and are aloof and withdrawn. At the same time, they are hypersensitive to criticism, and often behave very eccentrically. This condition is quite distinct from schizophrenia (see **XIV/1**).

Schizophrenia   One of the two main types of functional psychosis, the other being manic-depressive psychosis. See **XIV/1**.

Sciatica   A neuralgic disorder (see NEURALGIA). It takes the form of persistent PAIN in the buttock, back of the thigh, calf and/or foot, due to irritation of the spinal nerve roots of which the sciatic nerve is composed. Sciatic pain is a symptom and not a disorder in itself, which is why effective treatment is aimed at the underlying problem. The most likely cause is joint disease between the fourth and the fifth lumbar vertebrae. The DISC between these two bones may slip and press on the root of the nerve, or the passageway for the nerve fibres may become narrowed by arthritic changes.
  Sciatica can cause much distress and fatigue, one of the worst problems being the difficulty of finding a comfortable position. The pain is made worse by coughing, sneezing, bending and any type of physical straining, including straining to pass a motion. Skin sensation over the affected area is often blunted, and the muscles frequently become weak. The lower part of the back (the lumbar region) becomes stiff, and the spinal muscles go into SPASM.

Orthodox treatment
Bed rest is essential, on a firm mattress either placed on the floor or made firmer by putting boards beneath it. A hotwater bottle on the area and mild painkillers can help, and resistant sciatica can be helped by exercises and manipulation.

Osteopathic/chiropractic treatment
Manipulation, either osteopathic or chiropractic, is very helpful. Gentle daily stretch exercises are sometimes curative, certain yoga positions (e.g. the Coil) being especially beneficial (see page 477).

Scoliosis Sideways curvature of the spine. Scoliosis may exist for no apparent reason, or be due to muscular weakness on one side of the back; deformed vertebrae, for example after RICKETS; chronic lung disease, where the muscles on the affected side are clenched; a diseased hip joint; or SCIATICA. Scoliosis can cause chronic BACKACHE due to muscular strain.

Scurvy A disorder typified by abnormal bleeding below the skin, into the gums around the teeth and into the interior of joints, as well as by a tendency to succumb easily to infections and the opening of previously healed wounds. It is caused by a deficiency of Vitamin C, due either to a deficiency in the diet or to too heavy demands being made upon the supply that is normally ingested. The abnormal-bleeding tendency is due to a weakness that develops in the 'cell adhesive' which keeps cells 'sticking together' within a particular tissue. Tissues most commonly affected include (a) the small blood vessels (capillaries), whose walls therefore gape and ooze blood, and (b) connective tissue. The treatment is supplementation with Vitamin C.

Secondaries (**metastases**) Secondary deposits of malignant cell growth, arising from the initial (primary) site of a TUMOUR and developing in other body areas, which they reach either directly or by means of the bloodstream and lympathic system. Thus secondaries in the bones of the spine are often found as a result of a malignant lung tumour. See **XIII**.

Seizure A sudden CONVULSION resulting from FEVER in children, epilepsy (see **IX/1**), hysteria (see **XIV/6**), POISONING, or one of several other causes.

Selenium deficiency The mineral selenium and Vitamin E are described as 'synergistic', which means that they work together in such a way that the sum is greater than the parts. A deficiency of selenium causes a premature loss of stamina. A recommended daily intake of selenium, present in wheatgerm, bran and onions, is around 50–100mg.

Senility Mental deterioration resulting from changes in the brain brought about by the ageing process. Two main causes exist.
Firstly, nerve cells (neurones) are unable to regenerate, and the loss of brain neurones that occurs from adulthood onwards robs the ageing brain of much of its ability. In one recent experiment a decrease in the

number of neurones from 7,890 per cubic millimetre, at the age of 45, to 5,800 per cubic millimetre, at the age of 90 (a loss of 26 per cent), was recorded in the brain cortex.

The second, more important, reason for the development of senility is degeneration of the ARTERIES supplying the brain with resultant deprivation of blood and oxygen.

In the early stages of senile change, intellectual performance and agility are impaired, memory, concentration and time awareness are poor, and the elderly person frequently becomes intensely irritable, confused (see DEMENTIA) and anxious. As the condition progresses, speech becomes further impaired, behaviour may become abnormal or bizarre, and familiar personal care and domestic skills are lost. Communication becomes very difficult, and in the final stages the senile person may forget his or her own name. INCONTINENCE often occurs, the ability to walk is lost, and death usually occurs with the patient in a COMA.

It is important for the diagnosis of senility rather than DEPRESSION to be made by an expert, since the two disorders can easily be mistaken for one another in an old person. Tranquillizing drugs and alcohol worsen states of senile confusion.

Septicaemia (blood poisoning)   The presence of disease-causing bacteria in the bloodstream, particularly *Escherichia coli* (a frequent cause of DIARRHOEA), the meningococcus (a frequent cause of pyogenic, or pus-forming, MENINGITIS), and the pneumococcus (which also causes meningitis, and lobar pneumonia—see II/14). Appropriate antibiotic treatment is mandatory in septicaemia, as multiplication of pathogenic (harmful) bacteria in the bloodstream can easily be fatal.

Shingles (Herpes zoster)   INFECTION of a nerve root (usually spinal) by the virus *Herpes zoster*, producing a rash of BLISTERS. See IX/6.

Shock   Physical collapse resulting from impaired blood circulation. Causes include HAEMORRHAGE; serious plasma loss due to BURN injury; serious loss of body fluid, which in turn affects the circulation, due to profound DIARRHOEA and/or VOMITING, and ineffectual pumping of the blood around the body, following a CORONARY THROMBOSIS. Signs of developing shock include pallor, a fast thready pulse, sweating, NAUSEA, restlessness and anxiety (see XIV/4) and ultimately unconsciousness (see FAINTING).

First aid for shocked patients includes lying them down with their legs slightly raised and keeping them warm with light covers. When the circulating blood volume has been depleted it needs to be restored by means of intravenous fluid or blood replacement as a matter of extreme urgency.

Shortsightedness (myopia)   This is due to the lens of the eye focussing the rays of light from objects in the visual field in front of the retina, instead of upon it. This is corrected by suitable spectacles or contact lenses prescribed and prepared by orthodox practitioners.

Bates' eye training treatment
This is sometimes successful in improving the sight by natural means. The treatment includes eye exercises and hydrotherapy.

Siderosis   A lung disease belonging to the PNEUMOCONIOSIS group and caused by the inhalation of large quantities of iron-oxide dust.

Silicosis   One of the lung diseases in the PNEUMOCONIOSIS group.

Sinusitis   INFLAMMATION of the mucous membranes lining one or more of the sinuses connecting with the nose. See II/8.

Sleep disorders   These may be primary—i.e. arising spontaneously for no apparent reason—or secondary to any one of a number of possible causes. These latter include a disordered thyroid gland (see X/1), brain disease, alcoholism (see DRUG DEPENDENCE), and emotional problems.
   Primary INSOMNIA is usually treated with hypnotic drugs which induce sleep, the aim being the restoration of a normal sleep pattern by means of a brief course of drugs only. Primary narcolepsy (inability to stay awake) is often treated by means of stimulating drugs, such as one of the amphetamine-related compounds, with the same end in view. These drugs are known to be addictive and are best avoided.

Slipped disc   See DISC (slipped).

Sneeze   A protective mechanism consisting of the sudden, deep in-drawing of breath, followed by its violent expulsion. This action results from stimulation of the respiratory centre in the brain by nerve impulses arising in the sensitive membranes lining the nose. Agents include dust particles, poisonous fumes, bacteria, etc., as well as substances causing an allergic response in the nasal lining of susceptible people, such as pollen grains, animal fur, feathers, and certain perfumes (see ALLERGY).

Spasm   Sustained involuntary contraction of muscle, either 'voluntary muscle' which is used for everyday activities and which is normally under conscious control, or 'involuntary' muscle, such as that present in the wall of the gall bladder, bowel, etc. CRAMP in the calf muscles is a common form of spasm, whether it comes on during rest for no apparent reason or occurs during exercise (see CLAUDICATION). Intestinal spasm is the cause of the severe bowel pain (COLIC) experienced during an attack of gastroenteritis (see I/14), when the membranous lining of the bowel is inflamed and overstimulated.

Sometimes the word 'spasm' is used incorrectly to mean a CONVULSION or SEIZURE, or an attack of PALPITATIONS.

Spastic colon (irritable-bowel syndrome)   A disorder consisting of intermittent attacks of ABDOMINAL PAIN, DIARRHOEA and WIND, thought to be due primarily to stress (see STRESS REACTIONS). See I/30.

Spasticity   The loss or absence of voluntary movement, together with SPASM of the affected muscles. This results from damage to certain nerve cells in the outer layer (cortex) of the brain which are concerned with movement. Spasticity can occur following a stroke (see IX/7), the growth of a brain TUMOUR, or the development of multiple sclerosis (see IX/5), but the term 'spastic' is most often used in connection with the congenital handicap *cerebral palsy*, a developmental brain abnormality which gives rise to weakness and lack of coordination of the limbs. The various possible causes include MENINGITIS, oxygen shortage prior to birth, injury during birth, faulty development, and virus infection. Physiotherapy, surgery and often speech therapy are used to help sufferers.

Speech, disorders of   Slowness in a child's learning to speak may be due to DEAFNESS, lack of stimulation from adults, DYSLEXIA, extreme shyness or a low intelligence (see also STAMMERING). Speech difficulty can result from an injury to the tongue, throat or voice-box (larynx); or from poor control of the muscles involved in speaking, in which case it is known as DYSARTHRIA. This can feature in Parkinson's disease (see IX/3), and may also be due to brain damage following a stroke (see IX/7), a head injury or a TUMOUR.

Speech problems resulting from damage to the speech area in the brain are termed *aphasia* (speech loss) or *dysphasia* (speech difficulty). When speech is affected by a stroke, the problem may be partly muscular (i.e. dysarthric) and partly due to brain injury (i.e. dysphasic or aphasic). Usually, the ability to speak is at least partly regained, and sessions of speech therapy can help to achieve this. A partial or complete loss of speech can also be a neurotic condition—see discussion of hysteria (XIV/6).

Sperm, abnormal   See discussion of infertility (V/15).

Spina bifida   The condition that results from incomplete closure in the foetus of the tube of tissue that will form the future spinal cord, together with defective closure of the bony vertebral canal of the spine in which the cord is contained. The commonest site at which spina bifida occurs is the bottom of the back.

There are three types. *Spina bifida occulta*, the mildest, does not involve a defect of the spinal cord or its membranes; it is simply defective fusion of the vertebral arches in the affected region, and may never be suspected until it is observed on an X-ray of the back taken for other purposes. A *meningocoele* is more serious, and consists of a sac protruding through the defective bony archway. The membranes of which the sac is composed are those of the spinal cord (i.e. the meninges, which are an extension of the meninges covering the brain). More commonly, the membranous sac contains spinal-cord tissue or nerve roots, in which case it is called a *meningomyelocoele*. The last two mentioned types of spina bifida are associated in many cases with other congenital defects, such as HYDROCEPHALUS.

Sometimes badly affected babies are stillborn, or live for only a few hours. Others who survive may be mentally handicapped, incontinent of urine and/or motions (faeces), or have loss of sensation or muscular power in their arms and legs.

The underlying cause of spina bifida is not yet known, although leading experts are now almost certain that it is at least in part due to a deficiency of folic acid very early in pregnancy. (The doctors concerned stress that any folic-acid supplementation taken should be prescribed, and not merely bought over the counter.)

Any woman who has given birth to one affected baby stands an increased chance of doing so again. However, meningocoele and meningomyelocoele can now be established while the baby is still in the womb through the measurement of increased levels of alphafetoprotein in the fluid that surrounds the baby (amniotic fluid). A blood-screening test is also available for women known to have a higher-than-average risk of giving birth to an abnormal baby.

Splenomegaly   Abnormal enlargement of the spleen. There are many causes, including a number of INFECTIONS—e.g. malaria (see VIII/4), glandular fever (see **VIII/2**), TYPHOID FEVER—and certain blood disorders—e.g. leukaemia (see **VIII/3**).

Spondylitis INFLAMMATION of the vertebrae. In ankylosing spondylitis (bamboo spine) the joints between the vertebrae become more and more fixed and, in some patients, the associated ligaments become stiffened and hard, making it impossible to bend the back in the affected region. BACKACHE may be severe. For treatment, see discussion of rheumatoid arthritis (**VI/3**).

Spondylosis Osteoarthritis (see **VI/2**) of the vertebrae and their joints, in which the joint spaces become narrowed and small spicules of bone develop around the edges of the affected bones. Symptoms, if they occur, include pain and limitation of movement. The bony spicules can press upon spinal nerves as they emerge between the vertebrae, thus producing pain in the associated muscles.

Orthodox treatment
This may include painkilling drugs (e.g. aspirin, paracetamol), non-steroidal anti-inflammatory drugs (e.g. indomethacin [Indocid], piroxicam [Feldene]), and perhaps physiotherapy.

Manipulative treatment
Both chiropractic and osteopathy can help to free joints and improve mobility.

Sprain The complete tearing of a ligament (band of connective tissue supporting a joint). Although in itself a sprain is a minor injury, the pain can be severe, and swelling and bruising are often pronounced. A bad sprain must be distinguished from complete severing of the ligament concerned, and also from a FRACTURE. Ankles, knees and wrists are among the most commonly sprained joints.

Orthodox treatment
Cold compresses and elevating the limb help to reduce swelling. Bandaging helps to take the strain off the damaged ligament while it heals, and after an initial period of rest the joint should be moved and used.

Homoeopathic treatment
Arnica ointment on a sprain can speed healing.

Sprue (nontropical) The adult form of tropical COELIAC DISEASE, this is a MALABSORPTION disease found in tropical countries, with symptoms of anaemia (see VIII/1), muscle-wasting and DIARRHOEA. Its cause is unknown.

Squint (strabismus) A common condition in which the eyes do not remain parallel, due to one eye looking away from the direction of gaze. Some squints are corrected by surgical operation. In some cases it is claimed that Bates' eye exercises may help.

Stammering A speech disorder in which either (a) abrupt, sometimes lengthy, pauses occur while the person strains to 'get the word out', or (b) certain words or parts of words are repeated in a rapid, staccato manner. About one school child in every 100 stammers; the problem is commoner before the age of 10. In adults, men are much more frequently affected than women. Stammering is relatively more often found in left-handed and ambidextrous people, notably in those who have been born left-handed but have endeavoured to become ambidextrous. Stammering also tends to run in families.

The condition may embarrass sufferers greatly, and it is this which sometimes tends to make them appear withdrawn, since most stutterers are free from psychological disturbance in a causative sense. The outlook for sufferers is good, provided the correct treatment is provided.

Orthodox treatment
Speech therapy, the building of self-confidence, and the overcoming of any psychological problems that may have arisen due to the existence of the sufferer's defect. Obviously stressful situations should be avoided as much as possible until the sufferer has been taught to handle them successfully. Sometimes tranquillizing drugs and/or speech therapy are used.

Relaxation treatment
The teaching of relaxation exercises, possibly by the use of hypnotherapy, is by far preferable to the use of tranquillizers, and is a very useful adjunct to speech therapy.

Steatorrhoea The passage of stools with an excessively high fat content. These motions tend to be pale in colour and to float on the surface of the water in the toilet. See MALABSORPTION and COELIAC DISEASE.

Sterility The inability of a man to father children, or of a woman to bear a child. See discussion of infertility (V/15).

Stings Fish, insects and, among the arachnids, scorpions can have toxic stings.

Venomous fish carrying poisonous spines include the weaver fish, the stone fish, the scorpion fish and the lion fish. They lie concealed in shallow waters, in sand or hidden by rocks, and can be trodden upon without being seen. Fishermen are also sometimes stung when they remove their catches from lines and nets. Stingrays carry their stings in their tails, and drive them into their victims when disturbed. Jellyfish sting when touched accidentally by a swimmer or diver. The pain of these stings can be extremely severe, causing prostration, and death can occur in some cases.

Insect stings (by wasps, bees or hornets) are painful, and can cause serious and occasionally lethal reactions in people especially sensitive to them. Scorpion stings are more dangerous: the mortality rate may be as high as five per cent. Of course, swarming bees can very easily sting a person to death—but such cases are fortunately rare.

Orthodox treatment
This includes, for serious cases, the administration of antisera (specific antidotes) and the combating of SHOCK. Milder cases respond to antihistamine cream smoothed into the painful area, steroids to combat INFLAMMATION, and painkilling drugs.

Traditional/herbal treatments
Serious cases requiring professional attention should be taken to hospital as soon as possible, but less serious stings (and bites) can be treated with a strong cold solution of sodium bicarbonate in water, after the sting has been removed. The area should be wiped dry, and either some crumpled plantain leaves or a fresh slice of raw onion applied. Wasp stings, which are alkaline, can be treated with vinegar.

Homoeopathic treatment
For bee stings: *Apis Mellifica*; and for wasp stings: *Arnica Montana*.

Stitch A pain, sometimes severe, felt below the ribs on one side or another close to the attachment of the diaphragm muscle within. A stitch is probably due to SPASM of a portion of the diaphragm, and almost always follows periods of unaccustomed exertion when the breathing rate has been greatly increased. Rest is the best cure, but gentle massage of the 'stitch area' can ease the pain.

Stomach ache   A general term for ABDOMINAL PAIN which may originate from any of the abdominal organs, particularly the intestine and the organs of digestion.

Stomatitis   INFLAMMATION of the lining of the mouth. See I/1.

Stone (calculus)   A mass found in a hollow organ, such as the gall bladder, bile duct, kidney or urinary bladder. All these organs normally contain a number of substances in solution, such as cholesterol, calcium salts and uric acid. Under certain conditions, these chemicals precipitate out of solution and form a deposit or 'stone', just as the lining of a water pipe carrying hard water eventually becomes furred up with a deposit layer. See IV/4.

Strabismus   See SQUINT.

Stress reactions   Stress is any influence that upsets the body's natural equilibrium. Well known stress factors include physical injury, diseases, extremes of temperature, excessive demands on an individual's mental or physical resources, and emotional problems. Life events with high stress ratings include death of one's marital partner, child or parent; relationship problems; divorce; selling, buying and moving house; career changes; redundancy; sudden serious financial loss; examinations; and even Christmas.

The body's response to stress is largely regulated by the adrenal glands, which release the hormones they manufacture—adrenaline and noradrenaline (norepinephrine)—into the bloodstream. These hormones are responsible for the classic 'flight or fight' reaction which is especially noticeable when we receive a sudden fright—for instance, suddenly coming face to face with a potential mugger or rapist in a lonely street or isolated country area. Typically, the heart starts to beat extra fast, the mouth goes dry, and the trunk and limb muscles are primed with an extra supply of blood drawn from the skin and digestive organs. This provides the optimal conditions for either resisting attack or running away. At the same time, glucose is released into the circulating blood from the liver (where it is stored) to provide extra energy.

Besides adrenaline and noradrenaline, the adrenal glands produce the corticosteroid hormones, which help the body to overcome diseases and infections. They maintain the internal balance of fats, sugars and minerals, and help muscular tissue to incorporate protein into themselves for growth and repair purposes.

Prolonged stress eventually exhausts the body's ability to cope, and causes a damaging change in its internal environment, so that some type of physical or mental stress disorder results. Common ones include peptic ulcer (see I/9), HYPERTENSION, asthma (see II/15), eczema (see VII/2), migraine attacks (see IX/2), HEADACHES, ulcerative colitis (see I/29), depression (see XIV/3), anxiety (see XIV/4), schizophrenia (see XIV/1) and certain types of cancer (see XIII).

Orthodox treatment
Tranquillizing drugs are very frequently prescribed for stress reactions —e.g. diazepam (Valium) and lorazepam (Almazine, Ativan). Sometimes patients are referred to psychiatrists or to psychotherapists.

Naturopathic treatment
The naturopathic approach considers all aspects of the patient, and generally recommends a balanced, wholefood diet; adequate regular exercise; sufficient relaxation and rest; and specific stress-reduction techniques. Hypnotherapy, autogenic training, biofeedback and yoga are among the therapies/techniques that may well be recommended. Dietary supplements would be suggested—in particular, Vitamin C (1g daily) and a stress B complex (100mg strength, once or twice daily).

Stridor A harsh, rattling, snoring sound produced by breathing; it is fairly common in babies and toddlers and unlikely to be significant unless an infection is present—as in laryngitis and croup (see II/9)—but in older children and adults stridor can be symptomatic of a medical problem. Other causes may include an inhaled foreign body (e.g. a peanut, a bead, some vomited material), DIPHTHERIA (very unlikely in the UK), and TUMOURS of the voice-box (larynx), windpipe (trachea) or lungs.

Stroke (apoplexy) Sudden interference with the circulation of the blood in part of the brain resulting in some degree of impaired muscular function. See IX/7.

Stye (hordeolum) A BOIL in the follicle of an eyelash due to bacterial infection. Orthodox treatment consists of bathing the stye in warm water and applying an antibiotic eye ointment such as framycetin (Framygen).

Herbal treatment
An eyebath of a decoction of five chamomile flower heads to a litre of water.

Suicide In the UK suicide is as common as death on the roads, and attempted suicide by taking an overdose is now one of the most common causes for admission to hospital in most Western countries. Most successful suicides occur in people suffering from severe depression (see **XIV/3**)—an ailment which constitutes a medical emergency requiring urgent treatment, preferably in hospital. Suicide threats, and an admission even to contemplating the possibility of suicide, should always be taken seriously. Victims of failed suicide attempts should always receive adequate counselling and psychotherapy.

Sunburn The red, tender areas of skin, sometimes with blistering, that result from overexposure to the ultraviolet rays of the sun (see also HEATSTROKE).

Orthodox treatment
This consists of avoiding further exposure for the time being, and applying cold compresses and soothing creams to the affected areas.

Herbal treatment
Aloe vera gel on the inflamed areas of skin.

Sydenham's chorea See CHOREA and RHEUMATIC FEVER.

Syncope See FAINTING.

Synovitis INFLAMMATION of the fine (synovial) membrane lining the inner surfaces of a joint.

Syphilis The most serious of the VENEREAL DISEASES. INFECTION starts with the 'spirochaete' organism responsible (formal name *Treponema pallidum*) entering the body through a skin scratch or via the membranous lining of the vagina, mouth or penis. Within the body, the most likely structures to be affected are small blood vessels (capillaries), with consequent failure of the blood circulation in associated organs.
  Syphilis has three main stages. First is the appearance of a small hard lump (called a chancre), up to three months after initial infection. This may develop into an ULCER at the original site of entry into the body. It gradually clears up without treatment. The second stage, weeks or months later, is a non-specific illness with a skin rash and enlarged lymph nodes. This also disappears without treatment. The last stage usually affects the skin, bones and/or mucous membranes, although any part can be affected. A structure named a *gumma* (similar to a large

BOIL) might appear, and serious damage is often subsequently suffered by the heart and its main artery (the aorta) as well as by the nervous system.

Orthodox treatment
Penicillin is used, hopefully to cure stage one or stage two. The disease cannot be cured once it has reached the third stage, although its progress can be arrested.

–T–

Tachycardia   A pronounced increase in the rate of the heartbeat. Causes include exercise, emotional response, the sexual climax, certain drugs, anxiety states (see **XIV/4**), the SHOCK response to HAEMORR-HAGE, FEVER, heart disorders (see **III/1**, **III/3**), and certain other disorders, such as an overactive thyroid gland (see **X/1**).

Paroxysmal atrial tachycardia is a common form of tachycardia most often occurring in young people with healthy hearts. The pulse (i.e. heartbeat) rate can suddenly increase from normal (about 70–80 beats per minute) to as much as 150–250 beats per minute, but it remains regular. There is often a fluttery feeling in the chest, and the person experiencing an attack can become very distressed. The rate remains unaffected by rest, posture and exercise, and the way many doctors terminate an attack is by massaging an area of the carotid artery in the neck known as the carotid sinus.

An effective remedy which can be carried out at home is the Valsalva manoeuvre. Take a breath, and try to force it out against resistance —e.g. by closing the mouth and pinching the nose firmly. Although breathing out is impossible, the pressure inside the chest is raised, and the attack usually comes to an end, although a feeling of faintness may occur.

Tapeworm infestation (taeniasis)   See WORMS.

Teething problems   The soreness babies experience during teething is often accompanied by both fretfulness and mild FEVER, although it is essential to remember that cutting teeth may not be the cause of these symptoms: the baby should be carefully examined, as other disorders, such as an INFECTION, might be producing the fever. Successful potty training is likely to be temporarily disrupted when the baby has a sore mouth and raised temperature, and favourite foods and drinks may well be refused.

Orthodox treatment
This aims at supplying plenty of cool fluids, such as water and diluted fruit juice, and sometimes at reducing the fever using a small dose of aspirin or paracetamol. Soothing antiseptic oral jelly can also be smeared on the painful gum.

Homoeopathic treatment
When the child is irritable, with one cheek flushed and the other pale, and has diarrhoea: *Chamomilla*. If the condition is acute and the child is feverish: *Aconite*. When there is irritability, flushed cheeks and convulsions: *Belladonna*. When teething is delayed, and the child has slimy mucous diarrhoea: *Calcarea*.

Temperature, lowered   See HYPOTHERMIA.

Temperature, raised (pyrexia)   See FEVER.

Temper tantrums   These can arise in small children for a variety of reasons. They are especially likely to occur after the age of one year, when many children go through a recognizable phase of negative behaviour during which they rebel against parental discipline, however it may be applied. One reason for this behaviour is the frustration small children feel at their failure to communicate the growing complexity of their feelings and desires through the medium of coherent sentences. The interaction between toddlers (especially bright ones) and their environment increases their familiarity with simple objects and thereby their ability to master simple skills. It is also a source of great pleasure and excitement, and occasionally of confusion and irritation, all of which they would like to be able to express, and to share with their parents. Speech, however, develops relatively slowly in normal children, usually starting at around nine months, and it is not until they have reached the age of (usually) five years that they acquire a reasonably comprehensive vocabulary and the basic essentials of sentence structuring. Hence the—understandable—frustration.

Temper tantrums are also associated with the condition known as HYPERACTIVITY, and outbursts of uncontrollable behaviour and temper tantrums tend to occur not only in the small hyperactive child but also, in a more mature form, throughout his or her childhood and adolescence.

Very frequent temper tantrums occurring for no apparent reason in babies and especially in small children may, however, need expert advice. They may be an attempt to 'blackmail' the parents—and once given into are likely to be repeated at frequent intervals. On the other hand, they may indicate an emotional need or physical disorder which the infant has no other means of expressing.

Temper outbursts are also common in normal adolescents, who may be emotionally bewildered by the changing patterns of their feelings as they develop from child into adult. These feelings are made all the more complex by the adolescent's developing sexuality, his or her lack of self-confidence, and the demands of fitting in with the peer group. Adolescents may also be frustrated by a large store of pent-up physical energy which is finding insufficient outlet both at home and at school.

Temper tantrums in children of any age are distressing for parents, some of whom are tempted to combat them by using physical violence themselves. A smacked bottom, when warranted, is extremely unlikely to do a healthy young child any harm, and may well make a point that simple words fail to make. However, there is no excuse whatsoever for battering or assaulting children under any circumstances, and parents who are aware that they risk damaging their children should urgently seek counselling and help themselves—although the fact that they are aware of and worried about the situation is of course a good sign.

The best way to deal with toddlers' temper tantrums, generally speaking, is to attempt to understand what is infuriating them, and to explain to them, calmly and simply, the cause of the problem. It is very important—although often very difficult—to refrain from losing one's own temper, either during the tantrum or in other personal and domestic situations in which the child is the observer—children learn a great deal by imitation. At the time of the outburst as little fuss as possible should be made about it; while at home, it is often best first to see that the child cannot come to harm and then simply to allow him or her to scream and hammer the floor without the benefit of an audience —for a few minutes at least.

Adolescent temper tantrums are best dealt with in a calm, reasoning manner; while this attitude can be very difficult to achieve and maintain, it is worth remembering that most adolescents have pressures on them of which parents are quite unaware. Many will respond best when they are treated with respect and concern, as well as frankness and firmness of purpose. Above all, they need to be listened to, and treated with fairness and understanding.

Tendinitis INFLAMMATION, often painful, of the tendons (connective tissue cords binding muscles to bones). One form, which occurs at the shoulder joint, is known as the *rotator cuff syndrome*, referring to the muscles whose tendons are involved. The condition seems to be due to interference with the blood supply to the muscle tendons as a result of compression of blood vessels between the acromion (the top of the spine of the shoulderblade) and the head of the humerus (the bone of the upper arm).

Orthodox treatment
Orthodox doctors treat tendinitis with painkilling drugs, with non-steroidal anti-inflammatory drugs (NSAIDs) such as indomethacin (Indocid), and with steroid injections into the tendon sheath as a means of coping locally with the inflammation.

PEMF treatment
Pulsed electromagnetic field therapy has had a very high success rate in curing rotator cuff tendinitis.[30]

Tenesmus A persistent desire to open the bowels, resulting only in the passage of wind (flatus) and perhaps mucus and a little blood. Causes include ulcerative colitis (see I/29), dysentery (see I/31), diverticulitis (see I/32), piles (see I/34) and TUMOUR of the bowel. Other causes include impaction of the rectum with very hard faeces and, in children, infestation with WORMS.

Tennis elbow Pain and stiffness of the elbow joint. Possible causes include BURSITIS, nipping of the radial nerve at this joint, and torn muscle fibres. Uncustomary effort—for instance, with a screwdriver or in a hectic sports session of tennis, badminton, etc.—is usually responsible.

Orthodox treatment
This usually consists of an injection of hydrocortisone into the affected area. This treatment is very painful.

Alternative treatment
See discussion of alternative treatments for PAIN. TENS (see page 95) may be helpful.

Tension Nervous tension is one of the symptoms produced by the body and mind when stress is not being dealt with adequately (see STRESS REACTIONS).

Orthodox treatment
Psychotherapy; tranquillizers such as diazepam (Valium).

Homoeopathic treatment
Aconitum Napellus.

Testis, torsion of   A twisting round of the testis, with compression of the blood vessels in the spermatic cord. This is a very painful condition, and early surgery is essential.

Testis, undescended   The testis in the baby boy develops within the abdomen, close to the kidney. Normally, it descends into the scrotum before birth, but in about 10 per cent of babies it fails to do so. Often the testis descends a few weeks after birth; if not, it is brought down into its correct position in the scrotal sac by means of surgery.

Tetanus   See LOCKJAW.

Tetany   Twitching and SPASM of the muscles, especially those of the arms and hands. The condition is caused by an abnormally low level of calcium in the blood and tissue fluids, and is most frequently seen in small babies in association with RICKETS, prolonged VOMITING or disordered kidneys. Other causes include a deficiency of Vitamin D, malfunction of the parathyroid glands which help to control calcium metabolism, and HYPERVENTILATION. Tetany is treated by giving intravenous calcium gluconate, and extract of the parathyroid glands (parathormone) when these glands are at fault.

Thalassaemia (Cooley's anaemia)   An hereditary abnormality of the red, oxygen-carrying blood pigment (haemoglobin), most commonly found in Sicily, Greece and Sardinia. The symptoms in affected children are those of anaemia (see VIII/1) combined with JAUNDICE and enlargement of the spleen and the liver. Diagnosis is confirmed by examination of the blood for 'target cells' (abnormal red blood cells with a pale rim and a central spot of haemoglobin pigment).

Threadworms (pinworms)   See WORMS.

Throat, sore   A painfully inflamed throat, generally due to INFECTION of the pharynx or tonsils. See II/5 and II/6.

Thromboangiitis obliterans (Buerger's disease)   A chronic, recurrent vascular disease, primarily of the arteries and to a lesser extent of the veins. The affected vessels, especially those in the legs, become increasingly narrowed until finally the central hollow, or bore, becomes clogged ('obliterated') by blood clots. The symptoms of this condition are those of an inadequate blood supply—pain on exercising (see CLAUDICATION), a cold temperature, and inefficient healing processes. The skin over affected areas is likely to ulcerate, and GANGRENE can occur in the toes or feet.

Sufferers are typically men in their forties who smoke; while the cause of thromboangiitis obliterans is not known, tobacco smoking is known to make it a great deal worse. Treatment forbids the use of tobacco and centres at first on drugs that dilate the blood vessels, with, possibly, a 'sympathectomy' operation in which certain sympathetic nerve fibres are severed. This permits unaffected vessel tributaries to dilate and offer alternative routes for the flow of blood. Ultimately if gangrene occurs, amputation of parts of the lower limb may become necessary.

Thrombocytopenia A deficiency of platelets (thrombocytes) in the blood, giving rise to failure of the clotting mechanism: This condition frequently gives rise to excessive bruising.

Thromboembolism The obstruction of a blood vessel by a clot of blood which has travelled there from another part of the body. See THROMBOSIS and EMBOLISM.

Thrombophlebitis THROMBOSIS (clotting) in a vein following INFLAMMATION of the vein wall. Compare PHLEBOTHROMBOSIS.

Thrombosis The formation of a blood clot (thrombus) on the lining of an artery or a vein, thereby blocking the circulation in that area. This usually happens only when the lining of the vessel is damaged in some way which destroys its smooth, water-repellent quality. Thrombosis in veins is normally associated with THROMBOPHLEBITIS; in arteries with ATHEROMA. See also CORONARY THROMBOSIS.

Thrush An INFECTION due to the yeast-like fungus *Candida albicans*. This yeast is a normal inhabitant of our bowels and—in women—of the vagina. The infection arises when the *Candida* organism becomes much more active than usual, due in most cases to the immune defence system becoming weak. This can occur as a result of a number of circumstances, fatigue and STRESS REACTION being two prominent ones. The infection can be controlled by antifungal drugs such as nystatin (Nystan), but unless the immune defence system is strengthened the infection recurs.

Another factor that encourages the growth of *Candida* is the use of broad-spectrum antibiotics which destroy the helpful bacteria that normally keep *Candida* under control. When allowed to spread uninhibitedly, the yeast cells assume their 'mycelial fungal' form, growing roots which penetrate the tissue in which they are situated. When this is the intestine, the burrows made by the roots into the intestinal wall permit the entry into the bloodstream of yeast by-products and partially digested food. These 'foreign bodies' in the bloodstream cause a wide range of allergic symptoms, including emotional and mental disturbances. It is also thought that the yeast may produce the chemical acetaldehyde, which is highly toxic and capable of interfering with a number of biochemical processes.

Other drugs besides antibiotics which favour the spread of *Candida* include the contraceptive pill and 'immunosuppressive' drugs such as steroids. Also culpable is a diet containing refined food and a great deal of sugar and starch, since this provides the natural food of the yeast cells.

Some of the disorders believed by the two doctors who have researched *Candida* thoroughly (Truss of Alabama and Crook of Tennessee) to be probably due to this yeast infestation include digestive problems, especially copious flatulence after eating starch, as well as bouts of DIARRHOEA, cystitis (see **IV/5**), vaginitis (see **V/8**) and prostatitis (see **V/13**). Others include stubborn fungal infections, such as ringworm (see **VII/6**), vaginal thrush infection, many sorts of ALLERGY, lethargy, depression (see **XIV/3**), fatigue and a craving for sugar and alcohol.

Orthodox treatment

This consists of nystatin (Nystan) or clotrimazole (Canestan), but this should be regarded strictly as a short-term measure. Avoiding factors such as dietary items and drugs which aggravate thrush and choosing the right foods will ultimately bring it under control.[31]

Naturopathic Candida control

Besides dealing with STRESS REACTIONS and suggesting a healthier lifestyle all round, naturopathic practitioners recommend the foods discussed below as helpful, taken as part of a strictly wholefood diet which excludes refined, starchy and sugary foods. Foods based on a fermentation process (such as alcohol) and which contain mould (certain cheeses, mushrooms) are also banned. Wholegrains such as brown rice, whole wheat and pulses are acceptable. Fruits are forbidden during the first few weeks because of their sugar content. *Lactobacillus acidophilus* should be taken as a supplement—this is the useful bacteria killed by antibiotics which normally controls the spread of *Candida*. Recommended sources are acidophilus powder, sold as Superdophilus and Vital Dophilus; these can be up to 800 times more powerful than usual acidophilus products. Vital Dophilus is suitable for anyone sensitive to dairy products. For the first two weeks of treatment, up to 1g of one of these products should be taken daily, then 500mg daily for six months. Biotin (300–500mg tablet) should be taken after each meal; this is a B vitamin very helpful in controlling *Candida*.

Also helpful: garlic, either a whole raw head daily, or six odourless garlic capsules. Olive oil, helpful in a similar way to biotin, should be taken daily—two dessertspoonfuls of the cold pressed variety.

The amino acid arginine helps the immune system recover: take 1–2g daily on an empty stomach. This does not apply to anyone with a HERPES infection or with schizophrenia (see **XIV/1**).

Also advised are Vitamin C, one gram daily; a strong Vitamin-B complex from a yeast-free source; and 100mg of zinc orotate (B_{13} zinc). The drug nystatin (Nystan) can be taken for a brief period. If antibiotics ever have to be taken, the early use of high-potency acidophilus supplement helps repopulate the bowel with helpful bacteria, helping to protect against further spread of *Candida*. The diet as a whole should also be followed when antibiotics are taken.[32]

Thyrotoxicosis A toxic condition due to an overactive thyroid gland. See **X/1**.

Tic (habitual spasm) An involuntary twitch affecting a part of the body repeatedly and for no apparent reason. It is often an extension and exaggeration of a once-useful movement that has become habitual —for instance, an ill treated child who has been frequently cuffed around the side of the head may continue to jerk the head away in an habitual fashion after the ill-treatment has stopped.

Tics particularly affects nervous, highly strung people, especially when they are unwell or stressed, and may respond to psychotherapy or hypnotherapy.

The term 'tic douloureux' refers to spasm of the facial muscles due to the pain of trigeminal NEURALGIA.

Tinea See RINGWORM.

Tinnitus A ringing (or hissing or buzzing) sound in the ears. Causes include wax in the ears; a blocked Eustachian tube (which connects the middle ear with the throat); malfunction of the auditory nerve, concerned with transmitting sound messages to the brain (this can be due to irritation from various drugs, including aspirin and quinine); or Ménière's disease (see XI/3).

Manipulative treatment
Cranial osteopathy can relieve sufferers from this complaint.

Homoeopathic treatment
Graphites; *Salicylic acid*; *Rhus* Toxicodendron.

Tonsillitis   INFLAMMATION of the tonsils. See II/6.

Toothache   Pain in a tooth can be due to a mouth injury or to a disorder elsewhere from which the PAIN is referred. The commonest causes, however, are dental caries (decay—see I/4) and ABSCESS formation around the root. Decayed teeth are drilled and filled by the dentist. Although abscesses are often treated by extracting the relevant tooth, this can sometimes be avoided by the use of antibiotics and by drilling the length of the tooth and filling the cavity when it is clean.

Aromatheapeutic treatment
Application of clove oil to the root of the painful tooth. Tincture of myrrh is also very effective.

Torsion of the testis   See TESTIS (torsion of).

Torticollis   See WRY NECK.

Tracheitis   INFLAMMATION of the trachea (windpipe). See II/11.

Tranquillizers, dependence upon   See DRUG DEPENDENCE.

Travel sickness   See MOTION SICKNESS.

Tremor   A shaking or trembling of part of the body resulting from the alternating contractions of opposing muscle groups. Tremor may be a symptom of a disorder affecting the area of the brain and spinal cord concerned with movement, especially with the coordination necessary for a balanced posture and controlled muscular actions and locomotion. Disorders in which a tremor is characteristic, include Parkinson's disease (see IX/3); hyperthyroidism (see X/1); multiple sclerosis (see IX/5); disturbances of the cerebellar area of the brain, which is concerned with muscle tone, balance and the reflex adjustments of voluntary movements; and WILSON'S DISEASE.

Tremor can also result from the toxic effects of alcohol and drugs on the nervous system, and from emotional disorders. Treatment is directed at the underlying disorder, where possible.

Trichomonas infection   INFECTION of the vagina and bladder outlet (urethra) in a woman, or of the urethra in a man, by *Trichomonas vaginalis*, which is a single-celled parasitic animal. This condition is a form of VENEREAL DISEASE, and produces irritation and a characteristic bubbly discharge with a copious volume, a greenish colour and an offensive smell. DYSPAREUNIA (painful intercourse) is common.

Orthodox treatment
The usual drug for the treatment of this condition is metronidazole (Flagyl), which can be taken by mouth and also inserted into the vagina in the form of a pessary. The patient's partner might also require treatment to prevent re-infection.

Alternative treatment
It is an offence in the UK for anyone other than a registered medical practitioner to treat venereal disease. A doctor might choose *Sepia* as a homoeopathic remedy.

Trigeminal neuralgia   See NEURALGIA.

Trismus   SPASM of the jaw muscles, resulting from irritation of the motor branch of the trigeminal nerve concerned with conveying movement impulses to the side of the face. Mild trismus produces an unnatural grin, called 'risus sardonicus' ('sardonic smile').

The commonest cause of trismus is LOCKJAW. The condition can also accompany a dental ABSCESS, a QUINSY, incompletely erupted wisdom teeth, and neonatal JAUNDICE (i.e. jaundice of the newborn). In young babies the 'sardonic smile' may be absent, the only evidence of trismus being difficulty in feeding.

Treatment is aimed at the underlying cause of the trismus.

Tuberculosis   An infection due to the bacterium *Mycobacterium tuberculosis*. See **XII/8**.

Tumour   A growth. A tumour results from the abnormal multiplication of a group of cells to form a recognizable lump, and can be either benign or malignant. A POLYP is an example of a benign tumour; a tumour arising in the lining of the bronchus (air-tube), on the other hand, is extremely likely to be malignant. See discussion of cancer in **XIII**.

Typhoid fever An infectious disease caused by the bacterium *Salmonella typhi*, the usual source being drinking water or food contaminated with human sewage particles from an infected person.

–U–

Ulcer A persistent breach in the surface of the skin or of a body membrane, exposing structures normally covered by an intact lining or coating tissue. Causes of ulcers include poor circulation (e.g. leg ulcers; see discussion of varicose veins in **III/6**); repeated injury (e.g. an ulcer on the lining of the cheek, due to the eruption of a crooked wisdom tooth); chemical irritation (e.g. peptic ulcer due to action of stomach acid and the enzyme pepsin—see **I/9**); INFECTION (e.g. syphilitic ulcers—see SYPHILIS); unremitting pressure (e.g. BEDSORES); and malignant growths (e.g. RODENT ULCER).

Ulcerative colitis A disorder, probably autoimmune (see ALLERGY), of the colon, featuring severe chronic DIARRHOEA, blood and mucus in the motions, and loss of weight. See **I/29**.

Unconsciousness The loss of conscious awareness, combined with poor or absent response to painful stimuli. When unconscious patients are examined, the depth of their unconscious state is assessed by their response or lack of it to heavy pressure on the Achilles tendon immediately above the heel and to pinpricks in the skin. Causes include head injury (see CONCUSSION), general anaesthesia, a cerebral HAEMORRHAGE, or brain disease. See also FAINTING and COMA.

Undescended testis See TESTIS (undescended).

Uraemia A toxic condition which results from the accumulation in the bloodstream of protein-breakdown products, including urea, normally disposed of in the urine by the kidney. Symptoms of early uraemia include fatigue, lethargy, drowsiness and, later, mild CONFUSION. Patients normally have a poor appetite (see ANOREXIA) and are nauseous (see NAUSEA) and breathless. They may have abdominal or chest pain, and DIARRHOEA. As the condition worsens, they become weak and shaky, and have difficulty in walking. Psychological problems can occur.

Uraemia is a sign of malfunctioning kidneys. Wherever possible its underlying cause is treated, but sometimes an artificial kidney machine is needed to keep the patient alive, or a kidney transplant carried out if a donor becomes available.

Urethritis INFLAMMATION of the bladder outlet (urethra). This can occur for no apparent reason (*nonspecific urethritis*—usually some INFECTION is responsible) or exist together with cystitis (see **IV/5**).

Urinary frequency The symptom of passing small quantities of urine frequently. This can result from bladder INFLAMMATION (cystitis—see **IV/5**), inflamed kidneys (see PYELONEPHRITIS), or distortion of the bladder neck, which often occurs in pregnancy.

Urine, discoloured Bile pigments in the urine can give it a dark colour; they may appear in certain disorders of the liver—see JAUNDICE. Pink or reddish urine may contain blood, which suggests an abnormality of the kidneys or bladder. Alternatively, an unusual colour may simply result from edible dyes or natural pigments present in medicines or food. Beetroot can colour the urine pink, the condition being termed 'beetrooturia'.

Urine, infected This indicates a source of INFECTION in the kidneys, the ureter, the bladder or the bladder outlet (urethra). This can cause symptoms of cystitis, and is most often due to the bacterium *Escherichia coli*, normally present in the large bowel. See **IV/5**.

Urine, protein in There is no protein in normal urine. When the 'dipstick' test shows that albumen is present, no particular form of kidney malfunction is suggested, but further investigations should be carried out.

Urine, retention of Inability to empty the bladder can be caused by an obstruction to the flow of urine or by a neurological disorder. It can also occur for a short time after injury to the bladder, or following a pelvic operation—for instance, for an enlarged prostate gland.

Urine, smelly   Offensive-smelling urine is generally due to a bladder infection. Stale urine, on the other hand, smells of ammonia, due to the action of air and bacteria.

Urine, sugar in   When the 'dipstick' test shows the presence of a small amount of sugar (i.e. glucose), diabetes mellitus (see **X/2**) is not necessarily the cause, but further tests should be carried out to eliminate this possibility.

Urticaria (nettlerash)   See HIVES.

–V–

Vaccination, reactions to   Unpleasant reactions to vaccination can include FEVER, malaise, enlarged lymph glands, sore THROAT, and an ABSCESS or ULCER at the injection site. Arguments for and against vaccination are given in **XII**—consult the index.

Vaginal discharge (leukorrhoea)   All women have some degree of vaginal discharge—it becomes abnormal only when it is excessively heavy (sometimes called 'the WHITES'), has a bad odour or is coloured —either yellowish-green or blood-stained. The normal vaginal lubrication (or discharge) is colourless or faintly yellow, and has a 'normal' odour or none at all. Heavy, offensive-smelling discharge is a sign of an infection—see **V/7** and **V/8**.

Vaginal soreness   The vagina feels sore when it is infected (see vaginitis [**V/8**]) or when it is dry and intercourse is attempted. This is a common occurrence during and after the menopause, due to lack of lubrication from the degenerating lining cells. See **V/14**. A sore vagina is a common cause of DYSPAREUNIA.

Vaginismus   SPASM of the muscles around the entrance to the vagina, making intercourse difficult and painful (see DYSPAREUNIA) and sometimes impossible. Causes of vaginismus include anxiety (see **XIV/4**), dislike or fear of the male partner, loss of sex urge, VAGINAL SORENESS, or pain on attempted penetration due to a small vaginal opening.
    The condition responds to treatment for soreness of the vagina or

vulva. The entrance to the vagina can also be enlarged by employing special vaginal dilators which can be used at home. Psychological causes respond best to counselling (involving both partners) and psychotherapy, and sometimes to sex therapy. Patience and reassurance on behalf of the sexual partner are essential to progress.

Vaginitis   INFLAMMATION of the vagina. See **V/8**.

Varicella   Chickenpox. See **XII/1**.

Varices, oesophageal   See OESOPHAGEAL VARICES.

Varicocoele   Varicose swellings of the veins surrounding the testis. This condition is rarely of any significance.

Varicose veins   A disorder of the veins—most often those of the leg—in which they swell, stretch due to the back pressure of blood on their thin walls, and eventually become unsightly, prominent and knotted. See **III/6**.

Vasoconstriction   Reflex constriction of the muscular walls of arteries. This works selectively with VASODILATION to control the flow of blood to a tissue and to regulate skin temperature and blood pressure. Sometimes excessive vasoconstriction of arteries can cause problems, for example RAYNAUD'S DISEASE.

Vasodilation   Reflex dilation of the muscular walls of arteries (see also VASOCONSTRICTION). The body uses vasodilation to lower its temperature. The blood-flow through the skin is increased as a result of the widening vessels, so permitting a greater degree of cooling by the surrounding air. Conversely, body heat is conserved by vasoconstriction, as the vessels narrow and less blood flows through the superficial vessels. The skin, especially that of the face, tends to be flushed due to vasodilation in hot weather or after exercise, and pale in cold weather due to vasoconstriction.

Venereal disease (VD)   Infectious disease involving the genital organs and transmitted by sexual intercourse. Common varieties include GONORRHOEA, TRICHOMONAS INFECTION and genital herpes (see **XII/3**). SYPHILIS used to be far more common than it is now. Venereal diseases caused by the microorganism *Chlamydia*, which is in many ways like a bacterium but is only the size of a virus, are becoming increasingly frequent. It is illegal for alternative practitioners to treat venereal diseases.

Ventricular fibrillation   See FIBRILLATION.

Ventricular septal defect   See HOLE IN THE HEART.

Verruca   See WART.

Vertigo   A feeling of dizziness associated with an impression that either oneself or one's surroundings are rotating. The impression of rotation distinguishes genuine vertigo from attacks of light-headedness, QUEER TURNS and DIZZY SPELLS. In contrast to these, vertigo is due to disturbances in the balance mechanism of the inner ear (labyrinthitis —see **XI/4**) or in the auditory nerve, which is concerned with hearing and balance. NAUSEA, HEADACHE and VOMITING frequently accompany vertigo and, when Ménière's disease (see **XI/3**) is the underlying cause, there is concomitant TINNITUS and loss of hearing which fluctuates in severity. During a vertigo attack, most patients find that lying flat and the removal of any restricting clothing provide the most relief.

Sedatives are sometimes given; but the underlying problem should be determined. Possible causes, besides those mentioned above, include disease of the part of the brain (cerebellum) responsible for balance and muscular coordination; and the side effects of certain drugs (e.g. streptomycin). Vertigo can also result from MOTION SICKNESS, digestive upsets, and looking down from a height.

Vitamin deficiency   Deficiency of a particular vitamin occurs (a) when insufficient quantities are present in the diet, (b) when its absorption and use are prevented for some reason, and (c) when the body either has an increased need for it or excretes it in excessive amounts.

Examples of disorders likely to be encountered in the UK and involving vitamin deficiency include: the PREMENSTRUAL SYNDROME (Vitamin B_6); pernicious anaemia (Vitamin B_{12}—see **VIII/1**); Alzheimer's disease (see DEMENTIA), which may be associated with deficiency of the B-complex vitamin choline; XEROPHTHALMIA (Vitamin A); OSTEOMALACIA due to insufficient Vitamin D; and possibly some cases of infertility (see **V/15**) due to Vitamin-E deficiency.

A chart summarizing recommended vitamin requirements for adults and children can be found on page 436.

Vitiligo   The appearance of light-coloured patches on the skin or hair due to a loss of the pigment melanin. The cause is not known, and apart from the undesirable cosmetic effect the condition is harmless, although the depigmented areas are more prone to SUNBURN than those surrounding them.

Volvulus Twisting of a loop of bowel, usually around itself, in such a way that an obstruction occurs and the bowel contents are unable to pass further along its length. When the bowel loop becomes tightly twisted, the blood vessels also become obstructed, and GANGRENE can occur. The section of bowel deprived of blood circulation may have to be removed during the operation performed to untwist the loop and stabilize it.

Vomiting (emesis) The violent emptying of the stomach contents through the mouth, resulting from a reflex controlled by the vomiting centre in the brain; retching is a form of vomiting in which the stomach contents are not ejected. NAUSEA, sweating, pallor and TACHYCARDIA all frequently precede a vomiting attack.

A very large number of disturbances can cause vomiting. Some of the better known ones include: unpleasant sights and smells; emotional excitement and shock; MOTION SICKNESS; the early stages of pregnancy; excessive amounts to eat and drink and other gastric and intestinal disorders; and HEAD INJURY. Vomiting can also result from raised pressure within the skull, as when a brain TUMOUR is present or a stroke (see IX/7) has occurred. The vomiting centre is also stimulated by migraine attacks (see IX/2) and by MENINGITIS.

Orthodox treatment
Antinausea and antivomiting drugs (e.g. metochlopramide—Maxolon) can be given to abort an attack of vomiting; but when the cause is overindulgence in food and drink, or when FOOD POISONING is a likely explanation, it is usually better to permit the stomach to empty itself of its irritating contents.

Young children often vomit from excitement or when feverish, and babies are apt to vomit when given the wrong food or when they gulp too much air. Both babies and young children run a particular risk of serious dehydration and loss of essential salts if vomiting is prolonged. Water and salt should be replaced as a matter of urgency in all such cases. If the patient's stomach is unable to retain small sips of the replenishing fluid (see DIARRHOEA) it may be necessary to restore the fluid and salt balance by feeding it straight into a vein (i.e. by intravenous drip).

Homoeopathic treatment
For a simple vomiting attack with NAUSEA and DIARRHOEA: *Ipeca-cuanha*. When there is prostration, vomiting, a burning sensation in the stomach and cold extremities: *Arsenicum*. For chronic persistent vomiting (an expert should be consulted): *Kreosotum*. When the vomiting follows a period of dietary indiscretion: *Nux Vomica*.

– W –

Wart (verruca) Small, coarse-textured benign TUMOUR arising from the outer skin layer. Warts are caused by a contagious virus, and caught by direct contact with, for example, the floors of cloakrooms and changing rooms.

'Verruca' is the correct technical term for a wart wherever it occurs, but is often misused to apply only to warts on the soles (plantar surfaces) of the feet; the correct name for a wart in this region is 'verruca plantaris' (plantar wart).

Orthodox treatments
These include salicylic acid + lactic acid + flexible collodion (Salactol), and salicylic acid + podophyllum resin (Posalfilin), both of which are applied directly to the wart, which is then covered with a plaster.

Herbal treatment
Celandine juice or a slice of garlic applied to the wart, the surrounding skin being protected with a plaster.

Wart charming
Numerous ritual charms exist. They are often successful, and this has been attributed to the patient's implicit belief that the warts will disappear. This is an example of the power of the mind to heal the body.

Wasp stings See STINGS.

Water brash (water spring) The sudden filling of the mouth with a large volume of very watery saliva produced by the salivary glands and not regurgitated from the foodpipe or stomach. This is often a sign of peptic ulcer (see I/9).

Wax in the ears   See EAR WAX.

Weight problems   An adult is said to be obese if his/her weight exceeds that of an average person of his/her height, race and sex by 20 per cent or more. A child is considered obese if it weighs more than 20 per cent above that normally expected for its height, race, sex and age. Ideal weight can be assessed by consulting the tables of weight statistics provided by insurance companies, but 'body build' is a factor to bear in mind. Two healthy individuals of the same sex, height and race can differ considerably depending upon whether they are small-, medium- or large-framed, and one's ideal weight may differ by as much as 10 per cent from the average.

   Fatness can also be assessed by measuring skinfold thickness using specially designed calipers, but it is easy to get a wide variety of readings from the same skinfold unless the calipers are applied in precisely the correct way. For this reason, it is preferable in the first instance to have skinfolds measured by someone skilled in the use of the calipers.

   There are obvious social and cosmetic reasons which impel fat people to slim, but far more important are the health reasons. Excess body fat is associated with a higher risk of heart disorders (see III/1 and III/3), arterial disease (see hardening of the ARTERIES), diabetes mellitus (see X/2), GALL STONES, and kidney disorders (see IV/1–IV/4). Excess body weight (which need not be due to fat but can also be a result of OEDEMA [the accumulation of fluid in an unhealthy person] or of overdeveloped muscles, as in an athlete) also predisposes towards arthritis (see VI/1) and BACKACHE due to joint strain; breathing problems; fractured bones; HERNIAS; and varicose veins (see III/6).

   Many fat people attribute their overweight to their having 'heavy bones', malfunctioning 'glands', or the accumulation of body fluid. Healthy bone tissue weighs very much the same from one person to another, and bone size is taken into account by relating ideal weight to 'body build' (usually assessed by wrist measurement for a given height). Obesity due to glandular disorders is rare; and significant oedema is extremely unlikely to occur in an otherwise normal person. The basic reason many people are overweight (some estimates indicate that around 50 per cent of the adult population in the UK and USA are too fat), is that their energy intake exceeds their energy output; that is, they consume too many calories for the number they expend in their daily activities. Proper utilization of calories is related to the body's 'metabolic rate' (the rate at which food fuel is converted into energy), and people who find it very difficult to lose weight often have a problem with their basic rate of fuel consumption. This is why two people of the same race, sex and height can differ greatly in build while eating very similar diets. In fact the slim one can often eat a great deal more than the plump one, due to his or her greater capacity for burning up food fuel rather than storing it as fat layers.

Overeating at meal times together with between-meal 'snacking' on sugary snacks, processed carbohydrates and fatty fried foods is a neurotic problem and often associated with stress (see STRESS REACTIONS) and emotional insecurity. 'Comfort eating' is a problem commonly treated by psychotherapists and hypnotherapists; it can be dealt with effectively provided the patient really wants to relinquish the habit.

Orthodox treatment

Appetite-suppressant drugs have been available for years but do not have a high success rate since, as soon as a course of them finishes, the weight tends to reaccumulate. They are also frowned upon by many doctors and patients as most of them are related to the drug amphetamine and are capable of producing a sufficient 'high' for them to have become the subject of widespread abuse (see DRUG DEPENDENCE). Diethylpropion hydrochloride (Tenuate Dospan) is a well known example of this type.

Pharmaceutical companies are currently engaged in a race to produce a drug which increases the metabolic rate effectively but has no unhealthy side-effects.

In rare instances, surgery may be employed to remove excess weight.

Naturopathic treatment

The most effective way to lose weight is to increase the body's metabolic rate through regular aerobic exercise (i.e. exercise that makes noticeable demands on the heart and lungs) carried out four or five times weekly for at least 20 minutes, although many overweight people are extremely unfit (i.e. have low exercise tolerance) and have to build up to this achievement slowly. Most naturopathic doctors advise patients about suitable exercise or recommend that they get fit gradually—for instance, through learning yoga or T'ai Chi.

The diet most likely to be recommended to achieve an ideal bodyweight and optimal health is a wholefood one which is low in sugar, fat (especially animal fat) and salt, and contains a high proportion of raw fruit and vegetables. The healthiest form of carbohydrate is that present in pulses, grains and wholemeal-flour products, but even these should be taken in moderation by someone wishing to lose excess weight.

Dietary supplements

Naturopathic doctors may also recommend these. Certain amino acids have been found to stimulate the release of growth hormone from the pituitary gland. This hormone helps to convert stored fat into energy and to build up firm, healthy muscular tissue instead. The amino acids, together with other helpful nutrients, can be taken according to a daytime and night-time formula:

daytime	night-time
L-ornithine 3,000mg	L-ornithine 3,000mg
L-tyrosine 500mg	L-tryptophan 1,000mg
Vitamin C 1,000mg	glycine 4,000mg
Vitamin B_6 100mg	Vitamin B_6 100mg
	niacinamide 250mg

Low bodyweight

Before attempting to increase bodyweight it is essential to deal with any suspected underlying health problem responsible for weightloss or failure to gain weight. Certain glandular problems—in particular an overactive thyroid gland (see **X/1**)—may be the root of the problem.

Relaxation—e.g. yoga, meditation and autogenics—is helpful, as is a wholefood diet including all the items slimmers are encouraged to avoid. Complex carbohydrates—e.g. whole grains, wholemeal bread and pasta—can be included freely both in salads and in main meals. Cold-pressed olive oil, oily fish, whole-milk goats' yoghourt and cheese should be included, together with plenty of fruit and, occasionally, added honey. Between-meal snacks, of, for example, natural-dried fruit, wholewheat savouries, the occasional carob bar and nuts, are helpful. Drinks can include whole fresh goats' milk flavoured with blended bananas or other fruit.

To aid a poor appetite a half-hour walk in the fresh air every day can be very useful. If, however, overexercising might be contributing to an underweight problem, a physical-fitness expert should be consulted or the amount and/or intensity of exercise reduced for a trial period.

Wen   See CYST.

Wheeze   A whistling sort of sound suggesting a chest disorder and caused by the close proximity of the walls of the larger air passages. An asthmatic patient (see **II/15**) during an acute attack typically produces a high-pitched wheeze on trying to expel air from the lungs.

Whiplash injury The injury suffered when a vehicle in which a person is sitting is hit hard from the rear. The head and neck move violently forwards and immediately backwards in a similar fashion to a lashing whip. When the injury is mild, neck-stiffness—especially felt in the sternomastoid muscles—will result; occasionally a cervical collar is prescribed to limit the movements of the neck until recovery is complete. More severe injury can involve damage to the spinal cord and the brain.

Osteopathy and chiropractic
These can be helpful in reducing the PAIN and stiffness.

Whites (vaginal catarrh; leukorrhoea) A white, non-infected type of VAGINAL DISCHARGE.

Orthodox treatment
Treatment is not usually given when there is no suggestion of infection being present.

Herbal treatment
A douche of a handful of rosemary and a handful of thyme to two litres of water.

Whitlow (paronychia) A septic fingertip; a common type consists of an ABSCESS at the side of the nail. The pus is usually removed under local anaesthetic, and an antibiotic injection given.

Whooping cough (pertussis) An acute infectious illness of childhood, affecting the mucous membranes lining the air passages. See **XII/4**.

Wilm's tumour (nephroblastoma) This is one of the few cancers of childhood. Distension of the child's abdomen is the only early symptom.

Wilson's disease A rare hereditary disease in which there is cirrhosis of the liver (see **I/24**) and a TREMOR similar to that seen in Parkinson's disease (see **IX/3**). The fundamental abnormality is the accumulation of large amounts of copper in the cells of the liver and parts of the brain, with resultant toxic damage to those organs.

Wind A common cause of gas in the stomach is the swallowing of air, either as a result of nervous TENSION, through gulping food and drink, or by trying unsuccessfully to belch (bring up wind—see BELCHING). A common cause of gas in the bowel is the bacterial fermentation of food, particularly in constipated people. Eggs, beans and peas are broken down to sulphurous gases which have an obnoxious smell, and vegetable cellulose produces methane and hydrogen. These foods are best avoided by people especially troubled by flatulence.

Dietary approach
Exclude foods containing yeast and eat live, fresh goats' yoghourt. See also advice for spastic colon in I/30.

Worms In the UK the three major types of worms infesting humans are pinworms, roundworms, and tapeworms. *Pinworms (threadworms)* are the commonest of the three types, especially among schoolchildren. The adult worms are about 12mm long, or smaller. Eggs are laid outside the anus, the female coming out through the anus at night for that purpose. The area around becomes intensely itchy (see PRURITUS ANI). If the larvae, which hatch out after six hours, are swallowed (from fingers that scratch the area in sleep) the cycle starts again, since the worms inhabit the intestine. Eggs present in dust or dirt, at home or at school, also pass on the infestation if swallowed.

In girls, these worms can crawl out of the anus and enter the urethra and vagina, causing further irritation.

Roundworms are parasites found all over the world. The presence of a few produces no symptoms, but a large number of them cause a COUGH and SPASM of the air passages, since they spend part of their life-cycle in the lungs, air tubes (bronchi) and windpipe (trachea). Other symptoms they might cause are weight-loss, since they absorb food from the small bowel (where they spend the rest of their life-cycle), and VOMITING.

Orthodox treatment
Scrupulous hygiene and treatment with the orthodox drug piperazine (Antepar, Pripsen) should get rid of pinworms and roundworms (see below). All members of a family should be treated if one of them has pinworms.

Herbal treatment
For pinworms and roundworms: on waking, drink one glass of water flavoured with garlic by allowing three grated cloves of garlic to macerate overnight in 100ml of boiling water. An alternative (supposed to be more palatable) is two soupspoonfuls of syrup (30ml) made by

infusing 500g crushed garlic for an hour in a litre of boiling water and then adding 1kg of honey or brown sugar.

Tapeworms occur in most animal species; humans tend to pick up the infestation from eating infected beef and pork. The larvae are swallowed and develop and live in the small intestine, where they grow to adult worms, sometimes reaching 4–6m (depending upon species) in length. A single worm is unlikely to cause symptoms, but several will cause weight loss since they absorb nutrients from the small bowel. The species present in infected pork can cause a more serious condition (cysticercosis) if the eggs (present in the faeces of an animal or human sufferer) are swallowed. Partially digested in the stomach, the eggs hatch out as embryos with six hooks on their heads and penetrate the intestinal wall, enter the bloodstream, and finally come to rest in CYSTS in muscles, the brain and other organs. This condition is uncommon in the UK due to the standard of meat quality control and because pork is almost always eaten thoroughly cooked.

Orthodox treatment
This makes use of the drug niclosamide (Yomesan).

Aromatherapeutic treatment
An enema consisting of 300ml boiled water into which has been stirred a soupspoonful (15ml) of olive oil with 5 per cent essence of thyme; plus three drops of essence of thyme on a little brown sugar after each meal.

Wry neck (torticollis)   A condition in which the head is twisted to one side due to a defect of one of the two sternomastoid muscles. There are two such muscles, one on either side of the neck: they can be seen as the solid column of muscle when the head twists to one or other side. Each runs upwards from the upper edge of the breastbone (sternum) and a small part of the collar bone to be inserted into the mastoid bone of the skull on the same side.

The deformity can arise during birth, especially in a breech delivery, when fibres within the sternomastoid muscle may be torn. The formation of fibrous tissue and the subsequent shortening of the muscle produces the turning of the head towards the affected side.

'*Spasmodic torticollis*' is another form of wry neck and is found most commonly in middle-aged women. While some cases are rheumatic in origin, others are probably caused by psychological factors.

Finally, there is the intensely painful but usually short-term wry neck with which anyone—child or adult—can awake in the morning, without any warning. This is usually attributed—probably erroneously —to having slept in a draught.

For treatment, ice packs are applied to the area to ease the acute pain and the neck is very gently manipulated towards its normal position. Pain-killing drugs (e.g. paracetamol, aspirin) and muscle-relaxant drugs (e.g. diazepam [Valium], orphenadrine citrate [Norflex]) may be prescribed. The patient is advised to wrap the neck warmly in a scarf to avoid unnecessary exposure to draughts and to avoid jolting or jarring the head or neck.

–X–

Xeroderma   A congenital disorder which causes abnormal dryness and roughness of the skin. It is essentially a mild form of ICHTHYOSIS SIMPLEX.

Xerophthalmia   Dryness and sometimes opacity of the front of the eye, due to severe deficiency of Vitamin A.

–Y–

Yaws (framboesia)   An infectious illness found in the West Indies, Africa and parts of the Far East. (The name framboesia is derived from the French word *framboise*, meaning raspberry, and was applied to yaws because the skin lesions look like squashed raspberries.) The infection is due to a spiral-shaped bacterium, *Treponema pertenue*, very similar to the organism causing SYPHILIS, and it is spread either by direct contagion or by flies. After an incubation period of 14–28 days, the first skin lesion (known as the 'mother yaw' or 'mamanpian') appears. This is soon followed by other lesions over the surface of the body, which start as large lumps in the skin, and which, if not treated, are likely to break down into ulcers which erode the skin and bones.

Penicillin is the drug of choice, since it destroys the bacteria very effectively. The skin lesions shrink and disappear after several weeks, and a rate of recovery from yaws is high. Nevertheless, it remains one of the more dangerous debilitating tropical diseases, and can be devastating to chronically malnourished people, especially those already suffering from tuberculosis (see **XII/8**) or SYPHILIS.

Yellow fever   A dangerous viral INFECTION endemic in tropical Africa and the tropical Americas. Although the disease primarily affects monkeys and other forest-dwelling animals, it is spread to Man by means of *Aëdes* mosquitoes. It can cause serious epidemics in cities.

The first signs of illness appear after a 3–14 day incubation period; they include HEADACHE, muscular aches and pains and a FEVER, often combined with mental CONFUSION. These symptoms last for about 48 hours, but may return after a further 48 hours accompanied by the more severe features of kidney failure (see **IV/1** and **IV/2**), JAUNDICE, and signs of cardiac (heart) disorder. About 20 per cent of yellow-fever patients who become jaundiced fail to recover.

There is no effective remedy for yellow fever, but it can be prevented by vaccination and by control of the carrier mosquitoes.

–Z–

Zinc deficiency   Deficiency of the mineral zinc is very probably linked with a number of disorders, including stunted growth, failure of the male sexual organs to develop, increased tendency to develop cirrhosis of the liver (see **I/24**), childhood HYPERACTIVITY, NAUSEA in pregnancy, impotence (see **V/16**), amenorrhoea (absence of periods) and lack of ovulation, depression (see **XIV/3**), ANOREXIA NERVOSA, and acne (see **VII/1**).

The recommended daily intake of zinc for an adult is 15mg. This quantity should be increased in women by 5mg during pregnancy and by 10mg while breast-feeding continues. Foods rich in zinc include Atlantic oysters, herrings, clams, wheat bran, pig's liver and peas.

PART TWO

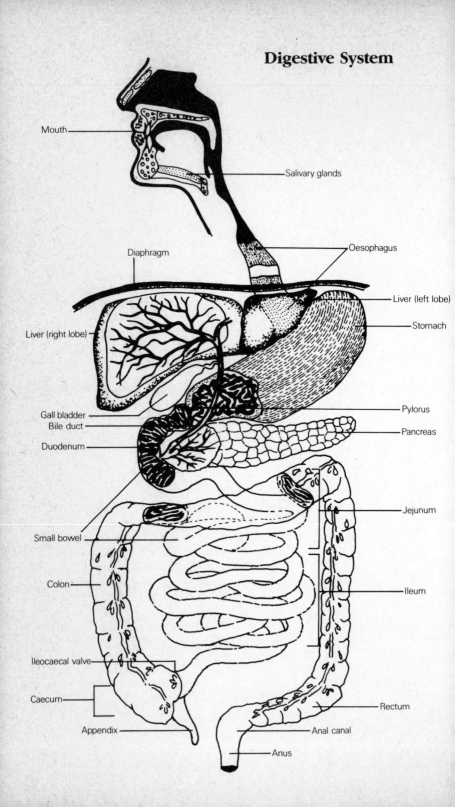

Digestive System

Mouth

Salivary glands

Diaphragm

Oesophagus

Liver (left lobe)

Liver (right lobe)

Stomach

Gall bladder

Pylorus

Bile duct

Pancreas

Duodenum

Jejunum

Small bowel

Colon

Ileum

Ileocaecal valve

Caecum

Rectum

Appendix

Anal canal

Anus

I Disorders of the Digestive System

The digestive system consists of a long tube which starts at the mouth and continues through the pharynx, foodpipe (gullet, oesophagus), stomach and bowels to the rectum. Also part of the digestive system are the liver and pancreas, which arise in the developing baby as offshoots of the first part of the small bowel (duodenum), and secrete substances into it to aid the digestive process.

The mouth extends from the lips to the back of the tongue, where the pharynx starts. Like the rest of the digestive tract, the mouth is lined with a mucus-secreting membrane, and this, combined with the saliva from the salivary glands, keeps the mouth moist, clean and infection-free; it also facilitates chewing and swallowing.

The pharynx is the passage extending from the back of the nose and mouth to the voice-box (larynx) and the entrance of the foodpipe. It contains the tonsils; and a specialized area of it (the nasopharynx) contains the adenoids.

The foodpipe is a muscular tube running down through the chest behind the heart to end in the stomach, which it reaches by passing through a hole in the diaphragm muscle separating the chest from the abdomen. At the point where foodpipe and stomach meet there is a valve-like ring of muscle fibres, the cardiac sphincter. This helps to ensure that there is no reflux of partially digested food from the stomach up into the foodpipe should one bend forwards after eating a meal.

The stomach sits in the middle of the upper part of the abdomen. It has thick muscular walls which contract to mix the food and liquid received from the mouth with digestive juices and mucus derived from its lining membrane. It finally squeezes its semi-digested contents through its lower end, the pylorus, which consists of a similar valve-like muscle ring.

The pylorus narrows into the duodenum, the first and shortest section of the small bowel, and the most common site for peptic ulcers. Ducts from the liver and the pancreas open into this part of the small bowel by a common opening; in addition, mucus is produced to help lubricate the contents. The duodenum continues into the next part of the small bowel, the jejunum, which leads to the final section of small bowel, the ileum.

The duodenum is a fixed structure, stuck to the back of the abdominal cavity by a layer of membrane (peritoneum) rather like a small light coil of rubber tubing might be placed against a wall and wall-papered over with a sheet of transparent plastic. It is shaped like a 'C'. Within its partial circle lies the head of the pancreas gland.

The jejunum and ileum, by contrast, hang freely in a loose drape of the membrane called the mesentery. The small bowel measures about 6m (20ft) in length, and has a calibre of about 3.8cm (1½in). Its mucous-membrane lining is arranged in millions of tiny inward projections—villi—which increase the total surface area enormously. It ends in the lower-right-hand quarter of the abdomen in a blind pouch, the caecum, from which the appendix, a long, thin blind tube, is suspended.

The large bowel consists of a soft, muscular tube about 1.2m (4ft) long (in an adult) and of calibre about 6.3cm (2½in). The muscle fibres in its walls run in several different directions, and it is capable of powerful propulsive activity. The first part of the large bowel, the ascending colon, runs straight up the right side of the abdomen from the caecum. When it reaches the underside of the liver it bends to the left, crosses the top part of the abdomen as the transverse colon, then bends sharply to become the descending colon running down the left side of the abdomen. It finally plunges downwards into the pelvis and becomes the rectum, which leads to the anus.

The liver lies under the shelter of the ribcage and immediately below the diaphragm in the upper-right-hand portion of the abdominal cavity. The liver has many functions. It receives, through the portal vein, all the blood from the spleen, the stomach and the small bowel, and extracts from it the substances digested and absorbed into the bloodstream from the food. The blood is then returned to the general circulation.

The liver's digestive secretion, the bile, is stored in the gall bladder, a pear-shaped sac suspended from the under-surface of the liver by the common bile duct. The bile either (a) runs through channels in the liver and straight down the bile duct into the duodenum or (b), when a surplus has collected, is squeezed out of the gall bladder by the muscular action of its walls in response to food reaching the duodenum.

The part of the pancreas lying within the 'C' of the duodenum is known as the 'head'; its 'neck', 'body' and 'tail' lie across the back of the abdomen behind the stomach. This gland has two main functions—it controls the level of sugar in the blood (see X/2), and it is also a digestive gland.

Digestion is the breaking down of large, complex food molecules into their smaller component units by the influence of chemical agents (enzymes) produced by the digestive tract and glands. The mucous membrane of the small bowel is able to absorb these simple molecules, which are then carried in the bloodstream to the liver, and there reassembled as required.

Digestion starts in the mouth where food is chewed into smaller pieces and mixed with saliva, which lubricates it, and with an enzyme, ptyalin (salivary amylase), which starts to break down any starch present into a sugar called maltose. The stomach continues the digestive process by churning around the food it receives and mixing it thoroughly with the gastric juice. This contains hydrochloric acid; the enzyme pepsin which starts the digestion of protein; and 'intrinsic factor', without which Vitamin B_{12} cannot be adequately absorbed (see **VIII/1**). The mucus produced by the stomach lining also fulfils an important function, protecting this delicate membrane from the breakdown effects of its own digestive juices.

The waves of muscular contraction (peristalsis) which occur throughout the digestive tract move the food and its residue along the tract's length, rather like toothpaste being pushed from the bottom to the top of a tube. Little by little, the mixture of partly digested food, liquid and mucus from the stomach reach the small bowel, and get thoroughly mixed both with the digestive juices produced in this region and with the bile and pancreatic juice. By the time the end of the small bowel is reached, digestion and nutrient absorption are complete. Most of the remaining fluid is reabsorbed in the colon, only a very little moisture remaining in normal stools. Severe DIARRHOEA can interfere with this reabsorptive process, and serious, sometimes fatal, amounts of fluid and salt can be lost to the body in this way.

I/1 STOMATITIS

Common causes of stomatitis (inflammation of the mucous lining of the mouth) include scalding with hot drinks and food, the eating of overspiced foods, and injury from badly fitting dentures or broken teeth.

Simple catharrhal stomatitis can occur in seriously ill people whose mouths are not cleaned regularly; when a fever is present; in association with severe dental and gum infection; and as a consequence of excessive tobacco-smoking. The gums and mouth are painful and dry, the mucous membrane is inflamed, the tongue is swollen and coated, and the patient usually has bad breath. The condition can be prevented or treated by adequate oral hygiene, especially when the patient is severely ill. A solution of 15 ml of glycerine and the juice of half a lemon in 300 ml (½ pint) of warm water can be used for rinsing and swabbing out the mouth.

Stomatitis can also occur as a result of a deficiency of vitamins—e.g. folic acid, riboflavin, nicotinamide (B₃), cyanocobalamin (B₁₂) and Vitamin C. It can feature in a number of blood disorders, including leukaemia (see VIII/3), agranulocytosis (a deficiency of granulocyte white blood cells) and PURPURA; and may arise as a local allergic reaction to chemicals present in toothpaste, mint sweets, etc., or to antibiotics. It can appear also as a symptom of certain viral INFECTIONS, such as herpes simplex (see XII/3), herpes zoster (see IX/6), and measles (see XII/5), and of metal poisoning by, for example, mercury, gold, lead, arsenic or bismuth. Some patients on the drug phenytoin (Epanutin, an anticonvulsant drug given to epileptics) suffer from stomatitis as a side effect.

In the UK a common infection causing stomatitis is THRUSH, infection with the fungus *Candida albicans* (see also I/2). Another common type of stomatitis is aphthous stomatitis, otherwise known as aphthous ulceration or mouth ulcers (see I/3).

I/2 ORAL THRUSH

This can occur after the use of certain antibiotics—e.g. chloramphenicol (Chloromycetin), tetracycline (Terramycin, Tetrabid etc.) —and after taking steroid drugs. It affects people whose immune defence systems are weakened, and is a feature of severely debilitating diseases such as cancer (see XIII) and tuberculosis (see XII/8), and it often affects patients with diabetes mellitus (see X/2). Meticulous oral hygiene can often prevent it from appearing in the severely ill adult. Oral thrush is also sometimes seen in newborn babies when the mother's nipples or the teats of feeding bottles are not being properly cleaned. Denture-wearers are prone to the ailment if their cleansing methods are inadequate. Other people especially prone to the condition are diabetics and anyone who uses an inhaler regularly.

Oral thrush takes the appearance of patches of white, curd-like slough covering areas of superficial ulceration on the gums, palate and cheek linings. Sometimes these patches extend to form a large membrane which can be easily detached from the underlying tissue.

ORTHODOX TREATMENT

This aims at killing the invading *Candida* cells. The superficial slough is removed by gentle swabbing, and hydrogen peroxide/saline mouth-washes given (a three per cent hydrogen peroxide solution added to an equal volume of warm saline solution). Specific treatment is with nystatin (Nystan) pastilles, which are held in the mouth in contact with the lesions and allowed to dissolve slowly; or with nystatin suspension (100,000 iu per ml), 1ml, four times daily, being dropped on the tongue and held against the affected mouth areas.

ALTERNATIVE THERAPIES

The alternative approach aims at strengthening the body's natural defenders against unwanted invasion—i.e. *Lactobacillus acidophilus*, normally present in the bowel, and the immune defence system.

Natural medicine

For discussion of nutritional therapy and helpful dietary supplements, see THRUSH.

Biochemic tissue salts   *Kali Muriaticum* is useful.

Herbal medicine

This aims at strengthening the body's defence mechanism against invading bacteria and other organisms. Herbal remedies for oral thrush include a warm mouthwash and gargle of a decoction of two pinches of aniseed, two pinches of burdock leaves, two pinches of sage flowers and two pinches of violet flowers to a litre of water.

Aromatherapy

A mouthwash made with lukewarm boiled water containing two per cent essence of lemon; or a mouthwash of equal volumes of pure lemon juice and water, enriched with ten drops of two per cent lemon essence per 100ml, and stirred well.

I/3 MOUTH ULCERS

These small ulcers are sometimes associated with gastric or intestinal upsets, and sometimes with fever and with periods of emotional strain (see STRESS REACTIONS). They may also appear (in susceptible people) for no apparent reason—although certain food items, differing from individual to individual, may spark off an attack.

Mouth ulcers can appear in groups of two or three or more on the lining of the cheeks, along the edge of the tongue, or at the tongue's root. They are very painful, particularly when they occur in an area where talking or eating irritates them further.

ORTHODOX TREATMENT

This aims at the symptomatic relief of the ulcers, and uses antiseptic mouth washes—e.g. Oraldene (hexetidine 0.1 per cent), soluble hydrocortisone pellets such as Corlan (hydrocortisone 2.5mg), and an oral paste of 0.1 per cent triamcinolone acetonide (Adcortyl).

ALTERNATIVE THERAPIES

Natural medicine

Nutritional therapy Wholefood diet, with emphasis on the importance of raw vegetables and fruit and their jucies. Cabbage juice is renowned for its peptic-ulcer-healing properties, and it is suggested that 250ml of fresh cabbage juice be prepared and drunk daily, each mouthful being held in contact with the mouth ulcers for 15 seconds before being swallowed.

SPECIFIC DIETARY SUPPLEMENTS

Tablets containing *Lactobacillus acidophilus* and L. *bulgaricus*, the bacteria traditionally used to culture yoghourt, have been found very useful. The dose is between two and four tablets four times daily, chewed and swallowed with milk, before or after food.

Daily doses of Vitamin B_2 (riboflavin), 10mg, together with Vitamin A, 7,500iu, are reported both to treat mouth ulcers effectively and to prevent their return.

Vitamin E, prescribed in daily doses of 1,600iu, has encouraged the healing of mouth ulcers, especially when used in conjunction with Vitamin E oil applied to the ulcers directly. Vitamin C in high doses of 20g or more may be prescribed by a nutritional expert.

Biochemic Tissue Salts *Kali Phosphoricum* for grey-coloured ulcers, and for their precipitating stress. *Kali Muriaticum* for white-coloured ulcers.

Herbal medicine

One remedy is tea made from the young leaves—fresh or dried—of goldenrod (*Solidago fragrans*); this can be drunk as well as used to rinse the mouth. Alternatively one can use the juice of, or powder made from, dried mouse-ear, a low-growing herb found in dry ditches and on ditch banks.

Aromatherapy

Remedies include geranium (*Geranium robertianum* or *Pelargonium odorantissimum*). The mouth is rinsed with a glass of lukewarm water to which a coffee spoonful of the alcohol preparation (90 per cent alcohol and 40g of the essence) has been added.

Sage (*Salvia officinalis; Salvia sclarea*) is an alternative. Oil of clary sage, which is derived from *S. sclarea* and is non-toxic, is generally used. The mouth is rinsed with distilled water containing 2 per cent of the essence.

Homoeopathy

Mouth ulcers, accompanied by bad breath and a metallic taste, are sometimes treated with *Mercurius Solubilis*.

I/4 TOOTH DECAY (CARIES)

Tooth decay consists of the demineralization of an area of tooth by the action of bacteria, followed by cavity formation. Bacteria normally present in the mouth (streptococci) attach themselves to the teeth and mix with protein present in saliva to form colonies. This mixture (plaque) soon covers the entire surface of the teeth, and can lead to gum disease (gingivitis—see I/5). When sweet food is eaten, the saliva becomes sticky as a result of bacterial action upon the sugar molecules, and the bacteria remain on the tooth-surface instead of being washed off by saliva. At the same time, acid is produced which attacks the crystals of calcium phosphate of which the tooth substance is composed. (The effect of fluoride is to bind with the calcium and reinforce the teeth against mineral loss.) The frequent consumption of sugar means that the saliva and plaque are maintained in an acidic condition for long periods of time, and the loss of minerals from the tooth is correspondingly high. Infrequent sugar consumption, on the other hand, allows the acid conditions in the saliva and plaque gradually to return to normal, and mineral loss is reduced. In fact, during the resting period remineralization can take place, minerals in the saliva replacing those lost from acid attack. (Fluoride encourages this to take place.)

Rather than drilling and filling early areas of decay, recent work shows that small changes in eating habits, plus increased use of fluoride toothpaste, can arrest tooth decay. Cutting down on sugar consumption is the most important measure that can be taken to protect teeth; the next most important are careful brushing with a fluoride toothpaste, the use of dental floss, and the use of disclosing agents that reveal plaque.

When a small area of tooth substance is eroded, no pain is experienced at first. However, as the destructive process encroaches upon the live nerve fibres within, the affected tooth at first becomes sensitive to very hot or cold foods and to pressure, and later starts to ache.[33]

Biochemic tissue salts   These can be given for dental decay: *Calc. Fluor.*; *Calc. Phos.*

I/5 GINGIVITIS

Plaque at the base of the teeth irritates the gum tissues and causes inflammation. This condition is called gingivitis, and it probably causes more loss of teeth than dental decay itself. Its commonest symptoms are the appearance of blood when the teeth are brushed or floss is used, and bad breath. Gingivitis can also be a symptom of disturbances elswhere in the body, including nutritional deficiencies, an abnormal metabolism and the herpes virus.

The plaque should be gently removed from the bleeding area and the correct dietary and oral hygiene measures should be followed. For details of further measures see under Periodontitis (I/6).

I/6 PERIODONTITIS

This is inflammation of the 'periodontium', the tissue in which the teeth are set. If gingivitis progresses unchecked, the bacterial plaque extends downwards into the space between the roots of the teeth and the gum tissue. The periodontal connective tissue fibres and surrounding bone are eroded, pus can form in the deepening periodontal spaces, and the teeth become loose in their sockets and eventually fall out.

ORTHODOX TREATMENT

If the condition has progressed to the stage where periodontal work is required, calcified deposits are removed from around the roots of the teeth and the pus pockets excised. Orthodontic appliances can be used to reposition teeth by stretching and squeezing the connective tissue (the periodontal ligament) anchoring them within their sockets. Compression of this ligament causes new bone formation and growth of the connective tissue, and strengthens the teeth within their sockets.

ALTERNATIVE THERAPIES

Natural medicine

The best diet for healthy teeth and gums, besides being wholefood and low in sugar, includes plenty of natural fibre since this offers some protection against the destructive effect of sugar in the meal and provides the teeth with chewing work to do. Calcium, phosphorus, Vitamin D and fluorine all promote sound teeth; good food sources are: green vegetables (calcium), fish, poultry, wholegrains and eggs (phosphorus), fish-liver oil, sardines, milk and dairy products (Vitamin D), and seafoods and gelatin (fluorine, as calcium fluoride).

Recommended supplements include chelated calcium tablets providing 1,000mg of elemental calcium daily; or dolomite, which combines calcium correctly balanced with magnesium and does not require Vitamin D for absorption—5 dolomite tablets provide 750mg calcium, so 7 tablets daily should be taken by an adult to provide 1,050mg calcium.

Vitamin D, if needed, 400–800iu daily. Most UK diets contain ample phosphorus, and supplements are unlikely to be needed.

Herbal medicine

A mouthwash of an infusion of the following: half a handful each of rose petals, sage, violet petals and bilberries to one litre of water.

PREVENTION

The surfaces of the teeth have natural dips and crevices (fissures) where neither toothbrush nor floss can clean. A new preventive measure called 'fissure sealing' can guard against decay or deal with it effectively if it has not progressed too far. The surfaces of teeth are coated with a special plastic to prevent bacterial and acid attack; any bacteria trapped inside the fissures die from lack of nourishment.

Fluoride applications are also used as a preventive measure.

I/7 HIATUS HERNIA (DIAPHRAGMATIC HERNIA)

This is the protrusion (herniation) of the upper part of the stomach into the chest, through the opening (hiatus) in the diaphragm normally occupied only by the lower end of the foodpipe (oesophagus). Middle-aged flabby women are especially prone to this kind of hernia, the immediate cause of which can often be traced to a recent increase in the intra-abdominal pressure. Chronic constipation necessitating hard straining to pass motions, or a chronic cough, are examples of likely causes. Other precipitating factors include recent weight-gain of more than a few pounds, and a late pregnancy. It is also thought that some weakness in the connective-tissue fibres anchoring the lower end of the oesophagus to its diaphragmatic opening, and of the cardiac sphincter, may contribute to the condition.

Symptoms are often absent, the hernia being discovered when an X-ray is taken for some other reason; but, when symptoms occur, discomfort below the breastbone after eating is common, due to distension of the hernial sac. HEARTBURN (a sign that the lower end of the foodpipe is becoming inflamed by the reflux upwards of acidic stomach contents) is another common sympton, and sometimes parti-ally digested food returns to the mouth if the patient bends over forward or lies down after a meal. This heartburn is associated also with the postural changes that take place when the sufferer strains to lift heavy shopping or bends over to make beds or sweep. It may come on when the sufferer lies down at night, in which case it occurs within an hour of lying flat in bed. In this respect it differs from the similar pain of a peptic ulcer which is not affected by changes in posture and typically wakes people up between 2 and 3 a.m. (see I/9).

Apart from the typical history, the diagnosis of hiatus hernia can be confirmed by X-ray. Endoscopy (inspection of the erea) shows evidence of regurgitated gastric contents, and the lower end and the inflamed foodpipe can become ulcerated.

ORTHODOX TREATMENT

A bland diet is recommended, and overweight patients are advised to lose weight. Night pain can be partially combated by the patient's mattress being raised by a wooden wedge at the head end, or by the head of the bed being raised on 15–20cm blocks to discourage reflux. It is also helpful not to take food or liquids within the three hours before retiring. The patient is advised also not to overeat, smoke or take alcohol.

Antacids are also prescribed, when necessary, to control the pain, and surgery is used when the symptoms have failed to improve after six months of conservative treatment.

ALTERNATIVE THERAPIES

Since the pain of hiatus hernia is due to the effect of acid stomach contents on the mucous-membrane lining of the foodpipe, and its subsequent (peptic) ulceration, the alternative treatment of hiatus hernia is considered under Peptic Ulcer (I/9). Specific advice applicable to a patient with hiatus hernia as opposed to a gastric or duodenal peptic ulcer would involve contributory factors such as chronic CON-STIPATION, persistent COUGH and overweight (see WEIGHT PROBLEMS).

I/8 CANCER OF THE FOODPIPE

This condition is associated with tobacco smoking—especially when the smoker also consumes alcohol. The commonest early symptom is dysphagia (severe difficulty in swallowing), followed by increasing pain and the regurgitation of food. Weight loss is usually pronounced.

ORTHODOX TREATMENT

This usually consists of surgical resection of the growth, and/or radiotherapy. Dilatation of the narrowing foodpipe in the region of the growth is sometimes performed. For further details of applicable therapies see Cancer (**XIII**).

I/9 PEPTIC ULCER

An ULCER in the mucous-membrane lining of those areas of the digestive tract exposed to gastric juice containing hydrochloric acid and the enzyme pepsin. The areas commonly affected include the lower end of the oesophagus (see Hiatus Hernia, I/7), the stomach (gastric ulcers —see I/10) and the duodenum (duodenal ulcers—see I/11). Therapies are discussed under I/11.

I/10 GASTRIC ULCER

This type of peptic ulcer is most likely to affect men in their 60s and 70s. It is associated with stress (see STRESS REACTIONS). Vomiting, which frequently features, relieves the ulcer pain, which usually starts within two hours of eating. Attacks last 2–8 weeks, interspersed by symptom-free periods of 2–12 months.

Factors associated with gastric ulcers include environmental ones (stress, cigarette smoking and the regular use of aspirin); an hereditary factor (a greater tendency to develop gastric ulcer exists among first-degree relatives of sufferers); chronic (atrophic) gastritis (see I/13); and arthritis (see VI/1), when aspirin and certain other drugs are used, e.g. indomethacin (Indocid), phenylbutazone (Butazolidin).

Two major diagnostic techniques are used by orthodox practitioners. The first is X-ray examination, including a barium meal; and the second is fibre-optic endoscopy, which views the interior of the stomach through a fibre passed into it via the mouth and foodpipe.

Gastric ulcers can cause anaemia (see VIII/1) through regular loss of small quantities of blood (see MELAENA; OCCULT BLOOD); they can perforate suddenly, with a heavy loss of blood (see HAEMORRHAGE); and can also cause an obstruction in the digestive tract, as the tissues involved in the ulcer-formation contract and form scar tissue.

I/11 DUODENAL ULCER

Duodenal ulcers occur in 10 per cent of the population, and symptoms are most frequently found in stressed male patients in their 20s and 30s. The commonest symptom is aching or boring ABDOMINAL PAIN in the upper central area of the abdomen in the midline, which starts within 2 hours of a meal and is relieved by alkalis (milk, sodium bicarbonate in water). WATER BRASH also occurs, but vomiting is uncommon.

The major factors associated with duodenal ulcers include cigarette smoking (environmental); first-degree relatives with duodenal ulcers, the blood group O, and the failure to secrete certain blood-group substances (hereditary); and cirrhosis of the liver (see I/24), chronic obstructive lung disease, chronic renal failure (see **IV/2**), and certain types of leukaemia (see **VIII/3**) (associated diseases). Diagnosis, as with gastric ulcer (see **I/10**), is confirmed by gastroduodenoscopy and by barium-meal X-ray.

ORTHODOX TREATMENT

The medical treatment for peptic ulcer has four goals: to relieve symptoms, to increase the rate at which ulcers heal, to prevent complications, and to prevent recurrence.

Histamine H-2 antagonist drugs (widely used at the moment) inhibit gastric-acid secretion. By contrast, the familiar 'anti-allergi' anthistamines (histamine H-1 antagonists)—e.g. mepyramine maleate (Piriton), prescribed for hay-fever symptoms—do not inhibit gastric-acid or pepsin secretion. They interfere with the release of histamine at other sites such as the smooth muscle in the air tubes (bronchi) and the second part of the small bowel (ileum).

Examples of histamine H-2 antagonists are cimetidine (Tagamet), which revolutionized orthodox peptic-ulcer therapy less than 10 years ago, and ranitidine (Zantac), which is very similar to cimetidine. The use of 1–1.2g of cimetidine daily over a four-week period results in healing of a duodenal ulcer in 70–80 per cent of patients (a placebo, by way of comparison, produces healing in 40–50 per cent of patients).

Antacids are still a popular method of relieving peptic-ulcer symptoms. Common examples are a suspension of oxethazaine together with aluminium hydroxide gel and magnesium hydroxide (Mucaine); and tablets containing dried aluminium hydroxide gel and magnesium hydroxide (Maalox Concentrate tablets).

Derivatives of hormone-like substances known as prostaglandins are likely to be the next drugs to rival the use of cimetidine and ranitidine in the treatment of peptic ulceration. As well as inhibiting the secretion of large amounts of gastric acid, the prostaglandins are thought to act by boosting the production of mucus and bicarbonate ions normally responsible for protecting the digestive tract from attack by its own hydrochloric acid and pepsin.

Bland diets are not particularly helpful, but patients are advised to stop smoking and to avoid cola-pop drinks, coffee, tea and large amounts of alcohol, since these stimulate the secretion of large quantities of gastric acid.

ALTERNATIVE THERAPIES

Natural medicine

Nutritional therapy Wholefood diet omitting coffee, tea, alcohol, highly spiced and very oily foods, with emphasis on fresh raw vegetables and fruit, and their juices. Cabbage juice may be useful, since it contains Vitamin U, believed to be an L-methionine methylsulphonium salt and reputed to help gastric ulcers to heal. 300ml of fresh cabbage juice twice daily is recommended, plus two kelp tablets and the daily vitamin and mineral regimen (see page 436). This latter precaution is because large amounts of raw cabbage can affect the function of the thyroid gland in people who are already iodine-deficient.

Specific dietary supplements The following supplements have been found useful in cases of peptic ulceration:

- Vitamin A, 25,000iu, one to three times daily for five days, then stop for two.
- Vitamin B complex 100mg (time-release), morning and evening.
- Rosehip Vitamin C with bioflavonoids, 1,000mg (time-release), morning and evening.
- Zinc sulphate, 100mg, three times daily with food.

Gastric ulcers are reputed to have responded to 150,000iu Vitamin A daily for four weeks. *This should be taken only under professional supervision.*

Biochemic tissue salts WATER BRASH responds to *Nat. Mur.* To treat symptoms of acidity: *Nat. Phos.*

Herbal medicine

Remedies include an emulsion made from the gel extracted from the *Aloe vera* plant: 30ml of the liquid is taken immediately before each of the three main meals, and a further 30ml before retiring.

Also used is a marshmallow infusion of 30g of dried leaves in 600ml boiling water. Strain and flavour with honey and drink.

Aromatherapy

The upper central abdomen, just below the breastbone, is massaged with warm olive oil and 10 per cent of essence. Also, three drops of essence of lemon on brown sugar after every meal.

Bach flower remedies

Homoeopathy

Severe heartburn is sometimes treated with *Lycopodium*. A very valuable homoeopathic remedy for peptic ulcers is *Ornithogalum*.

Acupuncture

Research work by Chinese physiologists has shown that acupuncture, the treatment of choice in China for peptic ulcers, can reduce stomach acidity. This probably accounts in part for its success in treating this disorder.

Manipulative therapies

Osteopathy can be useful.

Relaxation techniques

Biofeedback (for stress reduction and control), yoga, autogenic training.

Psychotherapy

Useful for the treatment of chronic anxiety (see **XIV/4**).

Spiritual therapy

Electrocrystal therapy; Aurasoma; art, music, colour therapy.

I/12 CANCER OF THE STOMACH

See **XIII**.

'Gastritis' is a term used vaguely to mean INFLAMMATION of the stomach; this can occur either as an acute attack or in a chronic form.

Acute gastritis can (a) be due to an irritant such as large volumes of alcohol, or drugs taken on an empty stomach; (b) be due to an infection elsewhere in the body; or (c) can accompany peptic ulcers (see I/9) or cancer of the stomach or small bowel (see **XIII**). It produces symptoms of anorexia (see **XIV/8**), NAUSEA, VOMITING, upper ABDOMINAL PAIN and giddiness.

Chronic gastritis is a condition found in patients who have repeated attacks of acute gastritis or suffer from a gastric ulcer (see I/10) or stomach cancer.

A condition known simply as 'gastric atrophy', which is not strictly speaking a true inflammation, is sometimes discussed together with gastritis. It occurs in patients with pernicious anaemia (see **VIII/1**) and in certain hormone disorders.

ORTHODOX TREATMENT

For acute gastritis, the patient is put on a fluids-only diet until the symptoms have disappeared; further contact with the causative irritant is avoided. Other measures are aimed at any associated condition such as peptic ulceration. Chronic gastritis does not usually produce symptoms apart from occasional DIARRHOEA when the stomach fails to produce hydrochloric acid (achlorhydria).

ALTERNATIVE THERAPIES

For the once-only attack due to a recognizable irritant, such as unsuitable food or too much alcohol, it is safe to treat the symptoms only (see below). Repeated attacks of acute gastritis merit investigation in the same way as other persistent disorders.

Natural medicine

Nutritional therapy   The recommended dietary regimen, apart from being wholefood and eliminating any known gastric irritants, would depend upon the underlying cause of the attacks of acute gastritis; the same applies to the application of other therapies. Many health practitioners would withhold solid food during an attack and probably recommend the patient to drink mineral water only; then later to progress to freshly squeezed vegetable or fruit juice diluted half-and-half with water, until eventually solid food could be tolerated again.

Specific dietary supplements   Treatment depends on the underlying cause.

Vitamin therapy   Treatment depends on the underlying cause. When achlorhydria is a feature of pernicious anaemia. Vitamin B_{12} cannot be absorbed through the stomach lining and must be given by injection.

Biochemic tissue salts   *Ferr. Phos.* relieves the symptom of vomiting up undigested food.

Herbal medicine

Treatment depends on the underlying cause. Herbal remedies to speed recovery include comfrey. A usual strength of tablet contains 270mg comfrey root per tablet, and the directions for use are: one tablet to be chewed at regular intervals to maintain a daily dosage of 12 tablets.

Slippery-elm bark powder: a dessertspoonful mixed in a little cold water to which are added a cup of warm milk together with a teaspoonful of honey.

Aromatherapy

As for peptic ulcer (see I/9).

Homoeopathy

Gastritis caused by too much alcohol: *Kali Bichromicum*. Gastritis following too much to eat: *Nux Vom*.

I/14 GASTROENTERITIS

This is INFLAMMATION of both the stomach and the small bowel (although, as with 'gastritis', the term 'gastroenteritis' is used vaguely). Its commonest cause is FOOD POISONING. Food can be intrinsically poisonous—e.g. the Death-cap fungus, often mistaken for an edible wild mushroom. Food can also be contaminated by traces of harmful chemicals. Alternatively, bacteria and their toxic products can be responsible. Two bacteria commonly responsible are *Staphylococcus* and *Salmonella*, the first frequently contaminating cooked fish, meat and dairy products and the second being found in a wide variety of food items.

The illness can start with little warning and produce violent VOMIT-ING, COLIC and DIARRHOEA resulting in physical collapse and severe DEHYDRATION if prolonged. Admission to hospital is sometimes necessary, especially in the case of babies and small children, since they become profoundly dehydrated (potentially fatally so) more rapidly than adults. Among babies and small children, about half of gastroenteritis cases are due to a viral organism called *Rotavirus*. Acute cases due to bacteria are highly infective.

Signs of dehydration to watch out for are loose skin (which can be picked up in folds), pallor, sunken eyes, a dry tongue and failure to pass urine.

ORTHODOX TREATMENT

In adults, symptoms usually clear up following bed-rest and fluid replacement, followed by adherence to a light diet. Should the symptoms persist for longer than 48 hours, the stools are usually examined for causative organisms.

Babies and children are treated for dehydration in hospital by means of an intravenous drip, followed, when they have stopped vomiting, by clear fluids given orally.

ALTERNATIVE THERAPIES

Alternative practitioners are unlikely to be consulted about the average attack of gastroenteritis or food poisoning since these are normally 'one-off' occurrences and, if dehydration did become profound, hospitalization offering intravenous fluid replacement would be indicated. However, various natural remedies may give relief from the symptoms and assist with recovery.

Natural medicine

Nutritional therapy   No solids by mouth, the fluid lost in vomiting and diarrhoea being replaced by small sips of a mixture made up as follows: to 600ml spring water add the freshly squeezed juice of one orange and one lemon; mix into the solution a large tablespoonful of liquid honey and a teaspoonful of finely ground rock salt.

Small quantities of simple whole foods should be slowly added once the patient can keep fluids down. Freshly squeezed fruit and vegetable juices, alone or diluted with water, are pleasant and easily assimilated.

Pure honey has been found valuable in treating mild infantile gastroenteritis, since it is bactericidal for many of the causative organisms —including *Salmonella*, *Shigella* and *Escherichia coli*; it is also a readily available source of glucose and fructose. It does not produce further diarrhoea when added instead of glucose to routine salt-replacement fluids, as it promotes sugar- and water-absorption from the bowel. The dose is 50ml honey per litre.

Specific dietary supplements   One gram of potassium divided over three meals.

Biochemic tissue salt therapy   Gastritis and pain, swelling and tenderness of the stomach, with vomiting of undigested food, can respond to *Ferr. Phos.*, alternating with *Kali. Mur.* For diarrhoea with foul-smelling stools and exhaustion: *Kali. Phos.*

Herbal remedies

For vomiting, see discussion under Gastritis (I/13).

For diarrhoea, two foot baths and hand baths daily of the following herbs: a handful of mallow flowers and roots, a handful of nettle leaves, and a handful of meadowsweet flowers to two litres of water.

Specifically for food poisoning: hot infusions of lime flowers to sip in the early stages. When the violence of the attack has lessened, a decoction of half a handful of artichoke leaves to one litre of water.

To deal with the infection: capsules of powdered propolis. These should be taken for about five days, after meals, in doses totalling 2g daily.

Aromatherapy

See discussion under Gastritis (I/13). Also, for diarrhoea: two drops of nutmeg essence on a little brown sugar after each meal, and rubbing of the abdomen with the aromatized oil (olive oil containing 10 per cent of the essence).

Homoeopathy

For vomiting: when there is constant nausea, *Ipecacuanha*; when there is an accompanying burning in the stomach, *Arsenicum Album*. For diarrhoea: *Arsenicum Album*.

I/15 CROHN'S DISEASE (REGIONAL ILEITIS)

Chronic INFLAMMATION of the gut. The chief symptoms include COLIC; pain in the lower-right-hand quadrant of the abdomen, in which area a tender mass can usually be felt; frequent DIARRHOEA; and either formed or loose stools which may be mixed with blood, mucus or pus if the diarrhoea is very severe. Mild fever, anaemia and weightloss are also quite common.

A typical barium-meal picture confirms the diagnosis, and shows that the tender abdominal mass consists of loops of inflamed ileum, bound together by ADHESIONS and sometimes segmented—i.e. interspersed with normal, healthy sections of ileum. FISTULAE often form between the loops of ileum, between the ileum and the abdominal wall, or between the ileum and tissues around the anus.

Crohn's disease is mainly found in young adults, and tends to undergo remissions and relapses over the course of years. In the early stages it is sometimes misdiagnosed as appendicitis (see I/16), and treatment is vital since the unchecked condition can result in ABSCESS formation and PERITONITIS.

No cause of Crohn's disease has been found, although many suggestions have been put forward, including those of an infectious or autoimmune origin. The symptoms are certainly made worse by emotional stress (see STRESS REACTIONS).

ORTHODOX TREATMENT

Acute phases of the disease are controlled by steroid drugs. Patients are also prescribed a high-protein low-residue diet, and drugs to control diarrhoea, bowel infection and nervous strain. Surgery is used only when necessary, as the disease can recur.

ALTERNATIVE THERAPIES

Natural medicine

Fasting during acute attack with deep breathing and hydrotherapy.

GENERAL NUTRITIONAL THERAPY

The aims of the diet are to provide adequate nutrition and to make good the calorie, protein, vitamin and mineral deficiencies from which most Crohn's-disease patients suffer, during or following a relapse. At the same time, it seeks to minimize stress on the inflamed and often narrowed segments of bowel. It also aims at maintaining the diseased small bowel in as healthy a state as possible between relapses.

These aims are shared with the nutritional plan devised by orthodox medical practitioners for Crohn's-disease patients. Where they are likely to differ is in the emphasis alternative practitioners would place upon all food eaten being wholefood, to the total exclusion of artificial dyes, preservatives, flavourings, etc.

The elimination of lactose-containing foods (milk, milk products) can produce remarkable improvement in those Crohn's-disease patients who lack the enzyme lactase. Similarly, patients with severe abdominal CRAMP and DIARRHOEA often benefit from a decrease in fibre-containing foods, and those with STEATORRHOEA can be improved by decreasing their daily fat intake to a total of 70–80g.

Specific dietary supplements   The best approach is for the individual's personal vitamin and mineral profile of requirements to be worked out by a health professional.

Herbal medicine

For herbal remedies for diarrhoea, see under Gastroenteritis (I/14).

For anxiety: two pinches of each of the following to one litre of hot water, steeped and drunk as a tea: vervain, mint, lime flowers and camomile.

Aromatherapy

For the treatment of diarrhoea, see under Gastroenteritis (I/14). For anxiety: three to four drops of essence of basil on a little brown sugar three times daily.

Bach flower remedies
Homoeopathy

For diarrhoea brought on by excitement and worry about forthcoming events (i.e. nervous tension): *Argenticum Nitricum*. For prolonged anxiety with periodic panic attacks: *Arsenicum Album*. Also, for underlying disease: *Podophyllum* or *Phosphoric Acid*.

Acupuncture

Crohn's disease is sometimes amenable to acupuncture, and this therapy can also be helpful in relieving anxiety.

Manipulative therapies

Osteopathy can be useful.

Relaxation techniques

Biofeedback (to combat tension and anxiety); yoga; dance therapy (also for gentle exercise).

Psychotherapy

Useful for treating chronic anxiety.

Spiritual therapy

Electrocrystal therapy; spiritual healing; colour, art and music therapies (where patient has much pent-up emotion).

I/16 APPENDICITIS

An acutely inflamed appendix. Although this is the commonest emergency in abdominal surgery, the symptoms can vary a great deal, and some cases go either undiagnosed or misdiagnosed (it is sometimes confused with Crohn's disease). A classical case of appendicitis generally begins with a poorly localized stomach ache around the navel (umbilicus)—see ABDOMINAL PAIN—together with NAUSEA and sometimes VOMITING. (Medical students are sometimes taught that, if DIARRHOEA accompanies a suspicious central abdominal pain, the diagnosis cannot be appendicitis, which is always accompanied by CONSTIPATION. However, exceptions prove the rule and some genuine appendicitis patients do have diarrhoea as a symptom.) After a few hours, the central abdominal pain shifts to the area immediately over the appendix, i.e. the lower-right-quadrant of the abdomen. The abdominal wall in this region then shows 'guarding', that is, it tightens to protect the underlying structures when pressed deeply. This sign later becomes one of 'rigidity', and the overlying muscles contract tightly, making examination characteristically difficult.

In addition to these signs, which the doctor finds on examination, the patient's temperature is usually slightly raised, the BREATH foul, and the tongue dry.

The only feasible treatment for appendicitis at the present time—and for the foreseeable future—is surgical removal of the appendix, although medical reports from China claim the successful treatment of acute appendicitis by acupuncture; however, in the UK this would be considered too risky a procedure. If the operation is delayed, the appendix is likely to rupture, causing PERITONITIS. Death may follow. Alternatively, the inflammation of peritonitis may become localized —i.e. confined to a small area—and an appendix ABSCESS may form; this will require draining later.

I/17 PANCREATITIS

INFLAMMATION of the pancreas. Like the inflammatory processes described elsewhere, this disorder can be acute or chronic. A 'subacute' form also exists, usually occurring as a complication of mumps, influenza or infective hepatitis. The symptoms include a mild fever, upper abdominal pain and general abdominal discomfort, and the patient usually recovers completely and quickly.

I/18 ACUTE PANCREATITIS

This is a serious condition, affecting both sexes primarily during their fourth to seventh decades. The cause is unknown, but about one patient in five with this disorder is an alcoholic. Some workers think that, due to an obstruction at their common opening, bile from the common bile duct is drawn up into the pancreatic duct where it activates the pancreatic digestive enzymes trypsin and lipase. Much of the pancreas can be destroyed by the subsequent 'autodigestive' process, and a localized or generalized PERITONITIS generally follows.

An attack starts with upper ABDOMINAL PAIN, which can be moderate to excruciating and which extends through to the back, coupled with NAUSEA, VOMITING, and signs of SHOCK. The abdomen becomes swollen and bloated, and later rigid as peritonitis develops. Some attacks are triggered by a bout of drinking or an especially heavy meal, and many patients remember recent bouts of INDIGESTION after eating.

It can be difficult to distinguish between a severe attack of acute pancreatitis and other medical and surgical emergencies such as a perforated peptic ulcer (see I/9), a CORONARY THROMBOSIS and acute cholecystitis (see I/26). The diagnosis, though, can be confirmed by a blood test measuring the level of pancreatic amylase, an enzyme which escapes into the blood-flow of the pancreas when autodigestion of the pancreatic tissue is in progress.

Patients are best managed in hospital, where bed-rest, intravenous fluids and pain relief are found to be far more satisfactory than surgery. There is no alternative therapy likely to be helpful in the management of an attack of acute pancreatitis.

I/19 CHRONIC PANCREATITIS

Symptoms of this disorder include repeated bouts of central ABDOMINAL PAIN; they may last for two or three days, and are often relieved by crouching. Poor digestion and absorption can cause weightloss, and lack of the appropriate digestive enzymes from the damaged pancreas can result in undigested meat fibres and an excess of fat in the stools, together with troublesome DIARRHOEA. The patient may suffer from jaundice (see I/22) and slowly develop diabetes mellitus (see X/2) and MALABSORPTION as the cells of the pancreas are gradually destroyed.

The usual causes of chronic pancreatitis include repeated attacks of the acute or subacute forms; persistent inflammation of the bile duct; and penetration by a chronic duodenal ulcer (see I/11). The factor all these have in common is that they result in recurrent bouts of inflammation in the substance of the pancreas, and the laying down of fibrous tissue which replaces the healthy, functional cells.

ORTHODOX TREATMENT

The patient receives a bland diet with little roughage, and frequent small meals. No alcohol is allowed, and fat intake is restricted. Most of the calories are supplied by protein and carbohydrate, and extra minerals and fat-soluble vitamins are given. Insulin is given if diabetes develops, and active pancreatic-enzyme extracts are given if STEATORRHOEA is present.

ALTERNATIVE THERAPIES

Natural medicine

Fasting on fruit juice to control acute attack. For general condition, a similar diet to the above, but wholefood. The individual's vitamin and mineral requirements should be worked out by a nutritional expert, and full supplementation given of the natural, organic variety. Similar substitution of live pancreatic enzymes.

Earl Mindell's recipe for a good pep-up protein drink useful in this context consists of 2 tbsp protein powder, 1 tbsp lecithin powder, 2 tbsp acidophilus liquid (*or* 1 tbsp acidophilus powder), 1 tbsp nutritional yeast. Blend with milk, water or fruit juice in a blender for one minute.[34]

Herbal medicine

Herbal remedies include, for the weakness and debility, foot baths and hand baths of the following ingredients: to 2 litres of water, a handful each of hawthorn flowers, sage leaves and flowers, and violets. This provides two baths daily. For the diarrhoea, see under Gastroenteritis (**I/14**).

Aromatherapy

For weakness and debility: four drops of sweet marjoram essence on brown sugar after each meal.

For diabetes and diarrhoea: raw onion to eat daily (if it agrees with the patient), to back up following alcohol preparation: allow 500g of chopped onions to macerate for two weeks in 500g of 60° alcohol. Strain and take one soupspoonful at the start of every meal.

Bach flower remedies

Homoeopathy

For exhaustion following the diarrhoea: *Arnica*, or *Arsenicum Album*.

Acupuncture

Used to counter diarrhoea, to boost energy levels and to speed recovery.

Spiritual therapy

Electrocrystal therapy may be helpful.

I/20 CANCER OF THE PANCREAS

This form of cancer affects men more than women, the peak age being 55—70 years. The symptoms depend upon which part of the pancreas is initially affected, but commonly include dull upper ABDOMINAL PAIN that bores through to the back, made worse by food and lying down and relieved by getting into the crouching position. Indigestion, loss of weight, poor appetite, flatulence and vomiting also occur, and sometimes jaundice (see I/22). This type of cancer produces SECONDARIES early, in adjacent organs and in the liver.

Orthodox treatment consists of surgery, which is often only palliative. See cancer (**XIII**).

I/21 ISLET CELL TUMOURS

Small, rare, benign tumours occur in the pancreatic cells responsible for manufacturing insulin (beta cells of the islets). They produce a higher than normal level of insulin and symptoms of spontaneous HYPOGLYCAEMIA occur.

I/22 JAUNDICE

This is not a true disorder but a sign that the liver is malfunctioning in one of three chief ways.

The word 'jaundice' refers to the yellow colour taken on by the skin, whites of the eyes and mucous membranes which become stained with the pigment bilirubin. This pigment is continually formed in the body from red blood cells which reach the end of their natural lifespan of about 120 days and are broken down into simpler parts. The iron in the molecules of haemoglobin (red pigment responsible for transporting oxygen around the body) is recycled for further use, and the 'globin' protein is retained, but the bilirubin fraction derived from the breakdown is no longer required and needs to be excreted.

One of the functions of a normal liver is to excrete the bilirubin in the bile. It is prevented from doing so, however, if its cells are injured—e.g.

by infection or poisons—and as a result bilirubin collects in the blood and stains the tissues. This condition is *hepatic jaundice*, and occurs in the infection YELLOW FEVER. Other symptoms include, in a late phase, dark urine and light-coloured motions.

When *obstructive jaundice* occurs, the bile is prevented from leaving the gall bladder by an obstruction such as a STONE in the bile ducts, or a TUMOUR in the ducts or in the pancreas. The consequence of this is that it is reabsorbed into the bloodstream, and the level of bilirubin rises. In obstructive jaundice, the motions are very pale and the urine dark.

Haemolytic jaundice occurs when extra-large numbers of red blood cells are destroyed, and the liver is unable to cope with the great quantity of bilirubin released from the haemoglobin pigment. Some spills over into the blood where the normal level rises. In haemolytic jaundice, the motions are dark and the urine normal in colour. Malaria (see **VIII/4**), poisons and circulating red-cell antibodies due to an incompatible blood transfusion all cause haemolytic anaemia.

Jaundice, as such, is not treated—always the underlying disorder causing it.

I/23 HEPATITIS

This is INFLAMMATION of the liver, generally due to a virus infection. There are two main types—infectious hepatitis (hepatitis A, also called epidemic jaundice) and serum hepatitis (hepatitis B).

Infectious hepatitis is chiefly spread from infected motions to the mouth by way of unwashed hands. Its incubation period is 4–6 weeks. *Serum hepatitis* has a longer incubation period, of up to six months, and is conveyed by traces of infective blood or serum (the fluid part of blood) on an unsterile hypodermic-syringe needle. Drug addicts are frequent victims.

The symptoms vary in severity. They can cause very little discomfort, or produce fever, nausea, loss of appetite, vomiting, headaches and aching muscles. Jaundice usually appears within a week or two of the other symptoms, and patients generally recover well although convalescence may be prolonged, and beset by depression (see **XIV/3**). A few patients later develop cirrhosis (see **I/24**).

ORTHODOX TREATMENT

The main requirements are bed-rest and complete abstinence from alcohol for at least six months.

ALTERNATIVE THERAPIES

Natural medicine

A short fruit-juice fast initially, with hydrotherapy.

Nutritional therapy Simple wholefoods are recommended, with mineral water or water/fresh juice to drink. Fats and oils should not be taken in large amounts, and the nausea and poor appetite should be overcome by offering the patient tempting foods attractively served in small quantities.

Specific dietary supplements Hepatitis due to viral infection (other, less common, causes do exist) may respond to very high doses of Vitamin C (25–30g) for a few days, preferably by injection. It can be given orally instead, at a dose of 5g every four hours. This should always be carried out under professional supervision. A high-potency multivitamin complex is also needed to replace the vitamins lost from the liver during and after hepatitis.

Biochemic tissue salts For bilious fevers, *Nat. Sulph.*; for aching muscles, *Silica*.

Herbal medicine

To purify the blood: a decoction of burdock root, made by boiling one teaspoonful of the root in one cupful of water for a few minutes. To relieve nausea: spearmint tea, made by infusing one teaspoonful of dried spearmint leaves and tops in one covered cup of boiling water for 10 minutes; strain and flavour with honey to taste, and drink warm or cold as often as required.

Aromatherapy

For jaundice: geranium, three drops of essence on a little brown sugar after meals.

Homoeopathy

For vomiting with persistent nausea: *Ipecacuanha*.

I/24 CIRRHOSIS

A chronic disorder of the liver for which many causes exist. Much of the normal liver tissue is destroyed, and fibrous tissue laid down in its place. Alcoholism is one cause of this condition; others include infection (hepatitis—see I/23), certain dietary deficiencies (e.g. of the amino acids cystine and methionine, or of the B vitamin choline), and long-standing congestive heart failure (see III/3).

Two chief consequences of cirrhosis are responsible for the clinical features associated with it. One of these is portal hypertension, a rise in the hydrostatic pressure of the blood within the liver which is delivered to it by the portal vein from the stomach and small bowel. This is due mainly to the obstruction of its flow by the thickened, fibrous liver tissue, and the symptoms include fluid in the abdominal cavity (ascites), poor digestion, and sometimes the formation of varicose veins at the lower end of the foodpipe (oesophageal varices).

The second important consequence of cirrhosis is liver failure, due to the inability of the few remaining normal liver cells to carry out the work of the entire organ. The attempt to do so causes the healthy cells to increase in size, and liver enlargement is a common sign of early cirrhosis. The results of this cellular failure include hepatic jaundice (see I/22) and a lowered level of blood proteins, which can cause OEDEMA and ascites and slow the blood's clotting rate. Pronounced mental changes (encephalopathy) leading ultimately to COMA can arise in advanced cirrhosis due to the escape of nitrogen compounds into the blood.

ORTHODOX TREATMENT

The most important measure that can be taken in cases of alcoholic cirrhosis is abstinence from alcohol, as this arrests the progress of the disorder. Steroid drugs can be useful in other forms of cirrhosis. Diuretic drugs are used to get rid of excess fluid, although ascitic fluid in the abdominal cavity sometimes needs to be tapped (withdrawn with a syringe). Portal hypertension is sometimes dealt with by surgery.

There are no special dietary restrictions unless the kidneys are retaining sodium or there is encephalopathy is present. In the first instance, the diet should be a low-sodium one; in the second the protein intake should be reduced to 20g per day, and at least 800–1,000 calories given in the form of a protein-free, high-carbohydrate drink supplement, such as Hy-cal.

ALTERNATIVE THERAPIES

Natural medicine

Specific dietary supplements   High doses of Vitamin B-complex plus the fat-soluble vitamins (A, D, E and K) to overcome deficiency due to the disease. Choline (up to 3,000mg daily) may be needed to prevent fatty infiltration of the liver, a disorder due to alcoholism that can occur alone or in association with cirrhosis.

Herbal medicine

A herbal remedy to help rid the liver of impurities, and to aid digestion is an infusion of a pinch of each of the following herbs in a cup of water, drunk after meals: anise, basil, fennel, mint, rosemary, savory and chervil. There is also substantial evidence for the protective power of the oil of the evening primrose flower (clinically used as Efamol) against liver damage caused by excessive alcohol.[35]

Aromatherapy

Four drops of essence of juniper on a little brown sugar after every meal. Also, rub the area of skin overlying the liver with olive oil containing 10 per cent of essence of Juniper.

Bach flower remedies

These might help where alcoholism is basic cause.

Acupuncture

This could be used to stimulate the healing process.

Spiritual therapies

Electrocrystal therapy may also accelerate healing.

I/25 CARCINOMA OF THE LIVER

While secondary deposits in the liver from malignant growths else-where are relatively common (see SECONDARIES), primary TUMOURS arising within the liver are fairly uncommon in the UK, although common in Africa and Asia. In the UK they are usually found in men past middle age with pre-existing cirrhosis. Symptoms include vague indigestion, weightloss, a protruding abdomen (due to ASCITES), weakness, pain over the liver area and often a fever. For treatment, see Cancer (**XIII**).

I/26 CHOLECYSTITIS

Acute INFLAMMATION of the gall bladder usually occurs when an obstruction such as a gall stone is present, preventing bile from escaping down its normal route. Swelling follows and the gall bladder may perforate, and it often becomes infected. Symptoms include NAUSEA, severe upper ABDOMINAL PAIN, and FEVER. The area over the gall bladder is very tender to the touch, and VOMITING is common. One patient in four becomes jaundiced (see **I/22**). Attacks can last a few days and be repeated every few months or years; but when the infection is severe and the obstruction to bile flow is complete, the gall bladder can become filled with pus and perforate, causing PERITONITIS and other complications.

The most usual treatment for acute cholecystitis is surgical removal of the gall bladder, either immediately on admission to hospital or after a lapse of 2–3 days, during which salt and water lost through vomiting are replaced and antibiotics are given.

I/27 CHRONIC CHOLECYSTITIS

Gall stones are the commonest cause of chronic gall bladder INFLAMMATION. They are commoner in women than men, and affect about 10–15 per cent of the population. Stones that remain within the gall bladder rarely produce symptoms, but those that obstruct the cystic duct cause recurrent infection, while those blocking the common bile duct can cause attacks of biliary colic and obstructive jaundice (see **I/22**).

The pain is usually severe, moving from the midline to below the right ribs. It often radiates through to the back and the tip of the shoulder blade, and is accompanied by FEVER, NAUSEA and VOMITING.

ORTHODOX TREATMENT

Some patients respond well to bed-rest, antibiotics and a suitable diet.

Others who suffer repeated attacks of biliary colic have their gall bladders and stones removed surgically.

The recommended diet is light and fat-free. In April 1984 a leading article in the *British Medical Journal* recommended that the best way to prevent gall stones is to 'keep slim, avoid sugar, drink a little alcohol, and perhaps, keep up a high fibre intake'.

One of the reasons why gall stones form is because the bile in the gall bladder is heavily saturated (i.e. supersaturated) with bile salts. Daily alcohol (in moderation!) considerably reduces this supersaturated state.

ALTERNATIVE THERAPIES

Natural medicine

Naturopathic practitioners frequently recommend a fairly long fast during which the patient takes only hot water and a little juice. In addition, enemas are given, and hot, soothing compresses placed on the abdominal area overlying the gall bladder. The object is gradually to dissolve large stones.

Other dietary approaches are adopted to deal with small gall stones capable of being passed down the cystic and common bile ducts to be excreted in the motions.

Nutritional therapy A low-calorie wholefood diet containing carbohydrates in their unrefined form, and thereby adequate fibre (e.g. wholegrain bread, wholewheat pasta, pulses, brown rice), and as little sugar as possible.

Specific dietary supplements Cholesterol is a major component of gall stones, and helps to form them by crystallizing out of solution when present in a high concentration in bile. Vitamin C is reputed to reduce the cholesterol concentration of the bile, thereby decreasing the likelihood of stone formation. One gram per day should be taken.

Magnesium helps to prevent the formation of gall stones. The recommended intake for an adult is 300–400mg daily. It is available in multimineral preparations (preferably in the chelated form), and as dolomite, which contains calcium too.

Lipotropic agents are substances which help to prevent the abnormal or excessive deposition of fat in the liver. They also encourage the liver cells to make lecithin, which helps to prevent cholesterol from forming into gall stones and from being deposited in blood vessels (see ATHEROMA). Examples of lipotropics include methionine, choline, inositol and betaine. Vitamin-B complex supplements often contain 50–100mg choline and inositol. Daily doses are generally around 500–1,000mg of choline and 250–500mg of inositol.

Herbal medicine

Herbal remedies include a hot compress for the gall-bladder area and foot and hand baths of the following ingredients: a handful each of artichoke leaves, grated dog's tooth roots, and poppy petals and seed capsules, plus half-handfuls of chicory leaves and roots, and dandelions. The compresses should be applied as needed and two or more baths taken daily.

Aromatherapy

Four drops of the essential oil of the Scots pine on brown sugar after every meal.

Homoeopathy

Chelidonium is often useful for gall-bladder problems. For severe pain, *Dioscaria* can be used.

Acupuncture

Chinese studies indicate that acupuncture can discharge large gall stones in the motions, including some which in the UK would normally, together with the gall bladder, be removed surgically. Further evidence is awaited with interest by Western physicians and acupuncturists.

I/28 CANCER OF THE GALL BLADDER

Primary CARCINOMA is this organ is not a very common type of cancer (see **XIII**), although years of chronic cholecystitis caused by gall stones may predispose to its development, especially in elderly women. The chief features of this illness are upper ABDOMINAL PAIN, gradually growing more severe, and fever, loss of weight and vomiting. Obstructive jaundice (see **I/22**) often occurs. Treatment is by surgical removal of the gall bladder.

INFLAMMATION of the colon. This is a chronic disorder, sudden attacks alternating with periods of remission of varying length. Symptoms include ABDOMINAL PAIN, which is mild and diffuse at first and then settles in the lower abdomen; poor appetite; and DIARRHOEA. The motions can be semi-formed or consist entirely of liquid, and may contain mucus and blood. Faecal incontinence can affect patients who normally have no trouble in this respect.

Weightloss affects sufferers of repeated attacks, and this is frequently a feature of *ulcerative colitis*, a type of colitis believed to be autoimmune in origin (see ALLERGY). In this disorder, the lining of the colon is riddled with ULCERS, and bleeds easily. Diarrhoea is especially troublesome, and attacks are often related to emotional problems and periods of worry and stress (see STRESS REACTIONS). Associated problems include anaemia (see VIII/1) from the frequent blood-loss; protein malnutrition, related to the persistent diarrhoea; strictures in the wall of the colon, due to the longstanding inflammatory process; and perforation of the damaged colon wall, producing an emergency condition needing immediate surgery. Patients with ulcerative colitis also have a greater than normal chance of developing cancer of the large bowel (see XIII).

Inspection with a isgmoidoscope (an instrument inserted via the anus), biopsy (tissue-sampling) of the colon lining, and a barium enema are carried out to confirm the diagnosis.

Often no cause can be found for non-ulcerative colitis, but possible factors include sensitivity to lactose, a sugar present in milk, an inherited tendency to the complaint, and bacterial INFECTION.

ORTHODOX TREATMENT

Mild cases of non-ulcerative colitis are treated symptomatically at home with, for example, an anti-spasmodic drug such as mebeverine hydrochloride (Colofac), or an anti-diarrhoeal, such as diphenoxylate hydrochloride (Lomotil).

Patients suffering from repeated attacks of ulcerative colitis, in whom dehydration and serious chemical disturbance can easily arise, are generally managed in hospital. A high-protein diet, replacement of lost salt and water, psychotherapy (where applicable) and antibiotics (to control any infection that arises in the inflamed colon lining) are all used. Steroid drugs are given for symptomatic relief. Surgery is sometimes employed, and can involve the removal of the entire large bowel, including the rectum, and the formation of an artificial opening of the end of the small bowel onto the skin (ileostomy).

ALTERNATIVE THERAPIES

Natural medicine

Nutritional therapy　For patients with non-ulcerative colitis it is often sufficient to avoid any foods that tend to worsen the condition, and to keep away from red meat, alcohol and stimulants such as tea and coffee until the attack starts to diminish. The diet should be wholefood, and drinks should consist of mineral water and freshly squeezed fruit and vegetable juices.

Sufferers from ulcerative colitis can benefit from a two-day fast on juice when an attack starts, followed by a bland wholefood diet. This should be very low in roughage during the first few days when the colon lining is at its most vulnerable, and then expanded to include raw fruit and vegetables. Baked jacket potatoes, nuts and dried fruit may be introduced gradually; dairy products, red meat (apart from offal) and tea and coffee should be avoided. Cereals should be taken only if the patient is certain that these never worsen his or her condition or bring on an attack. The diet should aim at replacing the lost protein; good sources for non-vegetarians are steamed, flaked white fish, poached or lightly scrambled eggs, steamed and minced chicken or turkey breast, and minced rabbit, lamb's kidneys or lamb's liver. Due to the advisability of avoiding unnecessary roughage during the early days of an acute attack of ulcerative colitis, vegetarians should obtain the protein they need from eggs and perhaps tofu, rather than from nuts, grains and pulses.

Specific dietary supplements　Orthodox drug treatment should be supplemented with a high-potency vitamin preparation, plus extra vitamins C and B_6 (pyridoxine) when corticosteroids are being used. In addition, to aid the healing process within the inflamed lining membrane and to make good the mineral deficit, the following are beneficial:

- Potassium, 100mg in its elemental form, one to three times daily.
- Iron, 320mg tablets, one twice daily.
- Sugarless cabbage juice for its vitamin U content (see discussion under Duodenal Ulcer—I/11), a 300ml glass three times daily.
- Mineral water, 6–8 tumblers daily.

- *Aloe vera* gel (for internal use), 1 tbsp three times daily.
- Acidophilus capsules, 3–6, three times daily.
- When the acute diarrhoeic episode and severe abdominal pain have been alleviated, 1 tbsp of bran flakes or 3–6 bran tablets three times daily.

Herbal medicine

A hot infusion of the following ingredients: two pinches each of lavender, lime flowers, marjoram and mallow to one litre of water. Drink two cupfuls daily.

Aromatherapy

For colic and colitis: five drops of essence of rosemary on a little brown sugar after meals. The area of the abdomen overlying the colon can be rubbed with 60° alcohol containing 3 per cent of essence of rosemary.

Bach flower remedies

Homoeopathy

For diarrhoea brought on by excitement and worry about forthcoming events: *Argentum Nitricum*. For prolonged anxiety, with periodic spells of acute panic: *Arsenicum Album*.

Acupuncture

Colitis, including the ulcerative form, is sometimes helped by this.

Relaxation technique

For stress reduction and physical control, biofeedback, yoga, dance therapy.

Psychotherapy

Hypnotherapy, for example, can be used to counter chronic anxiety.

Spiritual therapy

Colour, music, art therapy; Aurasoma; electrocrystal therapy.

I/30 Spastic colon (irritable-bowel syndrome)

This is the most commonly seen disorder of the digestive system. Its symptoms include ABDOMINAL PAIN, which is relieved by passing a motion; variable bowel habits (DIARRHOEA) may alternate with periods of CONSTIPATION); abdominal distension; and the production of large amounts of mucus. The abdominal pain can be diffuse throughout the lower or upper abdomen, or settle below the right or left rib margins. Persistent pain below the right ribs has often led to removal of the gall bladder, especially in patients known to have gall stones. INDIGESTION is also commoner in patients with spastic colon—HEARTBURN is frequently found; in a recent study, 73 per cent of spastic-colon patients complained of NAUSEA, compared with only 3 per cent of matched control patients.

Two main types of causes underlie the majority of attacks. One of these is overstimulation of the nervous and muscular activities of the bowel by irritating foods such as onions, cabbage, beer, orange juice, molasses and large volumes of coffee. The other consists of emotional factors; a 'typical personality' for a sufferer has been described whose chief features include over-conscientiousness, sensitivity, guilt and rigidity of character.

By no means all patients with spastic colon disorder, however, fit this personality description, and in many no trigger factors can be discovered. Nevertheless, stress remains the most commonly identified precipitating factor (see STRESS REACTIONS). Others include viral or bacterial intestinal infections, and certain drugs.

Spastic colon can affect people of any age from childhood onwards, although it occurs most frequently between the ages of 20 and 50. It was once thought predominantly to affect young women, but in fact there is no clear difference between its frequency in the two sexes.

The diagnosis of spastic colon can be made legitimately only when other, more serious disorders of the bowel have been looked for and excluded, such as carcinoma (see XIII), inflammatory bowel disease (Crohn's disease [I/15], colitis [I/29], and POLYPS.

ORTHODOX TREATMENT

Reassurance of the patient, together with an explanation of the disorder, is important. Attention should be turned to identifying and controlling any precipitating stress factors.

Single drugs seem to be less effective than a combination of several agents aimed at combating both aspects of the symptom complex.

Mebeverine (Colofac) relaxes the colon effectively. When nausea and upper-digestive-tract symptoms are troublesome, Stelabid (isopropamide and trifluoperazine) can be very helpful. In one study, the research doctors found that mebeverine and Motival (fluphenazine and nortriptyline, for anxiety and depression), together with an agent which gives the motions more bulk, such as granules of ispaghula husk (Isogel), represented the best combination.[36]

ALTERNATIVE THERAPIES

Natural medicine

Since spastic colon is a reaction to personal stress and does not imply actual disease of the large bowel, the emphasis lies in reassessment and possibly reorganization of lifestyle, plus possibly some dietary changes. Naturopathy fills this role very adequately; but remedies from some of the other therapies can be useful for the relief of symptoms without recourse to drugs.

Nutritional therapy A wholefood diet that excludes all items which may tend to aggravate the symptoms—possible culprits include cereals and dairy products. The emphasis can beneficially be placed on salads, raw fruit and vegetables, nuts, dried fruit, grains and pulses, with fish, white meat and two or three eggs per week to supply protein.

Specific dietary supplements The following vitamins and minerals are often very beneficial in the relief of anxiety (and depression), and so spastic-colon sufferers should make certain that their daily supplements include them: Vitamin B_1 (thiamine), Vitamin B_6 (pyridoxine), pantothenic acid, Vitamin C (ascorbic acid), Vitamin E (alpha-tocopherol), zinc, magnesium and calcium.

Herbal medicine

For anxiety, herbal expert Maurice Messegué recommends his special 'tea of happiness', to be drunk as required. To one litre of boiling water add two pinches of each of the following herbs: mint, vervain, camomile and lime flowers. A simpler one recommended by the same author consists of a fig, a prune and a pinch of hawthorn flowers, infused in a cup of boiling water for 10 minutes. This is probably best taken when any symptoms of diarrhoea have been brought under control.

For diarrhoea: two foot and hand baths daily of one handful each of the following herbs in 2 litres of water: mallow flowers and roots, nettle leaves and meadowsweet flowers.

Oil of peppermint has recently been used in a clinical trial to test its effectiveness in the treatment of spastic colon. It was administered in the form of capsules containing 0.2ml of oil, 3–6 capsules daily, and was found to be significantly more effective in relieving symptoms than was the placebo used as a control. The oil has its effect because it relaxes the gastrointestinal muscle.[37]

Aromatherapy

To relieve acute anxiety: three drops of valerian essence on a little brown sugar between meals. For intestinal spasm and diarrhoea: four drops of essence of savory on a little brown sugar after every meal. Also, rub the abdomen with 80° alcohol and 6 per cent of essence of sassafras.

Bach flower remedies

Homoeopathy

For diarrhoea brought on by excitement and worry: *Argentum Nitricum*. For abdominal pain associated with flatulence and colic after eating or drinking alcohol: *Nux Vomica*. Also of use are *Phosphoric Acid* and *Podophyllum*.

Acupuncture

Relaxation techniques

For stress control, biofeedback and meditation; dance therapy. Yoga is especially recommended.

Psychotherapy

For spastic-colon sufferers with deeply seated anxiety that remains unresponsive to biofeedback or yoga, psychotherapy, especially hypnotherapy, can be very useful.

Spiritual therapies

Aurasoma; electrocrystal therapy; art, music.

I/31 DYSENTERY

A diarrhoeal illness due to infection of the colon by bacteria or amoebae. The infection spreads as a result of food becoming contaminated with faeces in which the bacteria or amoebae are thriving. This comes about when the standards of sanitation are inadequate, and when infected people preparing food fail to wash their hands after going to the lavatory. Most sufferers display symptoms of dysentery, but others are 'carriers' and are unaware that their motions are infected. House flies are also responsible for spreading the infection.

The symptoms of bacterial dysentery (called 'bacillary' dysentery because the causative bacteria are bacilli) include COLIC, DIARRHOEA, and blood and mucus in the motions, and tend to be more severe in the tropics and subtropics due to the greater virulence of the bacteria involved. Dysentery in the West is less likely to produce severe dehydration, salt imbalance and collapse.

Symptoms of bacillary dysentery start to appear within 2–3 days following infection, and the diagnosis is confirmed by finding the responsible bacteria in a specimen of the patient's motions.

The amoeba responsible for amoebic dysentery is called *Entamoeba histolytica*. It is found worldwide, and thrives particularly well in undeveloped countries where poverty and poor sanitation abound. The symptoms of amoebic dysentery can vary in intensity from mild to very severe. Liver abscesses sometimes form and are liable to rupture, causing either an external abscess of the abdominal wall or even more serious problems within the chest or peritoneal cavity. The lining of the colon becomes ulcerated in a characteristic way, and its appearance, plus the existence of amoeba in the patient's motions, confirms the diagnosis.

ORTHODOX TREATMENT

The essential aspects of treatment, from whatever source, are the replacement of salts and fluid lost in violent DIARRHOEA. Sometimes oral fluids are sufficient; at other times intravenous fluid and salt replacement are vital. Suspensions of kaol in such as Kaopectate can give symptomatic relief, as can calcium sulphaloxate (Enteromide). Antibiotics are used in cases of bacillary dysentery, and amoebic dysentery is treated with emetine injections or with tetracycline (e.g. Terramycin) and chloroquine (e.g. Avloclor).

ALTERNATIVE THERAPIES

As mentioned above, the replacement of fluid and salt is vital. Alternative therapies can be useful if used in conjunction with this, and possibly as an adjunct to antibiotics and anti-amoebic drugs. The following remedies can relieve the symptoms of an attack, and speed recovery afterwards.

Natural medicine

A naturopathic doctor could review the patient's diet and lifestyle and point out changes in both that would enhance the strength of the body's personal defence system against infections.

Nutritional therapy   Initially a fluid fast consisting of mineral water; or water and fresh fruit or vegetable juice, half and half; or skimmed milk if no allergy to milk exists. When symptoms have abated, small meals of simple wholefoods can be introduced.

Specific dietary supplements   Potassium, 1g daily, divided over three meals. Special attention should be paid to an adequate intake of the whole Vitamin-B complex.

Herbal medicine

To ease the diarrhoea: an enema made up from a decoction of at least three handfuls of lime flowers to a litre of water. Also for the diarrhoea, foot and hand baths (two daily) of a handful of each of the following to 2 litres of water: mallow flowers and roots, nettle leaves, meadowsweet flowers.

Mark Bricklin, in his *Practical Encyclopedia of Natural Healing*, gives the following remedy for amoebic dysentery, but stresses that it should be made up by an experienced pharmacist (or herbal practitioner): to boiled skimmed milk add the active ingredients bismuth subsalicylate, salol, fennel, catnip and paregoric camphorata (no quantities given).[38]

Aromatherapy

Specifically for dysentery: essence of lemon, five drops on a little brown sugar after meals. In addition, rub the abdomen with warm olive oil and 10 per cent of the essence.

Homoeopathy

For diarrhoea brought on by FOOD POISONING: *Arsenicum Album*. For abdominal pain, with flatulence and colic: *Nux Vomica*.

Acupuncture

Studies on bowel infections carried out in China show that acupuncture can result in more rapid recovery and reduce the likelihood of complications developing.[39]

I/32 DIVERTICULITIS

The INFLAMMATION of small, blind fingerlike projections of the lining membrane of the large bowel which push through weak spots in the muscular wall. (The condition in which the projections exist but remain uninflamed is called diverticulosis.)

The symptoms of diverticulitis include episodes of ABDOMINAL PAIN in the lower-left-hand quarter of the abdomen, plus CONSTIPATION or DIARRHOEA. Acute attacks involve more severe pain, and often a fever. Associated complications are: narrowing of the affected segment of colon, due to the episodes of inflammation, sometimes leading to complete obstruction of the bowel; and perforation of one of the pouches, followed by HAEMORRHAGE and PERITONITIS; spread of inflammation to organs in the vicinity, such as the bladder, vagina, womb (uterus) and loops of small bowel, sometimes resulting in the formation of a FISTULA.

ORTHODOX TREATMENT

Patients with diverticulitis should adopt a diet with a high roughage and fibre content, sometimes aided in the early stages by a 'bulk' laxative such as ispaghula husks (Isogel) to help produce a bulky, soft motion. A wholefood diet, with emphasis on fresh fruit and vegetables, wholemeal bread and pasta, cereals, grains and pulses, is ideal for the diverticulitis patient. Refined sugar, and foods containing it, should be eliminated from the diet.

The aim is to prevent constipation and the development of high pressures within the interior of the colon. Fibre is believed to offer protection against the development of diverticulosis by increasing the bulk of the motions which, in turn, increases the diameter of the colon and thereby reduces the pressure inside it. The reasoning behind this is that the colon lining is thought to herniate outwards at weak spots in the wall, in response to a rise in pressure, as happens when the constipated patient finds it necessary to strain to pass a motion.

Pain due to spasm of the colon's muscular walls is treated symptomatically with an antispasmodic drug, such as mebeverine (Colofac). Antibiotics are prescribed for patients with pronounced abdominal tenderness and FEVER.

ALTERNATIVE THERAPIES

Natural medicine

The type of diet detailed above would be prescribed by most naturopaths.

Specific dietary supplements   Psyllium husks, 1–4 tsp or 3–12 capsules taken with water throughout the day.

Herbal medicine

To help relieve stubborn constipation, 1–2 cupfuls daily of an infusion of a pinch of each of the following herbs to a cup of water: anise, sage, camomile, vervain and basil.

Two foot and hand baths daily of the following ingredients to 2 litres) of water: a handful each of chicory leaves and roots, artichoke leaves, cabbage leaves, mallow flowers, thyme and violet, plus a large grated onion and a half-handful of camomile flowers.

Aromatherapy

For colicky abdominal pains: three drops of cinnamon essence on a little brown sugar, three times daily between meals. Supplement by rubbing the abdomen with olive oil enriched with essence of cinnamon (50g per litre).

Bach flower remedies

Homoeopathy

For abdominal pain and distension, with flatulence: *Lycopodium*. For nausea: *Ipecacuanha*.

Acupuncture

The inflammation of the diverticulitis may be helped by acupuncture.

Spiritual therapies

When condition is aggravated by inner tension, art, music, colour therapy; Aurasoma; electrocrystal therapy.

I/33 LARGE-BOWEL CANCER

Colorectal cancer (cancer of the colon and rectum) is, apart from lung cancer caused by smoking, the commonest cause of death from cancer in northern Europe, North America and Australasia. It is more prevalent in developed countries—environmental factors, especially diet, being most likely responsible. In particular, this disease seems to be encouraged by diets that are high in fats and low in fibre. High-fibre diets speed up the rate at which food and its breakdown products pass through the digestive system, so that any potential cancer-causing substances (carcinogens) are in contact with the lining membrane of the bowel for a shorter period of time than when the diet is low in fibre. In addition, the various components of the fibre may bind with (i.e. inactivate) any chemical carcinogens present and, by increasing the bulk of the food and motions as they form, dilute carcinogens as well.

There is also thought to be a direct link between the increased fat and animal-protein intake (particularly of beef) in the Western diet and the increased incidence of colonic cancer. It has been suggested that a high intake of beef and fat helps to establish in the large bowel colonies of bacteria capable of producing certain enzymes whose presence results in the increased metabolism of acids and sterol chemicals to carcinogens.

Studies are also being carried out to investigate possible mutagens (agents which can increase the rate of natural mutation in cells or organisms) in the motions which have been demonstrated in the faeces of people on high-beef diets, and may help to cause malignant change in the lining cells of the colon. A reduction in their ability to do so, and in the actual levels of nitrosamide (an example of such mutagens) in the motions, have been noted in patients taking large amounts of Vitamin C and alpha tocopherol (one of the Vitamin E chemicals).

Signs and symptoms of colorectal cancer depend upon the site within the bowel where the cancer occurs. Those occurring on the right-hand side of the abdomen (i.e. in the caecum and ascending colon) tend to produce OCCULT BLOOD in the motions, and rarely cause obstruction. Those on the left-hand side tend to cause DIARRHOEA or progressive though gradual CONSTIPATION, TENESMUS and smaller motions than usual, while those lower down in the rectum or anus are apt to produce pain, bright red blood when a motion is passed, and a change in bowel habits. General symptoms of malignant disease, such as weightloss, malaise and general debility are common. See Cancer (**XIII**).

I/34 PILES (HAEMORRHOIDS)

Piles are swollen painful veins around the anus. They are a type of VARICOSE VEIN, and can lie internally under the lining membrane of the rectum (*internal piles*) or lower down (*external piles*), where they are covered by the pain-sensitive membrane and skin of the anus.

The earliest symptom of piles is generally bleeding when motions are passed. Bright red blood is seen in the toilet water, 'on' although not actually mixed in with the motions themselves, and generally on the toilet paper as well. The anus is often itchy and uncomfortable, and great pain can result if the piles project downwards through the anal opening (*prolapsed piles*), where they get squeezed by the muscular anal ring contracting.

By the age of 50, 50 per cent of people in developed countries have piles, and numerous theories exist about why they occur. These include raised intra-abdominal pressure, as happens, for instance, in pregnancy and in chronic CONSTIPATION when straining is necessary in order to pass a motion. Other suggested causes are overweight, an hereditary predisposition to piles, the frequent lifting of heavy objects, insufficient exercise, and lack of dietary fibre.

ORTHODOX TREATMENT

Mild piles are treated symptomatically with a laxative such as Dorbanex (danthron plus poloxamer '188') to soften the motions, and a locally applied agent such as Lasonil (ointment containing heparinoid [50 units] and hyaluronidase [150 units] per gram).

Internal piles which prolapse or bleed can be ligated ('tied off' with a specially designed rubber band) or sclerosed (made to shrivel up by injecting the tissue immediately above them with 5 per cent phenol in oil). Neither of these procedures is painful, since they are not carried out on pain-sensitive external piles. When external piles thrombose—i.e. when a clot forms inside them—they can be cut out (excised) under local anaesthesia.

Severe piles can be removed surgically under general anaesthesia, and the remaining vessels tied off (haemorrhoidectomy). Piles can also be frozen (cryosurgery), or an 'anal stretch' operation can be performed under brief general anaesthesia to reduce the pressure on the varicosed veins and encourage them to heal.

ALTERNATIVE THERAPIES

Natural medicine

Hydrotherapy   Cold sitz baths.

Nutritional therapy   Wholefood diet, with emphasis upon fresh raw vegetables and fruit, wholemeal bread and pasta, brown rice, pulses, grains and nuts, and low in sugar, salt and animal fats. Coffee, chocolate and cocoa (as well as cola drinks) are reputed to aggravate the PRURITUS aspect of piles and are best avoided.

Specific dietary supplements   A high intake of bioflavonoids is recommended; e.g. lemon bioflavonoid complex plus rutin, up to 1,000mg per day, plus 1,000mg of Vitamin C daily. Three acidophilus capsules three times daily are likely to help relieve chronic constipation, as is additional bran—for example, one tablespoonful of unprocessed bran three times daily—but this ought not to be necessary on a wholefood diet.

Herbal medicine

Two hipbaths daily of a handful of each of the following in 2 litres of water: milk thistle leaves and roots, dog's tooth roots, and lavender flowers.

Especially to relieve itching, the anal area can be bathed with an infusion of a handful of chervil to one litre of water.

The following decoction relieves the pain and irritation of piles: Boil 30g of dried mullein leaves in 600ml of milk in a covered container for 10 minutes. Strain and flavour with honey if desired. Drink one wineglass three times daily.

Aromatherapy

Three drops of essence of cypress on a little brown sugar three times daily.

Homoeopathy

For bleeding, protruding and itching piles, *Calcarea Fluorata*. For the same when oozing dark blood, *Hamamelis*. For painful, protruding piles, *Ignatia*. For itching piles, *Nux Vomica*.

Acupuncture

Piles are said to be helped by acupuncture.

Exercise therapy

Dance therapy for the unfit. Yoga is reputed to help piles, in particular the asanas Fish, Plough, and Shoulder Stand.

Spiritual therapy

Electrocrystal therapy can speed healing of early piles, and of wounds after surgery.

II   Disorders of the Air Passages and Lungs

The respiratory tract consists of the route taken by the air which we breathe, in and out of the lungs, during the process of respiration.

The nose has right and left compartments separated by the sheet of bone and cartilage called the nasal septum. These two compartments meet behind the hard palate and form a single cavity, the nasal area of the pharynx (nasopharynx). Each nasal compartment has, as its outer wall, part of the skull bone called the maxilla which also forms the upper jaw. The floor of the nasal compartment is the palate; the roof is the underside of the skull. Three small ledges of bone (the conchae) protrude from the inner surface of the nasal septum into the nasal cavity. Tucked under the conchae are the openings into the sinuses.

The sinuses, spaces containing air and lined with mucous membrane, are situated inside the bones surrounding the nose. In addition to the sinuses, two other openings which deserve mention: (a) the Eustachian tube, which runs from the middle ear to the nasopharynx; and (b) the

Air Passages and Lungs

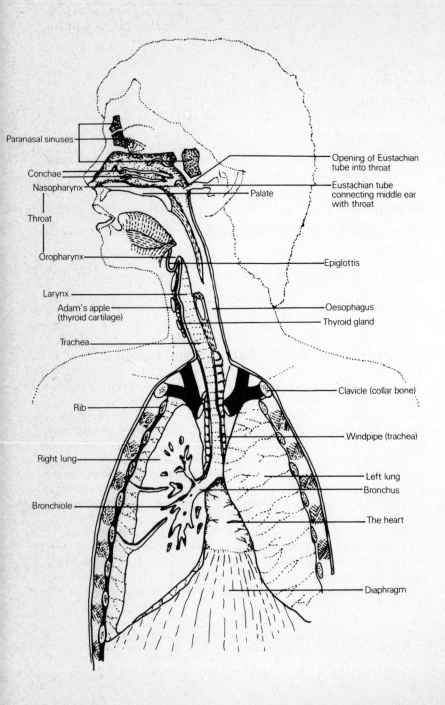

Paranasal sinuses

Conchae

Nasopharynx

Throat

Oropharynx

Larynx

Adam's apple (thyroid cartilage)

Trachea

Rib

Right lung

Bronchiole

Opening of Eustachian tube into throat

Eustachian tube connecting middle ear with throat

Palate

Epiglottis

Oesophagus

Thyroid gland

Clavicle (collar bone)

Windpipe (trachea)

Left lung

Bronchus

The heart

Diaphragm

nasolacrimal duct, which runs from the tear-forming glands in the eye to the nose.

The adenoids are situated at the back of the nasopharynx, and the tonsils are found between the pillars forming the arch of the palate. Both adenoids and tonsils are clumps of lymphoid tissue, and are involved in the defence against infection.

The pharynx proper runs from the back of the nasopharynx and the cavity of the mouth to the foodpipe (oesophagus) behind and the windpipe (trachea) in front. The voice box (larynx) is at the top of the windpipe. It is surrounded and supported by cartilage, which can be recognized in the front of the neck as the Adam's apple. The larynx contains the vocal cords and has a lid, the epiglottis, which closes off the passage through to the windpipe when swallowing occurs, to prevent saliva, liquids or food from entering the air passages.

The windpipe leads from the larynx down into the chest, where it divides above the heart into its two main subdivisions, the right and left bronchi—one to each lung. Horseshoe-shaped hoops of cartilage keep the windpipe open as air travels down it and up again during respiration.

The trachea and bronchi are lined by mucus membrane, which keeps them moist and helps to trap dust particles. The mucus is constantly swept upwards towards the larynx by tiny hair-like processes called cilia, but smokers lose this facility.

Within the lungs, the two bronchi divide into branches, three for the right lung and two for the left (the right lung has three lobes, the left only two). The branches divide further into smaller passages—segmental bronchi—10 on the right and 9 on the left. The segmental bronchi divide into smaller and smaller tubes, the narrowest and most prolific of which are the bronchioles. Each terminal bronchiole ends in a minute air sac (alveolus). The total expanse of alveolar membrane present throughout both lungs is referred to as the respiratory surface.

Respiration involves the exchange of gases at the respiratory surface, where oxygen in the air enters the bloodstream while carbon dioxide waste leaves. The oxygen is carried by the bloodstream to tissues throughout the body.

Air is drawn into the lungs (inspiration) by the diaphragm (a muscular sheet attached to the lumbar vertebrae and to the lower pairs of ribs) lowering itself by contracting, and the intercostal muscles (between the ribs) pulling the chest wall up and out. The net result of these two actions is to increase the size of the chest interior, so that atmospheric pressure forces air down into the empty space that results. Air is expelled from the chest (expiration) in a passive action: the muscles relax, and the elastic framework of the chest causes it to regain its original shape.

The act of breathing is largely a reflex one. The governing centre is the *respiratory centre* in the brain. This centre is controlled partly by the level of oxygen in the blood, but to a greater extent by the blood's acidity (pH), which is a reflection of the quantity of carbon dioxide dissolved in it. In fact, *any* acid in the blood (such as lactic acid that results from muscular activity) has the effect of stimulating the brains respiratory centre.

II/1 COMMON COLD AND INFLUENZA

These two disorders are being discussed here since, although neither of them is confined to the area of the nose, both often produce predominantly nasal symptoms. Together they are responsible for more lost working days throughout the world than any other disorder, including backache.

II/2 COMMON COLD

The common cold is a form of virus infection, and is especially liable to be spread in crowded conditions, because the cold virus is spread in moisture droplets sneezed and coughed into the atmosphere by infected people. Although we associate colds with cold wet weather, it seems that the link is that in cold weather we are more likely to be in crowded enclosed conditions—e.g. on public transport, in cinemas, or watching indoor sports, or working in centrally heated environments.

As with any viral infection, depression, chronic anxiety and stress predispose us to catching colds.

Common-cold symptoms include a prickling irritation of the nasal lining membrane, a shivery sensation, attacks of sneezing, and a 'running nose' requiring frequent blowing and wiping when the nasal discharge is clear and liquid. Sore THROATS and COUGHS are common accompaniments, and nasal stuffiness due to thick, yellow-green CATARRH often replaces the watery discharge. Mild colds last for a few days, more severe ones can last for two weeks or longer.

Therapies for common cold are treated under II/3.

II/3 INFLUENZA ('FLU)

Like the common cold (II/2), this is a form of viral infection. Passed on in a similar manner, it is best avoided by shunning crowded places as much as possible whenever bouts of infection are at large.

Influenza tends to make the sufferer feel iller than does a cold. A FEVER is more likely to be present, the malaise is greater, and aches and pains 'all over' are more severe. A COUGH, running nose or nasal congestion, a sore THROAT, ANOREXIA, and NAUSEA frequently figure, and post-'flu depression is well known.

Like the common cold, influenza predisposes the sufferer to bacterial infections by lowering his or her resistance. Because of these potential complications, influenza can have serious effects, especially upon the elderly, very young children, and individuals suffering from chronic heart or lung disease.

ORTHODOX TREATMENT

Antibiotics have no effect upon viral infections, and the majority of GPs do not prescribe them unless there is evidence of accompanying bacterial infection (or unless the patient is in a high-risk group, in which case they would be given for their protective action). Patients with a cold or 'flu are usually advised to keep warm, to rest in bed until feeling better, and to drink plenty of fluids. Aspirin is sometimes prescribed to treat the fever of 'flu or the muscular aches and pains. Throat lozenges and cough mixtures which suppress coughing or facilitate the bringing up of phlegm from the chest are also commonly prescribed.

Vaccines are produced frequently which provide a temporary immunity against known strains of influenza virus, but these offer no protection against the new strains which swiftly arise.

Doctors should be consulted about colds and 'flu that persist despite home remedies, or when signs of bacterial infection are present—e.g. a COUGH, often painful, which produces yellow and/or green phlegm; or a FEVER that persists for longer than three days.

ALTERNATIVE THERAPIES

Natural medicine

Advice would include bed-rest until symptoms began to clear, no food in solid form (or the Schroth cure), and plenty of liquids (water and fruit and vegetable juices). Hydrotherapy might be employed in the form of hot baths, followed by bed-rest under a thick duvet to help the body sweat out the accumulated toxins. Gargling with hot water relieves a painful throat; and steam inhalations and hot foot baths help.

Specific dietary supplements

- Vitamin C, 1g, three times daily. Vitamin A, 25,000iu, 1–3 times daily (take for five days and stop for two). Smaller doses for children: babies can suffer toxic side-effects if given more than 18,000iu of Vitamin A daily.
- Vitamin E, chewable, 400iu, 1–3 times daily.
- Acidophilus capsules, 3 capsules, three times daily.
- Zinc gluconate lozenges, which should be sucked and not swallowed or chewed, are effective in relieving colds. Treatment should start as soon as possible after symptoms appear. The recommended dose is: for adults and children weighing more than 27kg, one lozenge every two waking hours, not exceeding 9–12 lozenges daily; for children below 27kg, half a lozenge every two waking hours, not exceeding 6 daily. The treatment should be carried out for a maximum of 7 days.
- Propolis: coughs often respond to a propolis lozenge sucked as often as needed.
- Pollen has been shown to offer effective protection against colds and 'flu.
- Honey helps to relieve cold and 'flu symptoms. For a sore throat, mix 2 tbsp honey with the same amount of glycerine, 1 tbsp fresh lemon juice and a little ginger (either powdered, or the fresh root grated). Add a little whisky if you like. Warm the mixture and take a little whenever required.[40] Also, cold and 'flu symptoms may be relieved by drinking a mixture of two tsp of honey in a cup of warm water to which two tsp of organic cider vinegar have been added. A single teaspoon of warm honey will sometimes stop a cough effectively, especially at night.

Biochemic tissue salts   For symptoms of feverishness and sneezing that herald the onset of a cold or 'flu: *Ferr. Phos*. For a running nose and watery discharge: *Nat. Mur*. For white phlegm, stuffiness, congestion and a sore throat: *Kali. Mur*. alternated with *Ferr. Phos*.

Ionization therapy

An air ionizer can help to relieve a stuffy nose and catarrh.

Herbal medicine

A gargle made from red sage, steeped in hot water and used 3–4 times daily, relieves the inflammation of sore throats. For a heavy, chesty cough an infusion of ½tsp each of white horehound and marshmallow, left to stand for 10 minutes. Less serious coughs can be aided by taking a little of the following several times daily: finely sliced garlic added to 3–4tsp honey.[41]

For cold symptoms in general, hot elderflower tea, made by putting 1tsp of the flowers, fresh or dried, in a cup, adding boiling water, allowing to steep for 20 minutes or longer, and then straining. Add honey if you wish, and drink before going to bed.

Another long-established remedy mingles herbal medicine and hydrotherapy: a mustard foot bath. Its effectiveness is believed to be due to the antibiotic constituents of mustard, which enter the bloodstream through the surface blood-vessels of the feet. A tablespoon of dry mustard powder is placed in a bucket (the same quantity of kitchen soda should be added if the water is hard). The feet are placed in the bucket, and hot water added until it comes halfway up the lower legs. The feet are left immersed for 10–15 minutes—top up with fresh hot water when necessary. The feet are then dried and kept warm in bed or by wearing long slipper-socks.

Aromatherapy

An inhalation for stuffy nose and head colds: to 1 litre of boiling water add three soupspoonsful of the following alcohol preparation—1 litre of 90° alcohol, 30g essence of eucalyptus, 14g essence of thyme, 14g essence of pine needles, 10g essence of lemon and 10g essence of lavender.

For coughs: four drops of lavender essence on a little brown sugar half an hour before each meal.

Homoeopathy

For a head cold with watering eyes and streaming nose: *Euphrasia*. For head colds with a thick yellow-green discharge: *Eucalyptus*.

Manipulative therapy

Reflexology   Useful when the sinuses are infected. See Sinusitis (II/8).

Relaxation methods

Yoga is said to benefit people who suffer from recurrent colds. The Lion posture stimulates the circulation to the throat and tongue, and helps to relieve a sore throat. The Shoulder Stand encourages blocked sinuses to drain. Since people are more susceptible to infection by cold and 'flu viruses when stressed and anxious, positive relaxation—e.g. antogenics and biofeedback—would also be likely to help.

II/4 HAY FEVER

The term is a misnomer, since FEVER is not one of the symptoms of this disorder, and neither is it caused by hay! It is an ALLERGY to pollen and affects about 15 per cent of the population in the UK at some time in their lives; it is commoner in certain ethnic groups—e.g. West Indians —and in people with a personal or family history of allergic eczema or asthma. Symptoms include irritation of the nasal lining, with attacks of sneezing and a watery nasal discharge, followed by a blocked-up nose; red, watery eyes; and sometimes irritation inside the ears and over the roof of the mouth. They are most likely to start during the teens and 20s. City dwellers can be as badly affected as country dwellers, since pollen is windborne.

Hay-fever symptoms caused by tree-pollen allergy are the earliest to appear in any given calendar year, starting in February (alder, hazel) or slightly later, in March and April (birch). Symptoms due to grass pollen are produced between May and July; and attacks due to seasonal moulds affect sufferers in late summer or early autumn (all of these months are for the UK).[42] The severity of the symptoms varies from year to year, and is related to the pollen count.

ORTHODOX TREATMENT

This aims largely at suppressing the symptoms, and falls into two main classes: treatments applied locally to the affected membranes, and general (systemic) treatments applied to the patient as a whole.

Local treatment includes steroid sprays for mainly nasal symptoms (e.g. beclomethasone [Beconase] and flunisolide [Syntaris]). Possible side-effects include degeneration of the nasal membrane lining, with drying, crusting and bleeding; and candida infection (see THRUSH). Sodium cromoglycate (e.g. Rhynacrom) is likewise used locally. It is most effective for eye symptoms, and is used to prevent the onset of symptoms—it has little effect on them once they have started. Nasal decongestants like ephedrine can be bought from chemists; they are probably best avoided because they can be addictive.

Systemic treatments include antihistamines, such as the long-established chlorpheniramine (Piriton), which causes severe drowsiness in many users; and newer compounds such as terfenadine (Triludan) and astemizole (Hismanal), which are longer-acting and cause very little drowsiness. Steroids used systemically are a last resort and should be taken for short periods only; e.g. before an examination period.

Desensitization is favoured by many doctors, but should be used only for patients with severe symptoms due to isolated grass-pollen allergy found on skin test. The chief argument against it is that it can cause shock and collapse (in fact, it is potentially lethal) in highly sensitive individuals. Doctors are advised always to have resuscitation facilities available and to see that patients rest in the surgery under observation for half an hour after the injection.

ALTERNATIVE THERAPIES

Holistic therapists and orthodox doctors agree that the phenomenon of ALLERGY is a sign of a fault in the body's homoeostatic mechanism. Clinical ecologists[43] point to environmental pollution as the underlying causative factor in allergy generally. They maintain that unremitting bombardment of especially sensitive individuals by toxic material present in the atmosphere, water and particularly in food (chemical additives) disturbs that person's equilibrium. The result is that his or her immune defence system acts faultily, developing unnecessary antibodies to non-toxic environmental factors such as pollen (in the case of hay fever), house dust, cat fur and dog hair.

Nevertheless, the essential fault lies within the individual's homoeostatic mechanism: this is why, while a minority of us react badly to recognized allergens such as pollen, the majority of us remain unaffected.

Natural medicine

An acute attack may be treated with a fruit juice fast (2–3 days).

Naturopathic doctors, when encountering hay fever (and other allergic conditions) turn their attention to the underlying fault, and recommend restabilization of the patient's homoeostasis in a number of ways.

The well known naturopathic doctor Leon Chaitow suggests employing as many alternative therapies as are appropriate to a particular individual. In particular, he stresses the value of a strictly wholefood diet, relaxation methods, the reduction of stress and 'osteopathic normalization of spinal and cranial structures, etc.'[43]

Specific dietary supplements   High doses of Vitamin-B complex plus extra calcium pantothenate (100mg daily) and pyridoxine (Vitamin B_6)—100mg daily for badly affected people. Vitamin C, 500mg every six hours, is helpful because of its antihistamine effect. Vitamin E (300iu), chewable type, and bioflavonoids (200mg daily) may bring relief to some sufferers.

Pollen, as capsules, is also claimed to be helpful.

Biochemic tissue salts   Severe, acute attacks with congested membranes: *Ferr. Phos.* Copious thin watery discharge, sneezing, watery eye discharge: *Nat. Mur.* alternating with *Ferr. Phos.* Advanced stage with a discharge of white catarrh: *Kali Mur.*

Ionization therapy

This should give relief.

Herbal medicine

For the underlying allergy: an infusion of a pinch of each of the following to two cups of water—thyme, basil, rosemary, anise and vervain. Take a cup twice daily. To relieve cattarrh: an infusion of two pinches of wild thyme and two of garden thyme to 1 litre of water—3–4 cups daily, hot.

Aromatherapy

For inflammation of the nasal lining: an inhalation of niaouli (*Melaleuca viridiflora*) made according to the formula 1 litre of 80° alcohol, 10ml of essence of eucalyptus, 40ml essence of lavender, and 50ml essence of niaouli. You can also rub it on your chest.

Homoeopathy

Mixed pollen (potentized) is very useful in late summer attacks. To relieve streaming eyes and nose: *Sabadilla*. Much itching of eyes and nose, runny sore nose: *Allium cepa*.

Acupuncture

This is said to offer great benefit to hay-fever sufferers.

Reflexology

Foot massage aimed at stimulating the adrenals, ovaries, uterus, testes and prostate gland. Also, work applied to the reflexes of the organs manifesting hay-fever symptoms—e.g. for itching and aching eyes, on the eye reflexes; for an inflamed throat, on the throat reflex.

Manipulation

Osteopathy, cranial osteopathy, applied kinesiology.

Relaxation methods

Yoga, positive relaxation, autosuggestion, dance therapy.

Psychotherapy

Hypnotherapy.

II/5 PHARYNGITIS

INFLAMMATION of the pharynx, a common cause of a sore throat. This may be due to a virus (and often accompanies a head cold), or to bacterial infection, for instance when associated with tonsillitis. It can also be produced by irritation when excessive amounts of mucus are produced in the nasal cavity, due to infection or allergy, and pass down via the nasopharynx into the pharynx proper.

Inflammation of the pharynx can be due also to smoking cigarettes, sniffing glue or cocaine, irritation from a chemically polluted atmosphere, temporary reduction in the amount of saliva produced (e.g. in response to the drug propantheline [Probanthine] sometimes given for peptic ulceration), or to the nervous habit of frequently clearing the throat. If you suffer from a sore throat, either with or without difficulty in swallowing, that persists for no apparent reason for more than a few days, you should seek professional advice and a thorough examination.

ORTHODOX TREATMENT

Any treatment for pharyngitis, orthodox or alternative, depends on the cause. When an irritant is responsible, the best solution is removal of the source of irritation. Accompanying infections such as tonsillitis (II/6) or a head cold (II/2) might also require treatment. Relief can be gained by gargling with soluble aspirin; bacterial infections are usually treated with antibiotics. Antiseptic throat lozenges, some with an added local anaesthetic agent (e.g. Tyrozets), are common remedies.

ALTERNATIVE THERAPIES

See under Tonsillitis (II/6).

II/6 TONSILLITIS

Infected tonsils are a common cause of a sore throat, particularly in children. Small children, however, frequently complain of 'tummy-ache' rather than a sore throat, even when their tonsils are highly inflamed; other symptoms can include poor appetite, sometimes VOMITING, FEVER and enlarged lymph nodes in the neck. Streptococcal bacteria are the commonest cause of tonsillitis, and can make the patient feel very ill, with a high fever and very painful throat.

ORTHODOX TREATMENT

Antibiotics are an important form of treatment in a bad attack of tonsillitis, since streptococcal infections can lead to complications such as scarlet fever, rheumatic fever and kidney damage. Penicillin is usually given. A tonsillectomy is sometimes performed on patients who suffer several bad attacks every year. Throat lozenges and gargles are often prescribed or bought over the counter.

ALTERNATIVE THERAPIES

Natural medicine

This can be helpful in dealing with repeated attacks of tonsillitis, underlying nasal infection or ALLERGY, and the accompanying pharyngitis. A fruit juice fast (2–3 days) would help an acute attack.

Useful forms of hydrotherapy include gargling with hot water and mustard foot-baths for their antibiotic properties (see Common cold [II/2].

Nutritional advice for an acutely sore throat would suggest a fluid diet, including freshly squeezed vegetable and fruit juices and pure water, in the early stages, with little solid food. Fruit jellies and icecream made from wholefood ingredients (free from additives) would be useful as symptoms start to clear.

For a diet and lifestyle aimed at preventing repeated attacks of tonsillitis, a naturopathic doctor should be consulted. Good general advice is to follow a wholefood diet as described and to include plenty of naturally occurring Vitamin C, present in citrus fruit, berries, green leafy vegetables, tomatoes, cauliflower, potatoes and sweet potatoes. Effort should also be made to counter unavoidable stress by learning relaxation techniques.

Specific dietary supplements   Vitamin A, 10–20,000iu (less for children), 1–3 times daily for five days, then stop for two days; more than 18,500iu daily can cause toxic effects in babies, including rashes, nausea, vomiting and diarrhoea. Extra Vitamin-C complex, 1g morning and evening for an adult, 500mg three times daily for a child. Vitamin E, 400iu (as chewable tablets), 1–3 times daily for an adult, half this for a child. One or two dessertspoonsful of wheatgerm can be taken daily by children and adults in addition. Three acidophilus capsules, three times daily. Children who cannot take (or dislike taking) capsules, can have the contents added to cold drinks or can be encouraged to eat live fresh yoghourt.

Garlic can be usefully added to food, and garlic lozenges can be used for a few hours daily when infection is most likely to strike. Additional supplements include zinc and selenium: zinc orotate, 100mg daily for an adult (15–30mg for children), selenium 200mcg daily for an adult, 100mcg daily for a child.

Honey relieves the pain of tonsillitis: two tbsp mixed with same quantity of glycerine and a squeeze of lemon juice, warmed and sipped slowly.

Biochemic tissue salts   For tonsillitis, in the early stages, with a fever: *Ferr. Phos.* For chronic enlargement of tonsils, glands swollen and painful: *Calc. Phos.* For constant flow of clear saliva, swollen uvula: *Nat. Mur.* For suppurating tonsils or QUINSY: *Silicea.* Dose: four tablets hourly in the early stages of acute attacks, then two hourly.

Ionization therapy

This helps to relieve congestion of throat and nose.

Herbal medicine

Self-treatment remedies include red sage tea, which can be drunk and used as a gargle. Similar teas and gargles can be made with the following herbs: fenugreek, horehound and marshmallow. Honey helps to soothe a sore throat if added to the tea. Hoarseness is also said to be relieved by a syrup containing grated horseradish root, water and honey.

The following is recommended by Maurice Messegué as a preventative measure against tonsillitis: an infusion of two pinches of thyme in a cup of water, taken nightly.

Aloe vera juice, or the gel added to water, can help to relieve the pain and inflammation both of tonsillitis and of sore throats due to other causes. For tonsillitis: four or five drops of tincture of propolis on a lump of sugar three times daily, or one propolis lozenge to be sucked slowly three or four times daily. Propolis can also be used as a gargle: 4–5 drops of tincture of propolis is in half a glass of warm water, used several times daily when required.

Aromatherapy

To relieve a sore throat: four drops of savory essence on a little brown sugar after every meal. Also, frequent gargling with the following when lukewarm: half a coffeespoonful of 80° alcohol and 6 per cent essence of savory added to 100ml of hot distilled water.

Homoeopathy

When the sore throat follows exposure to dry winds: *Aconite*. When it is dry and burning: *Arsenicum Album*. When saliva is excessive: *Mercurius*.

Acupuncture

Tonsillitis, and pharyngitis arising from other causes, are claimed to respond to acupuncture.

II/7 ADENOIDS

Like the tonsils, adenoids swell in response to infection: this causes the patient—nearly always a child—to breathe almost exclusively through his or her mouth and to snore. Swollen adenoids are most likely to affect children between the ages of five and seven; later the condition gradually disappears.

ORTHODOX TREATMENT

Persistently troublesome adenoids are very occasionally removed, together with the tonsils when necessary.

ALTERNATIVE THERAPIES

Because the adenoids closely resemble the tonsils in structure and function, naturopathic treatment, nutritional therapy, specific dietary supplements and ionization therapy appropriate for tonsillitis are useful also for treating enlarged adenoids. The herbal remedies for tonsillitis (apart from gargles) and for Sinusitis (II/8) may also help reduce the swelling of enlarged adenoids.

II/8 SINUSITIS

Infection inside the nose sometimes spreads into the paranasal sinuses, and the sinuses' lining membrane becomes inflamed; sometimes the connecting channel running between a particular sinus (or several sinuses) and the nasal cavity becomes blocked. Head colds (II/2) and hay fever (II/4) are common causes. Symptoms of sinusitis can include HEADACHE, and FEVER due to the infection. Pain and tenderness over the inflamed sinus are due to the process of INFLAMMATION itself, and to the rising pressure inside the blocked sinus. The retained fluid and pus inside the sinuses usually show up on X-ray.

ORTHODOX TREATMENT

Antibiotics and steam inhalations are usually given for infected sinuses. Fluid retained within the sinuses is often drained surgically, and the sinus washed out.

ALTERNATIVE THERAPIES

Natural medicine

The acute attack would be treated by 2–3 days of fruit-juice fasting; and hydrotherapy in the form of steam inhalations. The recommended diet would be wholefood, excluding any items which might be responsible for an allergic reaction of the nasal and sinus linings. Food allergies may be investigated and possibly put right by means of applied kinesiology. Severe catarrh may be treated by the Schroth cure (see page 433).

Specific dietary supplements Mineral imbalance is capable of causing allergic puffiness of the nasal and sinus lining membrane. As well as the usual recommended supplementary programme, the following may well help:

- Vitamin C, 1g twice daily
- Vitamin E (chewable), 200iu twice daily
- Vitamin A, 10–20,000iu three times daily for five days, then cease for two days; repeat course if required
- Vitamin B$_6$, 50mg daily
- Zinc, 10–15mg three times daily
- Selenium, 200mcg daily

Biochemic tissue salts At the begininning of an attack of sinusitis, with fever, pain in the sinus area and congestion: *Ferr. Phos.* For nasal obstruction with watery discharge, loss of sense of smell, painful inflammation of infected sinus worsened by contact with cold air: *Nat. Mur.* For the chronic condition, with a thick, offensive discharge and chronic nasal catarrh: *Silicea.*

Ionization therapy

This can be helpful.

Herbal medicine

A herbal tea made from a tsp of each of the following to a cup of boiling water: horehound, mullein, eucalyptus, coltsfoot leaves and wild cherry bark. Honey can be added to improve the flavour.

Aromatherapy

An inhalation made up as follows: to one litre of boiling water add 3 soupspoonsful of this alcohol preparation—a litre of 90° alcohol, 30g essence of eucalyptus, 14g essence of thyme, 14g essence of pine needles, 10g essence of lemon, 10g essence of lavender.

Homoeopathy

For sinusitis producing catarrh and a stringy discharge: *Kali Bichromicum* For tearing pain in head, from root of nose to forehead, with nausea: *Natrum Muriaticum*. Pain beginning at the back of the head and settling over the eyes: *Silicea.*

Acupuncture

Sinusitis may respond to acupuncture.

Reflexology

This is said to aid sinusitis, the particular areas requiring massage including the big toe and the balls of all the other toes, the reflex of the ileocaecal valve, and the reflexes of the intestine if there are accompanying digestive problems.

II/9 LARYNGITIS AND CROUP

The voicebox (larynx) and the vocal cords inside it can become inflamed as a result of irritation or infection, or following a period in which the voice has been overused in some way. The inner lining becomes congested, and more mucus than usual is produced. Irritants capable of causing an inflamed larynx include noxious grasses and tobacco smoking (active or passive).

Infective laryngitis is usually caused by a virus, and can occur either alone, or together with a cold (II/2), influenza (II/3), pharyngitis (II/5) or tonsillitis (II/6). Symptoms include a weak, hoarse voice which sometimes disappears altogether, and often an irritating COUGH that fails to bring up phlegm. Speaking and coughing are painful, and often the throat is sore, although no discomfort other than hoarseness may be experienced. The symptoms are made worse by use of the voice, contact with cigarette smoke, other atmospheric pollution, and the excessively dry, warm indoor conditions resulting from an overactive central-heating system.

Croup is the name given to laryngitis in infants and small children. They have, besides a tiring cough, breathing which becomes partially obstructed by SPASM and mucous secretions and takes on a characteristic rasping quality. The chief danger is that the lining of the larynx may swell up enough to cause total obstruction of the air passage. For this reason, and because there is an accompanying fever and often vomiting and feeding problems, many croupy babies and toddlers are admitted to hospital for careful nursing during the acute stage of the illness. Signs to watch for are failure for the symptoms to resolve, a worsening cough and breathing noise, pallor and 'blueness' (cyanosis). It is important that even mild cases of croup are seen by a medical practitioner.

ORTHODOX TREATMENT

Immediate measures in dealing with croup (e.g. while waiting for the doctor's arrival) are to remain calm and reassuring to the child, who often panics when he or she experiences breathing difficulties.

A source of steam in the child's room will provide some moisture, which is most effective in aiding the swollen mucous membranes inside the larynx to return to normal. Once in hospital, he or she will be given moisturized oxygen, or placed in a steam cubicle.

Adults with laryngitis should rest their voices totally until the symptoms have subsided. Bed-rest is indicated if the patient feels particularly unwell; doctors may prescribe an antibiotic in the event that a bacterial infection is present, but the cause of the infection is most likely to be a virus. Similarly, croup is rarely treated with an antibiotic.

ALTERNATIVE THERAPIES

Natural medicine

Hydrotherapy would be used to provide steam, as mentioned above, as an inhalation. Hot-water gargling would also help a sore throat.

Dietary advice would be as appropriate for the underlying condition. If no infective cause is present, then a wholefood diet with emphasis of fresh raw fruit and vegetables. Smoking would of course be forbidden, and the patient would be advised to avoid polluted, overcrowded atmospheres and to rest the voice.

Applying a very cold compress around the child's throat, changing it as soon as it grows warm, is claimed to be most helpful in relieving the acute stage of croup.

Specific dietary supplements   As for pharyngitis (II/5) and tonsillitis (II/6). Also: cider vinegar, one tsp to half a glass of warm water every hour for seven hours. A little honey improves the taste if the patient has a sweet tooth, and is beneficial in its own right.

Biochemic tissue salts   For the painful hoarseness of laryngitis due to overuse of the voice, or from catching cold: *Ferr. Phos.* For loss of voice from a cold, a croupy cough which brings up thick, white phlegm: *Kali Mur.* Hoarseness after nervous strain and fatigue: *Kali phos.* Chronic hoarseness after excessive talking, accompanied by having constantly to clear the throat: *Calc. Phos.* (Dose: four tablets every hour while condition is acute, and less frequently as condition improves.)

For croup: The main remedy for croup, to control the swollen lining membrane and the acute coughing attacks: *Kali. Mur.* This ought to be given in alternation with *Ferrum Phos.*, which is used to treat the fever and the shortness of breath. For the spasmodic closing of the throat, and a suffocating cough: *Magnesia Phos.* (Dose for children: three tablets every 15 minutes, less frequently when breathing becomes easier.)

Ionization therapy

This can be helpful.

Herbal medicine

As for pharyngitis (II/5) and tonsillitis (II/6), and for common cold (II/2) and influenza (II/3) if accompanying laryngitis.

For the hoarseness aspect of laryngitis: a gargle of a decoction of these ingredients (one handful of each): cabbage leaves, lavender, mallow and violet to one litre of water. At the same time, drink an infusion of one pinch of each of wold thyme, anise and agrimony.

Aromatherapy

As for pharyngitis (II/5) and tonsillitis (II/6). Also for loss of the voice: 3 drops of essence of cypress on a little brown sugar three times daily. Also for chronic laryngitis, arising from frequent overuse of voice: inhalation of lukewarm essence of cajeput.

Homoeopathy

As for pharyngitis (II/5) and tonsillitis (II/6). Also, for loss of voice due to laryngitis: *Phosphorus.* For a very hoarse voice: *Carbo Vegetabilis* For laryngitis due to overuse of voice: *Kali Phosphoricum*

Acupuncture

As for common cold (II/2) or tonsillitis (II/6).

Manipulative therapy

Reflexology   Can be used for common cold if present. To strengthen vocal cords weakened by misuse of voice or an attack of laryngitis:

massage applied to the big toe and the portion nearest the second toe; also the throat reflexes; the patient himself or herself can massage the sides of his or her nose.

II/10 LARYNGEAL TUMOURS

These can be benign or malignant, the cancerous type being especially common in smokers. Any growth in this area will produce a number of characteristic symptoms and signs, and untreated malignant growths will cause progressive illness of a more serious kind (see **XIII**), as well as spreading to nearby lymph glands and other structures. The symptoms include increasing hoarseness, throat irritation, and a spasmodic cough producing a little clear phlegm.

The only satisfactory orthodox method of managing laryngeal tumours, benign or malignant, is to remove them surgically.

II/11 TRACHEITIS AND ACUTE BRONCHITIS

Tracheitis means INFLAMMATION of the windpipe or trachea, and bronchitis means inflammation of the bronchi, the tubes into which the windpipe leads.

Tracheitis can occur as a separate disorder, but it is more commonly found together with *acute* bronchitis. The two disorders are most often caused by pus-producing bacteria such as *Streptococcus pyogenes* or *Haemophilus influenzae*, following in the wake of a bad cold, an attack of influenza, or an infectious illness such as measles or whooping cough. This is because the viruses in each case predispose to later infection of the respiratory tract by bacteria. Attacks of acute bronchitis also commonly occur in patients suffering from chronic bronchitis (see **II/12**).

The inflammation spreads down the trachea into the two main bronchi and thence into their smaller subdivisions. Symptoms normally start with a hard, dry, painful COUGH, aching muscles, a mild FEVER, and often a sensation of tightness in the chest. The patient may be breathless and wheezy. After a day or two, the dry cough starts to be productive, and the PHLEGM is thick, colourless, difficult to shift and sometimes blood-streaked. Phlegm is soon produced in increasing amounts, and pus is apparent by its greenish-yellow colour. Most patients recover within 4–8 days, but occasionally the infection spreads further into the smaller airspaces, producing bronchiolitis (inflamed

216

bronchioles) and pneumonia (see II/14). This is most likely to occur in elderly, debilitated patients and very young ones.

Treatments for these conditions are discussed under II/13.

II/12 CHRONIC BRONCHITIS

This is in many ways a different disorder from acute bronchitis, and is the result of repeated irritation of the bronchi and their immediate subdivisions by pollutants. By far the worst offender is tobacco smoke, but other important ones include other types of smoke, industrial atmospheric pollution, dust and fumes. Symptoms of chronic bronchitis tend to be worst on waking in the morning, and include a persistent cough, tightness in the chest, wheezy breathing and breathlessness. There may be a great deal of phlegm or scarcely any, and its usual colour is white or greyish, sometimes with a few streaks of blood.

ORTHODOX TREATMENT

Acute bronchitis is treated with bed-rest in a warm room, inhalations to help loosen the phlegm, cough linctus to suppress night-time coughing, and antibiotics. If there are signs that the inflamed air-ways are constricted, a bronchodilator drug might also be given (see Bronchial asthma, II/15).

Chronic bronchitis may be treated in hospital when an acute attack develops. Treatment is likely to include supplementary oxygen, antibiotics, bronchiodilators, steroids and physiotherapy. Patients are encouraged to be up and about again as soon as possible, and also to try to elminate from their lifestyle any irritants to their condition. This applies especially to smoking.

Alternative treatments are discussed under II/13.

Inflammation of the bronchioles, the smallest branches of the bronchi, is known as 'bronchiolitis'. This, like croup (see II/9), is frequently due to a viral infection, and both are potentially life-threatening disorders in newborn and very frail babies. Bronchiolitis and bronchopneumonia (see II/14) in adults with chronic lung disease (such as chronic bronchitis or emphysema—see II/13) need careful hospital management.

Treatment for bronchiolitis is likely to include humidified air, oxygen, fluids as required, and antibiotics for additional bacterial infections. Severe croup and bronchiolitis are also treated on occasion with steroid drugs and with non-steroidal anti-inflammatory compounds.

'Emphysema' means an abnormal 'inflation' of body tissues with air. The type affecting lung-tissue is known as pulmonary emphysema, the underlying structural change being enlargement of the smallest air pockets, the alveoli. This results when the walls between adjoining alveoli break down and one or more alveoli merge together. The total amount of respiratory surface where gaseous exchange can take place is diminished by this breakdown process, and respiration is thus adversely affected.

Emphysema is commonly associated with chronic bronchitis (see II/12), and can also follow severe whooping cough (see XII/4) and other disorders affecting the lungs. The emphysematous patient is typically breathless, at first on exertion and then also when at rest.

It seems that some cases of pulmonary emphysema are associated with the congenital lack of any enzyme called alpha-one-antitrypsin. The job of this enzyme, present in most people, is to neutralize a second enzyme (trypsin) which breaks down protein. Trypsin released into the lungs from white blood cells during the process of inflammation, and when its action is unopposed by alpha-one-antitrypsin it attacks the protein walls of the alveoli and causes them to break down.

The chronic lung inflammation caused by tobacco smoke can bring on signs of emphysema in enzyme-deficient patients, or emphysema due to it can arise in middle age without years of chronic bronchitis having preceded it.

The lung damage of emphysema is not capable of repair by orthodox methods, and general measures of treatment include treatment of accompanying bronchitis and general advice about health.

ALTERNATIVE THERAPIES

Natural medicine

Advice for patients with acute infections (tracheitis, acute bronchitis, bronchiolitis) would include bed-rest; fluids and small quantities of wholefood if required; and steam inhalations to facilitate the coughing-up of phlegm when the chest is tight. Foot baths of hot water and mustard (see under Common cold, II/2) might be used for early cases of infection because of the antibiotic properties of the mustard.

The approach to patients with chronic bronchitis and emphysema would include a detailed scrutiny of lifestyle to try to eliminate chronic irritants of the underlying condition. Above all, patients would be advised not to smoke, and to learn and practise a method of relaxation, after identifying their own personal stress factors and tension points. Changes of work and/or living environment to avoid pollution would also possibly be suggested, although this is very often impossible.

Specific dietary supplements   For inflammation of the respiratory tubes:

- Vitamin A, 25,000iu, 1–3 times daily for five days, then stop for two days.
- Rose-hip Vitamin C, 1,000mg, morning and afternoon.
- Vitamin E, chewable, 400iu, 1–3 times daily.
- 3 acidophilus capsules, 3 times daily.
- Propolis—persistent, painful coughing can be eased by sucking a propolis lozenge as often as required. Propolis may also accelerate healing in the lining of the bronchi and smaller tubes, since there is evidence that it has this effect in the upper respiratory tract.
- Honey—an obstinate cough can be helped by equal quantities of honey, linseed oil and whisky. Dose: one tbsp, 3–4 times daily.

Biochemic Tissue Salts   For inflammation, fever and congestion: *Ferrum Phos*. This should be given in frequent doses to start off with when the cough is producing little phlegm, and then alternated with whatever remedy is indicated by the nature of the phlegm when it is eventually produced. For example:

- For thick, white, sticky phlegm: *Kali Mur.*
- For yellow, watery and copious, or greenish, slimy yellow phlegm: *Kali Sulph.*
- For thick, heavy and yellow phlegm: *Silicea.*

Dose: two tablets for children and four for adults every half-hour, less frequently when condition improves and fever lessens.

Ionization therapy

This would be likely to make breathing easier, especially at night when the cough is often worse.

Herbal medicine

To relieve bronchitis, an infusion of one pinch each of sage, thyme and nettles to a litre of water: 2–3 cupfuls to be drunk daily. An inhalation to aid bronchitis and tracheitis: a hot concentrated concoction of two handfuls of elecampane root to one litre of water.

Aromatherapy

For acute bronchitis and tracheitis: inhale the essence of cajeput, and take 5 drops of it on brown sugar three times daily.

For chronic bronchitis: on retiring, rub chest with the following cream: 1kg sweet almond oil, 250g white wax, 750g distilled water and 25g hyssop. Also the following gargle: one coffeespoon of alcohol preparation (90° alcohol with 5 per cent essence of hyssop) in 100ml boiled water, used lukewarm.

For emphysema: 3 drops of essence of garden thyme on a little brown sugar half an hour before every meal.

Homoeopathy

For bronchitis, when there is a rattling of mucus in the bronchial tubes: *Ipecacuanha*. When bronchitis is accompanied by hoarseness or loss of voice: *Phosphorus*. For breathing difficulty associated with a dry throat and chesty cough: *Bryonia*.

Acupuncture

Recent Chinese work has shown that about 50 per cent of patients with bronchitis are helped by acupuncture. The treatment has to be repeated regularly in order to maintain improvement.

Reflexology

Shortness of breath is said to be helped by reflexology done on the balls of the feet under the third and fourth toes. For emphysema: reflexes to the bronchial tubes, lungs, sinuses, adrenals, ileocaecal valve and coccyx.

Relaxation methods

Biofeedback and autogenics. Also, yoga is claimed to aid both bronchitis and emphysema. Besides the more general benefits of improved breathing techniques and stress control, specific postures are beneficial to both disorders. For bronchitis: the Mountain, the Shoulder Stand (drains out secretions), Fish and Locust. For emphysema: Complete Breath, Locust, Grip, Shoulder Stand.

Other possibly helpful relaxation techniques include meditation and positive relaxation.

Exercise therapy

For chronic cases, dance therapy.

II/14 PNEUMONIA

Pneumonia is consolidation of areas of lung tissue due to infection or chemical irritation. This occurs when the airsacs (alveoli) in the affected area(s) become filled with fluid and blood cells which leak into them during the inflammatory process. The membrane covering the lung often becomes inflamed as well, producing PLEURISY.

Two chief types of pneumonia exist: lobar pneumonia and bronchopneumonia. The first is confined to one lung, or to one lung lobe. The second, instead of being confined to a specific area, produces small areas of consolidation throughout the lung substance. Bronchopneumonia sometimes follows a bad bout of influenza (see II/3), and is the type of lung infection from which very frail, elderly or seriously sick people die.

Symptoms of the two types of pneumonia include pain when pleurisy is present; a cough; breathlessness; fever; and phlegm which may contain streaks of blood. Lobar pneumonia tends to produce more severe symptoms, and to begin suddenly. In children, the onset may be accompanied by vomiting or convulsions.

Aspiration pneumonia is a further variety. It results from an inhaled irritant—e.g. vomit—following a head injury.

ORTHODOX TREATMENT

This includes bed-rest, supplementary oxygen if required, pain relief if pleurisy is present, and antibiotics for bacterial pneumonias. (See also Tuberculosis, XII/8.)

ALTERNATIVE THERAPIES

Natural medicine

Naturopathic doctors would recommend bed-rest, additional oxygen for cyanosed patients, a fluid diet, warmth, and possibly steam inhalations to ease painful cough.

Raw juices especially recommended for the treatment of pleurisy: carrot 230g, celery 170g, parsley 55g.

Specific dietary supplements   Those recommended for inflammation of the respiratory tubes may help the recovery of inflamed areas of lung in pneumonia (see under II/13).

Biochemic tissue salts   In the early stages of the illness: *Ferrum Phos*. For thick white phlegm: *Kali Mur*. For hot dry skin, to promote perspiration, and for wheezing, rattling in the chest, with coughing-up of loose phlegm: *Kali Sulph*. For lung inflammation with clear frothy phlegm: *Natrum Mur*.
   Dose: two tablets for children and four for adults every half-hour, less frequently as condition begins to improve.

Ionization therapy

Can be used to promote easier breathing.

Herbal medicine

An elecampane infusion to inhale see under II/13. For pleurisy: a poultice of a mixture of fried white cabbage leaves, finely chopped leeks and a tumbler of vinegar.

Aromatherapy

For pneumonia: 5–6 drops of essential oil of Scots pine on a little brown sugar after each meal. Also, this inhalation: pour one coffeespoonful of the following preparation into 100ml of boiling water: 1 litre 90° alcohol and 15g pine-needle oil. The chest can also be rubbed with olive oil plus 5 per cent of pine-needle oil.

Homoeopathy

For chestiness with a dry painful cough: *Bryonia*.

Acupuncture

Said to be useful for 'mild pulmonary infections', so might be useful in the early stages of bronchopneumonia.

II/15 BRONCHIAL ASTHMA

The chief feature of bronchial asthma is (reversible) narrowing of the calibre of the small air-tubes (bronchioles) by inflammation and contraction of their muscular walls. This is responsible for the asthmatic symptoms most people know—difficulty in breathing, and a wheezing sound as air is expelled from the lungs. Asthma has recently been called by an expert 'probably the commonest chronic disorder in the country'. Estimates of its prevalence in the UK vary, but it is generally accepted that about 5 per cent of the total population (i.e. about 2.5 million Britons) have asthma.

Patients suffering an asthma attack are inevitably short of breath, cough frequently, and have to expend a lot of energy in drawing air into the chest and forcing it out again. They may be restless and panicky, pale in colour, and sometimes cyanosed. Prolonged attacks, known as 'status asthmaticus', can last for hours, and there is distinct danger of collapse and death from strain, exhaustion and anoxia. Sometimes asthma patients lack one or more of the familiar symptoms of their illness—when the obstruction in the small air tubes is slight, a persistent cough may be the only indication.

The causes of asthma are numerous and include both environmental and genetic factors; e.g. allergens, occupation, infection, emotional stress and changes in temperature. Common allergens include the house-dust mite, house dust itself, various kinds of pollen, animal fur, feathers, moulds and fungi and their spores. Viral infections commonly bring on an attack in susceptible people, and other common causes are unusual physical exertion, stressful situations and anxiety.

ORTHODOX TREATMENT

When asthma attacks are due to allergens, many attacks can be avoided if contact with the allergen(s) is reduced to a minimum. The commonest inhalent allergen in the UK is the house-dust mite, and the patient may be advised to take precautions against the collection of dust in the home. Diet alterations may also be necessary, as might the removal from the immediate environment of any cats, dogs, ponies or budgies to which the patient is allergic. Sometimes such measures are so emotionally stressful, however, that little benefit is gained in the long run.

Hyposensitization by injection has not proved to be very helpful to asthmatics, although it does help a number of hay-fever sufferers (see II/4).

The three classes of drugs used to treat asthma are the bronchodilators, the mast-cell stabilizers and the corticosteroids. Examples of the bronchodilators are salbutamol (Ventolin), available in a variety of forms including an aerosol, and ipratropium bromide (Atrovent), an aerosol. Examples of mast-cell stabilizers include 'SCG' and ketotifen (Zaditen); these help asthmatics by preventing the release from cells of chemical mediators known as mast cells, responsible for many of the symptoms of asthma. Examples of corticosteroids include prednisolone and hydrocortisone, and, as aerosols, beclomethasone (Becloforte, Becotide) and betamethasone (Bextasol). Corticosteroids have a variety of effects on asthma, one of which is the reduction of the inflammatory process.

ALTERNATIVE THERAPIES

Please see note under Hay fever (II/4). Clinical ecologists view asthma basically as a different manifestation of the same problem; other alternative practitioners agree in part but see the susceptibility of the affected individual as constituting the real problem.

Natural medicine

Wholefood diet, relaxation methods and stress reduction are all highly important in the management of asthma by natural means. Allergy to milk and/or wheat should be remembered as a possible cause of asthma. In addition, all tobacco smoking should be stopped immediately and weight reduction carried out if necessary. Applied kinesiology may be used to detect and possibly remedy food allergies and sensitivities.

A letter from a GP appeared in *Pulse* in June 1985 about the usefulness of the wholefood diet in the management of asthma: '... I have certainly found such a diet (i.e. one free from azo and tartrazine dyes), most helpful, not only in children who are overtly hyperactive but, more often, where one is using a natural, wholefood diet free of such dyes *and* of refined food—to treat asthma and eczema.'

Raw juices especially recommended for the treatment of asthma are:

- carrot 280g and spinach 170g
- grapefruit juice
- carrot 230g and celery 230g.

Specific dietary supplements Live yoghourt can be added to the daily diet to deal with the possible presence of *Candida albicans* as a cause of asthma, especially if numerous courses of antibiotics have been taken for chest infections. If symptoms do not improve, 1tsp of *Acidophilus* culture can be taken three times daily, as well as 2tsp of olive oil and a biotin supplement (about 300mcg). Additional daily supplements: zinc, 15–30mg; selenium, 100mcg.

Vitamins A, C and E, propolis and honey might also aid coughing and the inflammation of the bronchial tubes—see under II/13.

Cider vinegar treatment for asthma: 2tsp each of honey and cider vinegar in a tumbler of water, three times daily, have produced some remarkable results.

Biochemic tissue salts   For the difficult breathing of asthma, and for nervous asthma: *Kali Phos*. For thick, white, tenacious phlegm, difficult to bring up: *Kali Mur.*, alternating with *Kali Phos*. For spasm of the bronchiole muscles: *Magnesia Phos*. alternating with *Kali Phos*. Together with the other remedies, in all asthma cases (including children): *Calcarea Phos*.

Ionization therapy

This is useful in easing difficult breathing.

Herbal medicine

An infusion of the following ingredients: a clove of garlic, 2 pinches poppy petals, 2 pinches thyme, 2 pinches lavender and a pinch of aniseed to one litre of water.

Aromatherapy

Four drops essence of savory on a little brown sugar after each meal. For bronchial spasm and coughing: 3 drops essence of anise on a little brown sugar, three times daily.

Bach flower remedies

Homoeopathy

For difficult breathing, with the need to sit or bend forward: *Arsenicum Album*. For inflamed bronchial tubes with a rattling of mucus in the chest: *Ipecacuanha*.

Acupuncture

This can be highly effective in asthma, its effect being dilation of the narrowed muscular walls of the bronchioles. In one Chinese trial on asthma about 70 per cent of asthmatics gained 'good effect' from a course of acupuncture and moxibustion (about 10 treatment sessions) once yearly. Both frequency and intensity of asthma attacks were reduced.

Manipulative therapy

Reflexology This can help: work areas include solar plexus, reflexes to bronchial tubes, lungs, adrenals and thyroid, and possibly the reflexes to the testicles, prostate, ovaries and uterus. Patients are sometimes advised to hold their tongues lightly between their teeth for a few minutes every day.

Learning the Alexander technique can prove very helpful.

Relaxation methods

Biofeedback. Yoga is helpful for relaxation and stress-reduction; particularly helpful postures are the Corpse Posture, Shoulder Stand, Mountain, Fish and Complete Breath.

Spiritual therapies

Aurasoma; music, art, colour therapy; electrocrystal therapy.

III   Disorders of the Heart and Blood Vessels

The heart and blood vessels constitute the main circulatory system of the body, and are involved in keeping the blood constantly 'on the move' throughout its various parts.

If you follow your breast bone (sternum) downwards with your fingers from the base of your throat, you will detect a horizontal ridge 5–8cm from the top. This is known as the angle of the sternum, and it is level with the top of your heart, which lies centrally in the chest, tilted at an angle towards the left. The 'apex' of the heart points downwards, and is situated deep in your chest immediately below your left nipple.

The heart can most simply be described as a four-chambered pump. The two upper chambers are called the right and left atria and the two lower chambers into which they open are the right and left ventricles. Two one-way valves separate upper and lower compartments; on the right-hand side, the tricuspid valve lies between right atrium and ventricle, and on the left the mitral valve separates left atrium and ventricle.

The heart is made up almost entirely of muscular tissue (the myocardium), the walls of the ventricles being considerably thicker than those of the atria. The vertical dividing wall, or septum, between the right and left sides of the heart, however, is not composed of muscle; it is the pathway taken by a vital structure termed the bundle of His. Its fibres run the length of the septum and then branch out, running up in the walls of the ventricles on each side.

The insides of the atria and ventricles have a smooth lining, the endocardium, and the heart itself is enclosed in a fibrous tissue bag, the pericardium.

The main arteries attached to the heart are the aorta, which arches upwards from the left ventricle, and the pulmonary artery, which comes off the right ventricle.

The *aorta* is the largest artery in the body, and measures about 2.5 cm in diameter. It gives off major arterial branches to the head, neck and upper-limb regions, and then plunges downwards through the chest and abdomen, immediately in front of the backbone. The arteries supplying the head and neck structures are the left and right carotid arteries—you can feel these pulsating on each side of your neck, a little below the angle of your jaw. This pulse is sometimes easier to locate than the radial one at the wrist. At the level of the fourth lumbar vertebra, the aorta divides into a right and a left branch, the common iliac arteries, which supply the pelvic organs and the right and left leg. The aortic valve separates the aorta from the left ventricle. At the root of the aorta, just after it leaves the heart, the two main coronary arteries arise. These supply arterial blood to the muscular walls of the heart.

Compared with the aorta, the *pulmonary artery* is very short. Separated from the right ventricle by the pulmonary valve, it passes to the lungs. The pulmonary artery is the only artery in the body carrying deoxygenated blood, and the only one not to be directly or indirectly derived from the aorta.

Arteries can be defined as blood vessels carrying blood *away from* the heart. They divide and subdivide many times in order to supply all the

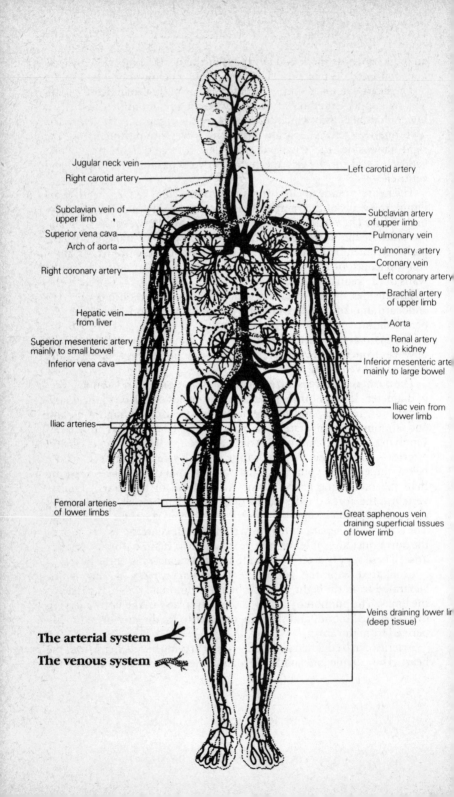

Jugular neck vein

Right carotid artery

Left carotid artery

Subclavian vein of upper limb

Subclavian artery of upper limb

Superior vena cava

Pulmonary vein

Arch of aorta

Pulmonary artery

Coronary vein

Right coronary artery

Left coronary artery

Brachial artery of upper limb

Hepatic vein from liver

Aorta

Superior mesenteric artery mainly to small bowel

Renal artery to kidney

Inferior vena cava

Inferior mesenteric arte mainly to large bowel

Iliac vein from lower limb

Iliac arteries

Femoral arteries of lower limbs

Great saphenous vein draining superficial tissues of lower limb

Veins draining lower lir (deep tissue)

The arterial system

The venous system

Heart and Blood Vessels

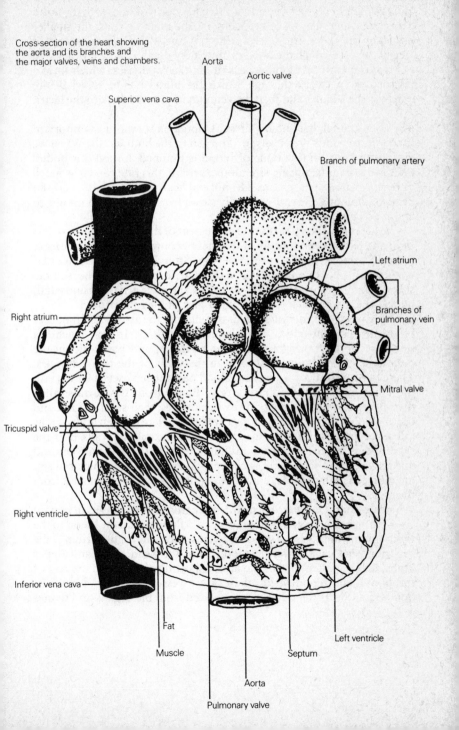

Cross-section of the heart showing
the aorta and its branches and
the major valves, veins and chambers.

Aorta

Aortic valve

Superior vena cava

Branch of pulmonary artery

Left atrium

Branches of
pulmonary vein

Right atrium

Mitral valve

Tricuspid valve

Right ventricle

Inferior vena cava

Left ventricle

Fat

Muscle

Septum

Aorta

Pulmonary valve

organs and tissues of the body with 'heart' blood (see below), and the pattern of their division is often likened to a tree, with the aorta being the trunk. The large branches are the main arteries, the smaller branches the lesser arteries, and the tiny twigs the minute vessels or 'arterioles' into which the arteries ultimately divide. The arterioles lead in turn to the tiniest blood vessels of all, the capillaries, which form a microscopic network through which the blood has to travel before reaching the venules and then the veins on its journey back to the heart.

The average adult has about 5 litres of blood, one of the most important functions of which is to transport oxygen to the body's cells. When we are resting, our total volume of blood is pumped around our bodies once every minute; during strenuous exercise, this rate can be as much as reach six times per minute. The normal heart-rate in adults is 60–80 beats per minute; the rate gradually slows from 120–140 in infants to about 80 at puberty.

The heart is responsible for the movement of the circulating blood, its right and left sides performing different but complementary activities in perfect harmony in the normal person. Stimuli causing its muscular walls to contract (a phase called systole) arise in a narrow, horseshoe-shaped area of specialized tissue called the sinu-atrial (orsinoatrial) node—the 'pacemaker'—in the upper part of the right atrium.

The wave of contraction spreads throughout the atria, which squeeze blood through the valves into the two ventricles. It then reaches a second node lower down in the right atrium, and passes down the bundle of His and along its fibres in the walls of the two ventricles. These in turn contract, squeezing blood past the next set of valves into the aorta and the pulmonary artery. Blood from the aorta is then distributed throughout the body by the arteries, their subdivisions, and the arterioles, finally reaching the capillaries. Here oxygen and various nutrients are able to filter through the thin capillary walls into the surrounding tissue fluid; from this fluid the cells absorb the oxygen and nutrients. At the same time, waste products of the cells' metabolism, including carbon dioxide, enter the capillaries and are removed from the area.

Venules, and later the veins, which are thin-walled vessels in certain cases furnished with valves to prevent backflow, return the blood to the right side of the heart. Two great veins enter the right atrium—the superior vena cava, carrying blood from the head, neck and upper limbs, and the inferior vena cava, transporting blood from the rest of the body. The blood inside these great vessels is 'body' blood (as opposed to 'heart' blood); i.e. it is derived from the organs and tissues and is therefore short of oxygen and nutrients but laden with carbon dioxide. This has to be removed and the blood refurbished with fresh oxygen for another trip around the body—this is accomplished by its circulation around the lungs (see pages 226–230).

Blood entering the right atrium is squeezed into the right ventricle during systole (the relaxation phase of the heart while it is refilling with blood 'between beats' is known as diastole). It then enters the pulmonary artery and circulates around the lungs, picking up oxygen. The blood leaves the lungs via the pulmonary veins, which carry it straight into the left atrium.

The walls of arteries are far thicker than those of veins. They are reinforced with both muscular and fibrous tissue to withstand the pressure which rises within them during systole. Arteries to various parts of the body also become constricted or dilated according to 'regional requirements'. For example, immediately after a large meal, extra blood is directed towards the digestive organs, to enable them to cope with their workload. Arteries in this region therefore dilate accordingly to accommodate this. Arteries elsewhere, however, at this time carry less blood than usual—for example, most people rest after eating a big meal and during this rest phase the arteries supplying the upper and lower limb muscles tend to constrict a little. This applies also to the arteries supplying the brain, and helps to account for the sleepiness many of us experience after eating a large amount. The behaviour of the arteries under these conditions is under the control of the autonomic nervous system (see page 346).

The commonest type of heart disease is ATHEROMA within the coronary arteries, rather than a disorder of the heart itself. Problems within the actual structure of the heart are of three kinds. Firstly, any of the four valves can be damaged and misfunction; the usual cause of valve damage is congenital valve disease; rheumatic fever is another common cause. Secondly, the electrical-impulse system can become disordered. Thirdly, the heart may have an anatomical defect due to maldevelopment, and misfunction accordingly; the possible developmental heart abnormalities with which a baby can be born are numerous—the commonest is HOLE IN THE HEART.

III/1 RHEUMATIC HEART DISEASE

Rheumatic heart disease arises as a complication of RHEUMATIC FEVER. Both the heart muscle and the valves can be affected, but the latter are more likely to suffer lasting structural damage and deformity. The valve most likely to be affected is the mitral valve; the next most likely is the aortic. The commonest problems are incompetence, in which the diseased valve leaks, and stenosis, in which the passage through it is narrowed and the flow of blood impeded.

When a valve is incompetent, some of the blood regurgitates back into the atrium against the normal direction of flow. Symptoms of incompetence depend upon the severity. They can include fainting, shortness of breath on exertion or in bed at night, angina and palpitations.

Stenosis occurs when the leaves (cusps) of the valves stick together as a result of the disease process. A similar circumstance arises when one attempts to squeeze sauce, cream, etc., out of a tube without having pierced the sealed metal top sufficiently thoroughly: a tremendous amount of effort has to be made to extract even a drop or two. Shortness of breath due to congestion of the lungs (due in turn to a build-up of back pressure in the lungs from the left atrium via the pulmonary veins) is characteristic of mitral stenosis, and typically occurs for the first time during the patient's 20s or 30s (depending upon when he or she had rheumatic fever). Palpitations, a cough, atrial FIBRILLATION and chronic fatigue are also common. Failure of the left atrium to overcome the problem of a narrowed mitral valve, despite the fact that it enlarges in its attempt to compensate and pump more strongly, can bring on attacks of pulmonary OEDEMA, and result finally in right-sided heart failure (see III/3).

Moderate to severe aortic stenosis ultimately causes the left side of the heart to fail in its task, despite the fact that the left ventricle can and often does enlarge enormously in its attempt to pump more vigorously. Symptoms tend to come on later in life than those of mitral stenosis, and to include fainting spells, angina and heart block. Sudden death can occur.

ORTHODOX TREATMENT

Surgery is the only really satisfactory form of treatment for damaged heart valves. They are either repaired or replaced with an artificial valve, according to their condition.

ALTERNATIVE THERAPIES

Since surgery is the only satisfactory treatment for cardiac valvular defects, the orthodox management remains the treatment of choice. However, alternative management of the symptoms (possibly combined with orthodox treatment) is indicated for patients who are unsuitable for repair or replacement operations; this is discussed for appropriate symptoms under heart failure (III/3).

III/2 CONDUCTION DEFECTS

Disorders of cardiac conduction can arise from a wide variety of causes. The rate of rhythm impulses are controlled by the autonomic nervous system; they can be affected by emotion and by reflexes within the sympathetic nervous system (see page 346). They are also affected by reflexes involving the vagus nerve, which arises in the brain and travels down the neck to the chest, where it acts as a 'brake' upon the heartbeat, preventing it from pumping too rapidly.

A number of chemical substances—e.g. adrenaline—alter the heart's rate. A patient given a life-saving injection of adrenaline will have a greatly increased pulse-rate. Similarly, our pulses start to pound if we get a fright—this is due to the adrenal glands secreting adrenaline into the bloodstream as part of the 'flight or fight' mechanism.

Obviously, if any part of the conduction apparatus of the heart is diseased the rhythm of the heart will be affected. This can occur when ATHEROMA is present in the right coronary artery, since a small branch of it supplies arterial blood to the atrio-ventricular node and the bundle of His. A reduced blood supply can seriously impair healthy impulse conduction.

The chief conduction disorders are EXTRASYSTOLES, atrial FIBRILLA-TION and atrial FLUTTER, HEART BLOCK and Stokes-Adams attacks (i.e. temporary losses of consciousness due to ventricular loss of heartbeat or ventricular fibrillation).

III/3 HEART FAILURE

This term refers to one or other side of the heart (sometimes both) working inefficiently; i.e. 'failing' to pump the blood adequately around the lungs (right side) or around the rest of the body (left side).

There are several possible causes for cardiac failure, the commonest being diseased coronary arteries, high blood-pressure (see III/5), or diseased heart valves (see rheumatic heart disease, III/1). Any one of these conditions would be likely to cause left-sided heart failure. Right-sided failure might be expected as a sequel to longstanding lung disorders; e.g. chronic bronchitis (II/12) and emphysema (II/13).

Symptoms characteristic of a failing left ventricle include excessive fatigue, shortness of breath (especially apparent on exertion and when lying down) caused by back pressure and congestion of the veins in the lungs, and a cough.

Attacks known as 'paroxysmal nocturnal dyspnoea' sometimes occur at night, waking the sufferer with a feeling of extreme breathlessness and an urgent need for fresh air. Characteristically, the sufferer sits up gasping, or gets out of bed, gasping for breath, goes to a window, opens it and leans out. This symptom is caused by extra-severe lung congestion, due to two factors. One is having been asleep (the reflex that reduces the lungs' capacity in the presence of left-sided heart failure is less readily stimulated during sleep); the other is that extra tissue fluid that accumulates during the day (see OEDEMA) tends to be reabsorbed at night, and pulmonary oedema—fluid in the lungs, due to the congestion—becomes more severe.

With right-sided heart failure there is a back pressure upon the small blood vessels in the extremities, due to the pressure that builds up on the right side of the heart and is transmitted to great veins draining into the atrium. The result of this back pressure is the formation of oedema, the site where it forms depending upon gravity and the position of the patient.

A patient confined to bed will get 'presacral' oedema, a pad of swollen fluid-laden tissue forming immediately above the buttocks. The patient who is up and about, or sitting up in a chair, will get ankle-swelling. Also due to back pressure from the right side of the heart, the patient's liver may become congested and swollen. This is rare in adults.

ORTHODOX TREATMENT

Rest and digitalis-related compounds are the mainstay of treatment. The value of the rest on a heart that is failing to cope satisfactorily is self-evident. The value of the drugs is basically threefold. Firstly, digoxin (or whichever equivalent is chosen) improves the efficiency with which the heart acts—it causes it to beat more strongly, thereby conserving energy rather than wasting it on inefficient action. The ventricles empty more completely during systole, the output of blood from the heart is increased, and as a result the pressure in the veins is lowered. Secondly, digitalis compounds slow the rate at which the heart beats, and this also helps to improve its function. Thirdly, the drugs have a 'diuretic action' on OEDEMA caused by cardiac failure, due to the improved blood-supply to the kidneys which results from the drugs' action on the heart muscle. Other diuretics may be added to the regimen. The recommended diet for overweight patients would be a reduced-calorie one, since obesity puts extra strain upon the heart. Other measures might include the administration of oxygen and the withdrawal of any fluid that had collected in the chest or abdomen.

ALTERNATIVE THERAPIES

Since the treatment of heart failure depends a great deal upon the underlying cause(s)—the commonest circulatory ones of which are coronary artery disease and hypertension—the reader is referred to III/4 and III/5. Discussion here is limited to alternative ways of promoting general cardiac health, and of managing specific aspects of the symptoms of heart failure as such.

Natural medicine

The attitude of naturopathic practitioners to patients with heart disease depends upon the type of disorder and its underlying cause(s). As with other disorders, naturopaths are less inclined to treat the immediately apparent symptoms than to consider what the symptoms mean in terms of a basic, underlying problem. They generally concede that surgery is advisable in patients whose heart failure is due to valvular disease; they may agree that a bypass operation was desirable in a victim of severe coronary arterial disease causing the heart to malfunction severely; and they may condone the use of drugs to treat cases of left-sided heart failure due to raised blood pressure (see III/5).

Encountering a patient with right-sided heart failure secondary to chronic lung disease, naturopathic practitioners would turn their attention directly to attempting to correct the lung problem. This does not mean that they would deny the usefulness of orthodox drugs in any case of severe cardiac failure, nor that they would counsel seriously ill patients to forgo hospitalization or drug therapy. But it does mean that they, more than most people, are aware that much heart disease results from overindulgence in the 'wrong' foods, from failure to combat stress by effective relaxation methods, and from too little exercise. Seeing a patient in a state of cardiac failure, the naturopath would therefore advise him or her either to consult his doctor or possibly a practitioner of herbal medicine for immediate treatment; but would help the patient as soon as the symptoms started to respond to drugs or herbs by reviewing his or her lifestyle and diet and by suggesting methods by which he or she could learn to relax (and to give up smoking if this applied).

Treatment might well commence with the Grape Cure (see page 433). Subsequently the recommended diet would of course be wholefood, and would start by eliminating saturated animal fats and replacing them by small quantities of polyunsaturated fats and plant oils; oily fish would be thoroughly recommended for their protection against heart disease, and the inclusion of eggs and dairy products would be reduced to an absolute minimum. The diet, moreover, would be high in complex carbohydrates (pulses, wholegrains, unpolished rice, natural cereals, wholemeal bread and wholemeal-flour products, fresh fruit and fresh vegetables). An emphasis might very well be placed upon raw fruit and vegetables for their natural enzyme, vitamin and mineral contents and their fibre. Refined processed foodstuffs, red meat, sugar, coffee and tea would be banned entirely.

Certain foodstuffs are known to lower the blood level of cholesterol, one of the components of the fatty plaques present in atheromatous arteries (see ATHEROMA and III/4). These foods include onion (cooked and raw), aubergine, garlic, yoghourt (even when made from whole milk), soya beans and pectin (present in apples and in the white pith of citrus fruit).

Recommended raw juices to aid heart function: carrot, 280g, and spinach, 170g; or carrot, 200g, celery, 110g, spinach, 85g, and parsley, 55g.

Many heart patients are overweight—cider vinegar can aid slimming if taken as part of a wholefood calorie-controlled diet. Recommendations: start the day by sipping 2tsp of cider vinegar in a glass of cold or lukewarm water, and sip a tumbler of water containing 2tsp of cider vinegar during each main meal, trying to make the drink last throughout the meal.

Royal jelly as a supplement is said to contribute to a healthy heart.

Honey as a supplement may help a little in two ways: taking 5–6tsp daily is claimed to have a relaxing and calming effect upon highly strung individuals who are inclined to aggravate underlying cardiac conditions by their response to stress. A mixture of honey and fresh lemon juice may be helpful for a troublesome 'bronchial' cough, due either to chronic bronchitis (see II/12) or to congestion of the lungs secondary to heart failure.

The amino acid taurine has proved of value in treating congestive cardiac failure. A controlled trial[44] was carried out in which 58 patients with this condition received, for a four-week period, either a placebo or 6g of taurine daily in three divided doses. Following administration of taurine, the following symptoms improved significantly: breathlessness, palpitations and oedema. Improvements were seen also on X-ray examination and in everyday function. The taurine was effective whether or not the patient concerned was on digitalis. By contrast, there was no significant improvement due to the placebo. Patients with diseased coronary arteries and valvular heart disease were improved on taurine.

Herbal medicine

For the treatment of OEDEMA, a diuretic effect produced by foot and hand baths (two daily) of the following: a handful of celandine leaves, a bunch of cress, a grated onion, a bunch of parsley and a handful of meadowsweet to 2 litres of water.

The following infusion may also benefit patients with a mild to moderate degree of chronic cardiac failure because of its mixture of stimulant and diuretic properties: one pinch to a cup of water of each of anise, savory, mint, fennel and chervil.

Aromatherapy

For the lowered urine output which can occur in severe right-sided or combined heart failure: four drops of essence of juniper on a little brown sugar after every meal.

Bach flower remedies

Homoeopathy

For troublesome breathlessness, accompanied by a need to sit forward: *Arsenicum Album*. As a heart tonic in cases of heart failure: *Crataegus*.

Acupuncture

Some patients with rheumatic heart disease develop arrhythmias, a common one in this situation being atrial FIBRILLATION. This can occur also in patients with hypertension (III/5) and coronary artery disease (III/4). Acupuncture can sometimes restore the heart's rhythm to normal. In established atrial fibrillation it affects few cases (about 1.5 per cent), but in some recently acquired arrhythmias it can be effective in up to 70 per cent of cases.

Manipulative therapy

Reflexology For general condition of the heart, benefit is claimed from massaging the reflex to the heart on the left foot; the reflex to the shoulderblade; and the fifth toe and seventh cervical vertebra. If the reflex to the colon is tender, this also should be massaged. Reflexologists claim that some heart disorders can result from the pressure pocket in the colon.

Relaxation techniques

These can be immensely helpful in both the prevention and the treatment of established heart failure, and in the maintenance of a healthy heart and blood vessels generally. Rest is one of the two main principles of the orthodox management of heart failure, but restraint upon physical activity is of limited benefit unless the body and mind are relaxed. Any of the following (or a combination) could be usefully employed: autogenics, self-hypnosis and autosuggestion, yoga, meditation, biofeedback.

Exercise therapy

Very gentle dance therapy can help the chronically unfit and the overweight.

Spiritual therapy

Aurasoma, electrocrystal therapy.

III/4 CORONARY ARTERY DISEASE

Known also as ischaemic heart disease, or IHD, the basic disease process affecting the coronary arteries is that of atherosclerosis (see ATHEROMA). As the interiors of these vessels become increasingly clogged with fatty deposit, the blood supply—and thereby the oxygen supply—to the heart muscle becomes correspondingly reduced.

Anginal chest pain results (see ANGINA) and the condition may progress to total blockage of one of the arteries, either through further accumulation of fatty plaque material, which ultimately cuts off altogether the blood supply in that artery, or through a blood clot obstructing the already narrowed channel (see CORONARY THROM-

BOSIS). The resulting damage to the heart is called an infarct (see INFARCTION).

THERAPIES

The following breakthroughs have been made on the nutritional and exercise fronts:

- Lecithin and oil with a high linoleic-acid content (combined in the correct proportions) are believed to be capable gradually of dissolving atheromatous plaques in arterial walls—the recommended combination[45] is given on pages 244–5.
- Vitamin E can improve the circulation through its effect upon blood viscosity (blood with a high viscosity clots too readily). A frequent reason for this type of clotting is that the platelets are too sticky; this problem is seen most frequently in diabetics and in patients with an impaired absorption of fats.[46] Vitamin E also helps to reduce clotting by inhibiting the manufacture within the body of Vitamin K, which is normally responsible for promoting the beneficial clotting of blood —e.g. after an injury.

Vitamin E supplements are recommended for patients with diseased coronary arteries and/or an increased proneness to thrombosis. The dosage is 400–800iu daily.

- Octacosanol, the active ingredient in wheatgerm oil, has been shown to increase stamina, endurance and vigour, to help resist the effects of stress and—among other things—to improve the function of muscle, including heart muscle. Improvement was also shown on ECG heart tracings that 'suggested an improved nutritional state of the heart myocardium [muscle], and a strengthening of the contraction action voltages [the 'force' with which it beats]'.[47]
- The beneficial effects of aerobic exercise on diseased coronary arteries have been well tabulated. Exercise plays an important part in the four-step programme used at the California Heart Medical Clinic (Huntington Beach, California) to stop the progression of atherosclerosis and, hopefully, to reverse the process.[48] Besides a diet designed to lower the cholesterol level in the blood, in order that the fatty plaques themselves can then surrender their cholesterol content, the patients are given supplementary vitamins and minerals, oxygen therapy and moderate exercise carefully tailored to their individual requirements and capabilities. The prescribed diet is very

low in total fat, which provides only 10–15 per cent of the daily total calorie intake (the average for most people is 42 per cent). The emphasis is upon wholegrain breads, high-fibre cereals such as oatmeal, fresh fruit and vegetables, rice, beans, corn, lentils and other pulses. On average, the patients achieve a cholesterol fall of 25 per cent in only 12 days. Other benefits are a fall in blood pressure (nearly always), improvement in anginal pain, and weightloss.

The oxygen therapy consists of the patients receiving an increased level of oxygen for 1–2 hours daily while at the clinic; sometimes this therapy continues at home. This measure is based on recent research which suggests that raising the oxygen level in the blood will speed the process of healing atheromatous arteries.

The exercise, which consists of brisk walking or slow jogging, cycling or swimming, is aerobic. Aerobic exercise has been found in numerous studies to improve the oxygen-carrying capacity of the blood, to stimulate the development of new blood vessels to the heart, to lower the undesirable types of fat levels in the blood, and to raise the level of healthy cholesterol.

- The food substances and supplements described below are frequently recommended for inclusion in the diet of patients especially at risk from heart disorders and diseased coronary arteries, since they measurably decrease the tendency of the blood platelets to aggregate and form blood clots. There is, it would seem, every reason to include them in a normal diet, for their potentially protective effect: bromelaine (an enzyme that breaks down protein), sold as Ananase and derived from pineapples; codliver oil; evening primrose oil (Efamol); garlic oil; Vitamins B_6, C and E. Also increasingly recommended is EPA (eicosapentaenoic acid), a marine lipid found in fish oils and producing many valuable effects including the control of blood viscosity and clotting, the control of arterial spasms and the lowering of blood levels of cholesterol (especially the LDL [dangerous] cariety) and of other lipids called triglycerides.[49]
- The amino acid carnitine has the job of transporting fatty acids into the mitochondria, the power centres of our cells within which fatty acids (and glucose) combine with oxygen to generate essential energy. The heart-muscle contains a high percentage of carnitine, one of the reasons being its dependence upon long-chain fatty acids as an energy source—it uses them for 48–70 per cent of its total energy requirement.

Reports have suggested that carnitine may well have protective value to the heart muscle of people with diseased coronary arteries. Its beneficial effects during a recent trial, in which it was given intravenously to 18 patients with coronary artery disease, included improved utilization by the heart of fatty acids and decreased accumulation of lactate during trial exercise (i.e. better exercise tolerance).[50] Other beneficial effects have included improved mental alertness and better muscular function in intermittent CLAUDICATION. No adverse side-effects have been reported.

Carnitine is recommended by Leon Chaitow, commenting upon a report of the above trial, as 'part of the safe, firstaid type measure employed by nutritionally orientated practitioners in conditions involving myocardial distress'.[50]

- Two other amino acids, histidine and taurine, have been found to have beneficial effects in patients suffering from coronary artery disease. Histidine has been used to improve the circulation in the coronary arteries, and to lower blood-pressure through vasodilation. Taurine (see also pages 236–7) was found by research workers at the University of South Dakota to be involved in regulating the responsiveness of heart tissue to stimulation, and to have an anti-arrhythmic effect.[51] It also helps to keep cholesterol in solution in the blood (rather than precipitating out of solution to form plaques).

Chelation therapy

This is available in the USA and Holland. It was first used to treat coronary heart disease in 1948. Several hundred medical articles have been written about its successes since 1950, yet it has still to achieve the popularity it deserves.[52] It consists of giving the patient an intravenous solution of an artificial amino acid known as EDTA (ethylene diamine tetra-acetic acid) which has the ability to reduce the calcium content of the atheromatous plaques and in other areas, without affecting the calcium content of the bones. It does so by joining up with the calcium and forming a compound with it which can then be excreted through the kidneys or the intestine by the liver. Clinical studies have shown great improvement in anginal and other types of ischaemic pain (for instance, intermittent CLAUDICATION) and in the circulation and resultant organ function throughout the body.

Chelation seems certainly to be a feasible alternative to the coronary-artery-bypass operation, and it paves the way for the patient with very severely diseased coronary arteries to take full advantage of the cholesterol-mobilizing techniques and other benefits associated with a corrected diet, exercise and behaviour-modification. Chelation therapy also offers some protection against a number of degenerative functions, including the effects of 'free radicals' which can badly injure arterial walls.

Antioxidants

Besides the facts now established about the roles cholesterol, blood fat, obesity and insufficient exercise have in generating coronary artery disease, a further factor is now being discussed in terms of free radicals. These are unstable atoms and compounds sometimes formed during the body's utilization of oxygen as well as under other conditions. One of their chief characteristics is a tendency to react in an undesirable way with other compounds.

Some free radicals are necessary for the body's metabolism; but they have to be kept under control—normally exercised by two chemicals we make for this purpose, glutathione and superoxide dismutase.[53]

When too many free radicals are formed, they can damage the cells of the walls of the coronary arteries. As a result, atheromatous plaques and blood clots form. Free radicals also cause damage to cells in other areas of the body. In addition, they can suppress the formation of a substance called prostacyclin, or PG_{12}, lack of which encourages the formation of blood clots on arterial walls.

It is a good idea to provide the body with supplements which help it to deal with free radicals and to control the rate at which they are produced. Antioxidants, substances which put a brake upon the rate with which oxidation proceeds, have this effect—antioxidants include Vitamins A, C and E; several amino acids, including cysteine; glutathione; zinc; selenium; and Vitamins B_1, B_5 and B_6. A wholefood diet, as suggested above and on page 236, supplies many of the antioxidants we need. Nevertheless, supplementation is a good idea (to be on the safe side); any supplement programme for patients with heart disease, especially involving the coronary arteries, ought to include the above vitamins, minerals and amino acids.

Stress

Stress which remains uncounterbalanced by regular and thorough relaxation is known to contribute significantly to coronary artery disease, high blood pressure and a tendency to suffer ANGINA, STROKES and CORONARY THROMBOSIS. Some individuals, however, have been found to be more predisposed to these disorders than others, and the common personality traits they share have been designated 'type-A behaviour' (TAB). Coronary-prone behaviour seems to appear in two main patterns: (a) typical TAB characteristics, which include impatience, overactivity, fearfulness and chronic anxiety, ambitious strivings, easy arousal to hostile and aggressive behaviour, and a sense of time urgency; and (b) the combination of depression (see **XIV/3**) and neurotic behaviour. It is probable that when these two patterns co-exist in one individual, the risks are enhanced.

In order to modify TAB, patients exhibiting this behaviour complex and who have experienced at least one myocardial infarction have been helped under trial conditions by counsellors working in small groups. In particular, the sufferers learn how their attitudes and behaviour have harmful physical consequences. When the trial was set up, it was intended to continue over a five-year period, during which the TAB patients receiving behaviour counselling were compared with two other groups of TAB patients. The first of these was helped with diet, exercise and medication guidance but no behaviour counselling, and the other received no counselling of any type but was examined and interviewed annually. After three years, changes in TAB occurred in the counselled group, and their total reinfarction rate (rate of repeat myocardial infarctions) was so much lower than that in the other groups that the five-year programme was halted, bringing the two control groups into the behavioural counselling programme so that they might benefit similarly.

As Leon Chaitow remarked in his 'Comment' following the report of the relevant paper in the *Journal of Alternative Medicine*, 'the fact that by insight and awareness, such individuals can alter their attitudes and behaviour and therefore avoid hazardous health complications vindicates the basic natural health concept of dealing with basic causes rather than effects and symptoms'.[54]

ORTHODOX TREATMENT

Orthodox doctors treat coronary artery disease by supplying drugs for ANGINA and by counselling patients about the suitability of their type of employment, about the avoidance of unnecessary or sudden hard physical exertion, and about losing weight and giving up smoking where these are applicable. Underlying problems such as hypertension (**III/5**) are treated with drug therapy; moderate exercise is encouraged; and a coronary-artery-bypass operation is considered for suitable patients.

A 'heart attack' involving a myocardial infarction may be treated with pain-killing drugs, measures to combat shock, rest, oxygen if necessary, anticoagulants to avoid further thrombosis, and drugs to restore the normal rhythm of the heart if this is disturbed.

ALTERNATIVE THERAPIES

Much of this has been discussed above, but the following should be mentioned.

Natural medicine

Initial treatment may start with the Grape Cure or the Rice Diet (see page 433). The patient's lifestyle would be reviewed in detail, and advice given about losing weight, ceasing to smoke, combatting stress, and eating a wholefood diet along the lines described on page 236. The following factors tend to raise the blood cholesterol-level and should be avoided wherever possible: tobacco, coffee, stress, refined sugar, the Pill. The following tend to lower the cholesterol level and should be included in the diet wherever possible: aubergines, onion (raw and cooked), garlic, yoghourt, pectin (apples, white membrane of citrus fruit), soya beans.

Also as part of a wholefood diet, with an emphasis upon fresh raw fruit and vegetables and their juices, fresh undiluted beetroot juice (300ml), for instance, can be mixed with an equal volume of freshly squeezed carrot juice and drunk daily. Beetroot juice is said to be an excellent solvent for organic calcium deposits, and to aid high blood-pressure and heart disorders associated with 'thickened' arteries (calcium is frequently deposited in the fatty atheromatous plaques within arteries). Carrot juice supplies potassium, necessary to the heart's normal functioning, and to all other body cells, and produces a feeling of vigour and well-being.

Specific dietary supplements   It is best to consult a nutrition expert who can advise you about your personal requirements with respect to supplementation, but the following is a guide:

- Vitamin A, 10,000iu daily
- Vitamin-B complex, containing 100mg of B_1 and B_6
- Vitamin B_5, 250mg
- Vitamin C, 3–4g daily
- Vitamin E, 400–800iu daily
- minerals: zinc, 50mg; selenium, 200mcg

- amino acids: carnitine, 200mg, three times daily, increasing after a week to 400mg, three times daily; histidine, 1g, three times daily (take in conjunction with some of your daily Vitamin C); taurine, 100mg, three times daily.
- EPA (eicosapentaenoic acid): 2–3g (available as Max-EPA capsules from chemists and healthfood shops); codliver oil, 20ml; bromelaine (Ananase), 2 tablets; salmon oil, 60–80ml; garlic oil, 25mg; evening primrose oil (Efamol) 2–4g.
- Lecithin granules: 2tbsp daily, plus safflower oil, 1tbsp daily
- Octacosanol: 6,000mcg daily, preferably in the chewable form
- Honey: this can be a useful addition to the diet of an overactive 'workaholic' TAB sort of person, for its natural medative effect —1tsp, 6 times daily.
- Tradition has it that propolis is helpful in heart complaints, so a propolis capsule a day might add a little benefit; certainly its antiseptic properties can be readily utilized to help prevent infections of the upper respiratory tract from developing into bronchitis.
- One patient quoted in *Hanssen's Complete Cider Vinegar* claimed that 2tsp of cider vinegar in a tumbler of water, sipped during the day, helped relieve the severity of angina attacks; it certainly has a reputation for helping with slimming (see page 236).

Herbal medicine

For atheromatous arteries, two foot and hand baths daily of 2 crushed heads of garlic and one handful each of hawthorn flowers, celandine leaves and broom flowers to two litres of water. Also: an infusion of one pinch each of marjoram, sage and mint to a cupful of water. To prevent the development of atheromatous arteries, eat plenty of garlic.

Aromatherapy

To treat atheromatous arteries: add garlic to raw salads. Before meals, take five drops of the alcohol preparation on a little brown sugar. (Allow 200g of crushed garlic to macerate in one litre of 60° alcohol; after a fortnight, strain and store in a glass bottle away from the light.)

Bach flower remedies

Homoeopathy

For angina pectoris, worsened by exercise: *Cactus*. As a heart tonic, when there is a degree of cardiac failure: *Crataegus*.

Acupuncture

Chinese trials have shown a marked increase in the functional ability and efficiency of the heart muscles after acupuncture. This is supported by clinical work which shows that about 80 per cent of patients with angina have improved following acupuncture treatment. The usual routine is for a course of treatments to be given, followed by booster sessions every 4–6 months.

Manipulative therapy

Reflexology Angina is treated by working on the reflexes to the solar plexus, heart, lungs, bronchial tubes, shoulders, pituitary gland, adrenals and the thyroid gland. The shoulder muscles are also massaged by gentle kneading.

Relaxation techniques

Learning to relax is a large part of the success secret connected with the counselling of the TAB personality. Tense anxious patients who show no other TAB characteristics are likely to become more so once they develop angina or experience a heart attack, so any techniques which teach the patient to relax and let go of inner tension are likely to be beneficial.

Yoga, as well as being a therapeutic exercise physically, induces serenity and calms inner turmoil when practised properly—especially when combined with a meditation session. Relaxation can be learned also through autogenics classes, and hypnotherapy can teach the individual to relax and encourage the practice of relaxation on a daily basis between treatment sessions.

In a recent trial[55] 192 high-risk men and women were randomly assigned either to a control group or to one in which relaxation, meditation, breathing techniques and stress control were taught in weekly sessions lasting one hour each. Both groups were supplied with literature explaining the dangers of smoking and high blood pressure and the importance of reducing animal-fat intake. After two months and after eight months, the treatment group had significantly lower blood pressures (systolic and diastolic) compared with the control group. Four years later these differences were maintained, although the reductions in smoking habits and in cholesterol levels noted at two and at eight months had not been maintained. The treatment group produced fewer cases of angina and of hypertension and its complications.

The control subjects also showed a higher incidence of atheromatous coronary arteries, fatal heart attacks and ECG evidence of poor coronary blood-supply. It was considered that, if a larger study showed similar results, then the health-care and financial implications would be tremendous.

Exercise therapy

Yoga and T'ai chi can both help the overweight at-risk patient who has not exercised for years to start exercising again in a manner that imposes no strain and yet increases flexibility and muscular control.

Psychological therapies

Biofeedback is likely to help by reducing tension and helping the patient to gain control of his own reactions to stressful stimuli. In addition, counselling and group therapy can help in the way discussed above in connection with TAB patients.

Spiritual therapies

Aurasoma; electrocrystal therapy; art, music and colour therapy.

III/5 HYPERTENSION (RAISED BLOOD PRESSURE)

About 80 per cent of hypertension arises for no apparent reason, and is termed essential hypertension. The remaining 20 per cent of cases (secondary hypertension) are associated with an underlying causative disorder affecting the arteries, the kidneys or the adrenal glands. Many people with hypertension are symptom-free, at least in the early stages, and a raised blood pressure is commonly discovered for the first time during a routine check-up. When symptoms are present they can include HEADACHES, especially noticeable on waking; DIZZY SPELLS; breathlessness; PALPITATIONS; and blurred vision. Further symptoms are likely to be present when the hypertension is secondary to another disorder.

Patients with symptomless hypertension are often reluctant to receive treatment of any kind; but the reason doctors and health therapists are concerned to normalize a raised blood pressure is that there can be deleterious effects on vital organs of the body. Hypertension predisposes the patient to coronary artery disease (see III/4) and also to

CORONARY THROMBOSIS. STROKES are also more likely to occur, and any underlying cardiac disorder, such as valvular defects due to rheumatic heart disease, is likely to be exacerbated.

ORTHODOX TREATMENT

Treatment is directed at any underlying causative disorder, and also at the state of hypertension as such. Weight reduction will be suggested if the patient is overweight, as this is an additional risk factor with relation to heart attacks and strokes; moderate degrees of hypertension often respond to weight reduction alone in obese people. Advice is also given on the subjects of tobacco smoking, diet, and personal stress and tension. Unfortunately, tranquillizers are often prescribed at this point in order to try to control the blood pressure. In other cases (or if tranquillizers do not work) specific 'antihypertensive agents' will be prescribed in most cases. Drugs used include diuretics (e.g. cyclopenthiazide [Navidrex]) or a diuretic used in combination with a beta-blocker—i.e. a drug which blocks what are known as 'beta receptors' in the walls of small arterial blood vessels, causing them to relax and dilate. An example of a beta-blocker drug used for raised blood pressure is propranolol (Inderal).

ALTERNATIVE THERAPIES

Natural medicine

Naturopathic doctors regard hypertension as a sign of an underlying disorder that requires correction, not as a disease process which must be artificially submerged by drug therapy. Attention would be focused upon the patient's diet, lifestyle, personal stresses, ability to relax, and the amount of exercise taken. Dietary advice would be based on wholefood principles (bearing in mind the need for calorie-control in the case of overweight patients) and on eliminating salt in cooking and at table. Exercise would be carefully regulated to suit individual needs, abilities and tastes, and some regular relaxation therapy would be instituted—together with suggestions for counselling and/or psychotherapy in the case of TAB individuals.

Specific dietary supplements   Special emphasis on the following supplements:

- Vitamin E, 100iu daily, building up to a dose of 400iu daily over a

period of eight weeks (i.e. an increase in dose of 100iu every two weeks)
- Vitamin C, 1g daily, in combination with bioflavonoids
- Lecithin, 2tbsp daily, and one of cold-pressed safflower oil
- Magnesium has been found to be helpful in reducing blood pressure —two chelated magnesium tablets should be taken three times daily with food, reducing to one three times daily with food as the blood pressure drops.

Raw juice therapy   At least ½–1 litre daily is recommended of two or three of the following: celery, grapefruit, orange, pineapple, pear and cucumber. After two weeks, two or three others can be chosen.

Honey: to calm the nerves, 1tsp, 6 times daily. Cider vinegar drink (2 tsp cider vinegar to one tumbler of water) three times daily has been reputed to help. This is also helpful in weight reduction.

Pollen

This helps the body tissues to resist the ageing process.

Herbal medicine

Two foot baths and hand baths per day of the following ingredients, one handful of each to 2 litres of water: hawthorn, celandine and broom flowers, plus one head of garlic.

Aromatherapy

Three drops of ylang-ylang essence on a little brown sugar after each meal.

Bach flower remedies

Homoeopathy

For nervous strain, due to overwork and worry about the future: *Argentum Nitricum*.

Acupuncture

Acupuncture can lower the blood pressure, but it is not known whether these effects are temporary or longlasting.

Reflexology Massage to the solar plexus, then determination of which reflexes are tender; these should then be attended to.

For appropriate exercise therapy, psychological therapies and relaxation techniques, see Coronary artery disease (**III/4**).

III/6 VARICOSE VEINS

Varicosity, the process of vessel-wall stretching and dilation, most commonly occurs in the superficial veins of the legs but can also occur in the veins around and within the anus (piles), at the lower end of the foodpipe (see OESOPHAGEAL VARICES), and by the spermatic cord which suspends the testis in the scrotum. The common factor in all these cases is back pressure of blood upon the thin walls of the veins, which stretches them out of shape.

In the case of the leg veins, this is caused by inefficient return of blood to the heart and a consequent build-up of back pressure due to the force of gravity and to pelvic masses (as in pregnancy). Under normal conditions, blood is able to flow up the leg veins against the pull of gravity; the flow is helped by one-way valves inside the veins preventing the blood from running back down again. Also, the veins situated deep within the leg among the muscles, into which the veins at skin-level drain, are massaged by the squeezing action of our calf and thigh muscles as we walk and run. The act of breathing-in also helps. When we enlarge our chest capacity by lowering our diaphragms, a negative pressure develops within our chest and our lungs expand accordingly, drawing air in. This same factor encourages the flow of blood towards our hearts, with every breath we draw.

The return of vein blood ('venous return') from our legs becomes impaired when the one-way valves become weak and incompetent (this can be an inherited tendency), and when the flow in the deep veins receives insufficient muscular massage to encourage the upward flow. Blood in the deep veins can then run backwards along the connecting or 'perforating' vessels to the veins at skin-level, and cause back pressure on the ascending columns of blood within.

Other factors contributing to varicose veins include: disturbances in the nervous and hormonal control of venous return; long periods of standing still, uncompensated by sufficient leg exercise; constipation and straining (this makes the return of blood upwards into the pelvic veins an even greater problem while straining is taking place); WEIGHT PROBLEMS; the contraceptive Pill; being a woman and having children (the more, the greater the chance of varicose veins); and our modern, processed diet, in particular the lack of sufficient fibre. Other, less common, causes are thrombosis in a vein, and pressure inside the pelvis obstructing the flow of blood upwards from the leg—examples of factors are advanced pregnancy, large fibroids, or a pelvic tumour.

Symptoms of varicose veins, besides the appearance of knotted, enlarged veins, include aching throbbing legs and feet, and swelling of the feet and ankles. 10–20 per cent of the world population have varicosed leg veins, but the changes in the leg tissues preceding damage to the veins is even more widespread. When the venous return has been impaired for long enough, a reversible state called *chronic venous insufficiency* sets in, and many patients experience the RESTLESS LEGS SYNDROME. Complications of pronounced varicose veins include HAEMORRHAGE resulting from a superficial injury to an area of dilated vein; varicose ECZEMA; varicose ulcer; and thrombosis or clot-formation inside a varicosed area.

PHLEBITIS refers to INFLAMMATION of a vein, and is likely to occur in varicose veins following an infection or injury. When a clot forms within and sticks to the inflamed vein lining, the condition is known as THROMBOPHLEBITIS. The affected part of the leg is red, tender and swollen, and the patient may have a fever.

ORTHODOX TREATMENT

Varicose veins are treated by elastic support stockings or bandages; by injections which cause inflammation and ultimately scarring which puts the affected vein out of action; and by surgical removal ('stripping') and tying. A drug containing oxyrutosides, called Paroven, is sometimes prescribed for chronic venous insufficiency and for early varicose veins.

Varicose eczema is a sign of chronic venous insufficiency, and is likely to be treated with Paroven and locally applied creams and ointments. Varicose ulcers are treated in a variety of ways, including dressings (e.g. Sofra-Tulle—lanoparaffin gauze impregnated with Soframycin anti-biotic) and wound cleansers that help to remove slough (e.g., Aserbine, a combination of several ingredients). Paroven might be prescribed to combat the chronic venous insufficiency.

ALTERNATIVE THERAPIES

Since the basic problem—chronic venous insufficiency—underlies both varicose veins and their various complications (such as phlebitis and varicose ulcer), the same alternative therapies are applicable to all of these.

Natural medicine

The best diet for varicose vein sufferers is a wholefood one high in natural plant fibre, with an emphasis on daily or twice-daily salads of fresh vegetables and fruit. Lightly cooked vegetables, pulses and wholegrains are excellent; bread, pasta and other flour products should be wholewheat.

Weight reduction, giving up tobacco smoking, daily exercise involving the legs in particular, and going barefoot wherever safe to do so would all be likely lifestyle changes to be recommended. Painful varicose veins and phlebitis can be helped by splashing the affected area with cold water after bathing or washing with warm water; by wearing elastic support hose; by 'marching on the spot' leg movements, carried out even when having to remain stationary (for instance, when queuing); and by elevating the legs whenever sitting down. A 13cm block placed under the foot of the bed encourages nightly drainage away from the damaged vein area.

Raw juice therapy   Carrot juice, 170g, celery juice, 170g, and parsley juice, 60g.

Specific dietary supplements   A B-complex preparation, containing 50–100mg of these: B_1, B_2, nicotinamide (B_3) and pyridoxine (B_6); Vitamin A, 10,000–25,000iu daily for five days, then stop for two days; lecithin granules, 15g daily; 50–100mcg Vitamin B_{12}; 400–600iu Vitamin D; Vitamin E, 800–1,000iu, working up to that dose by starting with 200iu daily and increasing it by 100iu every two weeks; 2,500mg Vitamin C; 500 mg bioflavonoids; 50mg rutin; 25mg hesperidin.

Minerals: phosphorus, 900mg; potassium, 1,200mg (double the potassium during menstruation, if you drink coffee, or eat refined sugar); calcium and magnesium, which are in the correctly balanced proportions in dolomite tablets, five of which supply 750mg calcium (take 7–10 tablets daily); zinc, 15–25mg; selenium, 100–150mcg; chromium, 100–150mcg.

The Vitamin-E oral supplement is likely to help prevent phlebitis and to encourage it to disappear if already present. It is equally likely to help relieve varicose eczema and aid the healing of a varicose ulcer.

Vitamin-E cream can be applied beneficially either to the eczematous skin or to the ulcer or to an area of phlebitis.

Honey was recommended as an application to help ulcers heal by Hippocrates in the fourth century BC; but probably a better application of a bee product to varicose ulcers consists of a lanolin and propolis ointment applied twice weekly until healing is well established. This ointment is then replaced by an application of propolis tincture, and the ulcer covered with sterile gauze to encourage drying and further healing.

Cider vinegar has been reputed to help relieve the pain and swelling of varicose veins. The following drink, taken three times daily, also aids weight reduction when taken as part of a calorie-controlled diet: one tumbler of water, to which is added 2tsp of cider vinegar.

Biochemic tissue salts   *Calc. Fluor.* is recommended for varicose veins and varicose ulcers, in a dose of 4 tablets, 6 times daily, gradually reducing in frequency as the condition improves.

Herbal medicine

Hand baths (not foot baths) of the following ingredients in two litres of water: one handful each of hawthorn, broom flowers, yarrow and rose petals. Alternatively, an infusion of a pinch of each of the following to one large cup of water: vervain, mint, sage and basil; drink one large cup daily.

For varicose ulcers: comfrey, a warm poultice made of mashed roots of the comfrey plant; or an ointment made from including some strong infusion of comfrey root with some Vitamin-E cream.

Aloe vera gel, applied to varicose leg ulcers, can be most useful in bringing about healing.

Aromatherapy

To treat varicose veins, the following ointment: 1,000g sweet almond oil, 250g white wax, 30g tincture of benzoin, and 25g oil of cypress. To treat a varicose ulcer: wash the ulcer with distilled water and 2 per cent essence of cloves.

Homoeopathy

Hamamelis tincture, applied locally when acute. When condition follows childbirth: *Pulsatilla*. When the circulation is poor: *Carbo Vegetabilis*.

Acupuncture

This is said to be able to improve a poor circulation.

Manipulative therapy

Reflexology Massage of the reflexes to the adrenal glands and the parathyroids—the adrenals regulate muscle-tone. If digestion is a problem, work is applied to the reflexes of the intestines, and on the forearms and elbows on the places that directly correspond to the affected areas on the legs, the zones being estimated as accurately as possible. Phlebitis and varicose ulcers are believed to result from both impaired circulation and quite often a malfunction of the colon.

Exercise therapies

Dance therapy can help the patient to regain a degree of suppleness, if proper exercise has not been taken for years. Yoga is likewise beneficial —a particularly useful posture for varicose veins is the Shoulder Stand.

Ultrasound

This is known to help the healing of certain inflammatory conditions. Tested in a hospital trial against a group of control patients[56] it was applied to the problem of varicose ulcers. Both control and 'ultrasound' patients continued to receive drug therapy and ulcer dressings and, to obviate the placebo effect of the real untrasound, the control patients received a dummy variety of this therapy. The 13 patients who were treated with ultrasound (three times weekly for four weeks) experienced a 35 per cent reduction in the size of their ulcers. No such improvement was experienced by the control patients on dummy ultrasound.

IV   Disorders of the Kidneys, Ureters and Bladder

Our kidneys are two bean-shaped structures 'plastered' to the back wall of the abdomen amid a surrounding layer of fat and below a covering of the abdominal cavity's lining membrane, the peritoneum. Each kidney weighs about 150g, measures just over 10cm in length, and has a 'dip' along its inner border called the hilum. It is at this point that the renal artery (a branch of the aorta) enters to supply the kidney with blood, and here also that the renal vein leaves to drain into the inferior vena cava on its way back to the heart. Also leaving the hilum is the tubular ureter, carrying urine from the hollow renal pelvis, just inside the hilum, down into the bladder within the pelvis proper. Sitting on top of the upper pole of each kidney is an adrenal gland.

The urinary bladder lies deep within the pelvis. In a man it lies in front of the rectum; in a woman it is separated from the rectum by the womb (uterus) and vagina. It has a muscular wall, and, in an adult man, an average capacity of about 500ml. The bladder is usually emptied when it contains around 300ml of urine; when it contains approximately full capacity pain is felt and the desire to pass urine becomes urgent.

The bladder leads into the urethra, from which it is separated by a ring of strong muscle which is in a state of permanent constriction until the bladder is emptied by the contraction of its muscular walls. A man's urethra is far longer than that of a woman, as it runs through the prostate gland situated at the neck of the bladder and along the length of the penis before opening to the exterior.

Each kidney contains around one million nephrons, which are its microscopic 'work units'. Each nephron consists of a cup (Bowman's capsule) and an attached renal tubule. The cup itself contains a minute bunch of capillary blood vessels (the glomerular 'tuft'), and the renal tubule, after following a winding course, joins one of the larger collecting tubules leading into the hollow renal pelvis.

Our kidneys are among our most important 'built-in' homoeostatic mechanisms. The word 'homoeostasis' here refers to the maintenance of balanced, harmonious chemical conditions within the body, of optimum suitability for the overall functioning of our cells and their millions of metabolic processes.

Kidneys, Ureters and Bladder

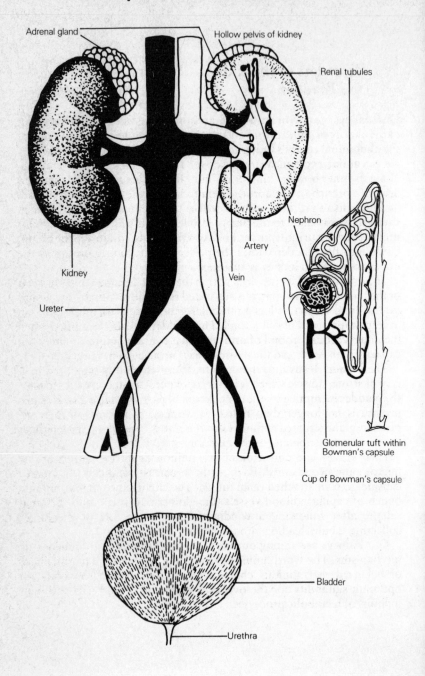

Adrenal gland

Hollow pelvis of kidney

Renal tubules

Nephron

Artery

Vein

Kidney

Ureter

Glomerular tuft within Bowman's capsule

Cup of Bowman's capsule

Bladder

Urethra

Our kidneys contribute to inner biochemical balance by regulating water and salt output and acidity; and by excreting waste material, in particular urea, produced as a breakdown product by the digestion of proteins. They also help to regulate blood pressure, and produce a hormone called erythropoietin which controls the rate of red-cell formation in the bone marrow.

The earliest stage of urine production begins as the blood speeds around the capillary blood vessels in the glomerular tuft under pressure. The result is that about 120ml of dilute fluid per minute filter out of the capillaries and across the membrane of the Bowman's capsules into the renal tubules. This filtrate consists of water, salts, glucose and waste products, but no proteins.

Clearly we cannot afford to lose fluid, salt and other nutrients at such a rate, so selective reabsorption of the materials we need to conserve takes place through the walls of the renal tubules. Here they re-enter the blood circulating through surrounding capillaries, thus altering the composition of the fluid until, as it flows into the renal pelvis and down the ureter into the bladder, by the time the renal pelvis is reached the fluid has become urine proper. Much water is conserved in this way, only 1ml of urine being formed per minute on average from every 120ml of the original filtrate. Glucose is reabsorbed; and salt is reabsorbed, or excreted in the urine, depending upon our need for it or excess of it under prevailing conditions. Thus, if the weather is very hot and we play a game of tennis and lose a lot of salt in sweat, very little will appear in the urine passed during the next few hours. If, on the other hand, we eat a very salty meal and the level in the blood rises as a result, the urine will subsequently get rid of as much salt as it can until we are in salt-balance again—i.e., until homoeostasis has been regained. This mechanism is governed by the adrenal glands, which (to simplify) secrete a hormone called aldosterone in response to our need to conserve extra salt, or withhold aldosterone when we have extra salt to get rid of.

The normal acidity-alkalinity balance of the body (pH around 7.4) is inclined to fall from its state of mild alkalinity to a more acidic state. The kidneys help to retain the necessary balance by both (a) combining excess acid with phosphate and excreting it in the urine, and (b) buffering the extra acid with bicarbonate.

How much urine we pass depends upon our water balance. The average volume for an adult is in the region of 1.5 litres daily, but if for instance we go for hours without drinking, and perhaps lose extra fluid through sweat, a VOMITING attack or a bout of DIARRHOEA, then the body fluids lack sufficient dilution and our kidneys correspondingly conserve fluid by allowing us to pass only very small quantities of concentrated urine. The reverse happens if we drink more fluid than usual. This response is governed by a specialized area in the brain called the hypothalamus, which is sensitive to small alterations in blood dilution (other reflexes are also involved). It is stimulated by extra loss of fluid from the body, and in turn stimulates the pituitary gland above it to secrete a hormone called ADH (anti-diuretic hormone). In response to this the renal tubules reabsorb more water than usual from the highly dilute glomerular filtrate. The reverse occurs when excess fluids are drunk, and ADH secretion is suppressed.

IV/1 ACUTE RENAL FAILURE

Apart from kidney cancer (see **XIII**), the main disorder, associated with the kidneys is renal failure, which can arise from a variety of causes and take either acute or chronic forms (see **IV/2** for the latter).

The function of the kidneys can fail suddenly and dramatically following a loss of blood sufficiently great to affect the normal renal blood flow of 70 litres per hour. This can occur as a consequence of sudden HAEMORRHAGE, loss of plasma following a severe burn, or SEPTICAEMIA, especially when due to the bacterium *Escherichia coli*. Acute renal failure can also follow heavy fluid-loss from the intestine due to prolonged VOMITING and/or DIARRHOEA, or from the skin during a HEATSTROKE.

The early signs of acute renal failure are a reduction in the normal amount of urine passed and the gradual accumulation of urea in the blood. Prompt treatment to restore the blood-volume to normal is essential, blood or saline solution being given by an intravenous drip. If the volume of urine fails to return to normal, or production ceases altogether and the blood level of urea continues to rise (see URAEMIA), the kidney tubules are assumed to have suffered damage. The symptoms of uraemia include anorexia, nausea, vomiting, mental confusion and muscular twitching, followed by drowsiness, COMA and HAEMOR-RHAGE. This phase can last for 1–3 weeks. If the patient survives the renal tubules gradually heal and urine production increases, while the concentration of urea in the blood starts to fall.

Treatment (for further discussion of which see under **IV/2**) consists of attention to the underlying cause, providing a protein- and salt-free diet, and replacing only the daily amount of fluid normally lost in urine and through the skin and lungs. Protein is withheld so as to reduce protein digestion (and thereby urea formation) to a bare minimum; minerals are withheld since none are being excreted.

A typical diet would be 100–300g of lactose dissolved in 500ml of water, since 100g sugar daily spares utilization of the body protein and allows the body to make use instead of its own fat store as a source of energy. A light diet with a little protein and sufficient water to cover the amount lost in the urine is given once the kidneys start working again.

IV/2 CHRONIC RENAL FAILURE

In contrast to the acute form (IV/1) chronic renal failure progresses without producing symptoms until the point at which the kidneys have suffered extensive damage. A raised blood-pressure (i.e. secondary hypertension—see III/5) might be the first indication of the disorder, perhaps accompanied by the passage of large volumes of very dilute urine (due to the kidneys' failure to concentrate the urine as they normally do). The blood's acidity and content of both potassium and sodium salts may be disturbed. As the disorder progresses the urine volume is likely to become reduced and URAEMIA to arise.

ORTHODOX TREATMENT

The orthodox approach includes a restricted protein intake, sufficient liquids to balance the urine produced, and treatment of any complications. These can include congestive cardiac failure (due to the hypertension), anaemia (due to failed erythropoietin production—see page 339), and bone disorders resulting from a disturbance in calcium and Vitamin-D metabolism. Kidney dialysis and transplantation offer the best hope to many patients. The commonest cause of chronic failure of renal function is GLOMERULONEPHRITIS; the second most common is kidney infection (PYELONEPHRITIS). Others include damaged renal arteries (e.g. by ATHEROMA) and congenital disorders such as polycystic kidney.

ALTERNATIVE THERAPIES

Natural medicine

The regulation of diet plays as important a part in the naturopathic approach as it does in the orthodox approach—and for an additional reason. The naturopath would very probably agree the sense of withholding protein under certain conditions (e.g. when the kidneys obviously cannot cope with excreting the waste products of protein metabolism, as evidenced by a rising level of urea in the blood). But he or she would see the underlying cause—especially of chronic renal failure—in a different light. He or she would attribute the failure of, say, the body's homoeostatic mechanisms to control infection (e.g. in pyelonephritis) to a faulty lifestyle, imbalanced diet or excessive stress. The orthodox physician, conversely, would accept as a satisfactory explanation the ascent of bacteria from a bladder predisposed to a degree of retention of the URINE and therefore stagnation (e.g. in an elderly man with enlargement of the prostate gland—see below).

Diet therapy—orthodox and naturopathic—would therefore be similar; but the naturopathic doctor would stress the need for all food items to be whole and completely free from artificial chemicals. He or she would also seek to identify and help the patient deal with personal stress factors, and to avoid toxic pollutants such as tobacco smoke.

Raw juice therapy For disorders of the kidneys and urinary tract generally, the following to be taken twice daily between meals: ½tbsp parsley juice, 1tbsp dandelion juice, 3tbsp spinach juice, and 6tbsp carrot juice. (This would be contraindicated wherever sodium and potassium salts were supposed to be withheld.)

Specific dietary supplements All of the following, including the biochemic tissue salts, should be given to patients with acute or chronic renal failure only under professional supervision. In addition, the patient's requirement of vitamins and minerals should be worked out by a qualified nutritionist working in collaboration with the orthodox and naturopathic doctors.

Pollen tablets have been reported as useful in benign enlargement of the prostate gland,[57] sometimes a contributory cause to kidney infection (see PYELONEPHRITIS) and thereby of chronic renal failure. Pollen used alone, or in conjunction with royal jelly, has been effective in helping to relieve stress symptoms,[58] which naturopaths view as a probable contributory factor in the development of kidney and other urinary-tract infections.

For kidney infections, the following dose of propolis is recommended: 3g for the first 3 days, followed by 2g daily for the next 8 days.

Biochemic tissue salts For the presence of albumen in the urine, *Kali Phos.* or *Calc. Phos.* For pain over the kidneys (as occurs in pyelonephritis): *Ferrum Phos.* For excessive flow of very dilute urine: *Natr. Mur., Ferrum Phos.*

Herbal medicine

For kidney disorders generally, hipbaths of the following ingredients, a handful of each to two litres of water (2–3 baths daily): dog's tooth roots, maize tassels, mallow flowers. *Or* an infusion of 2 pinches to a cupful of water of each of vervain and the inner bark (or new wood) of the lime tree.

Horseradish is useful when excessive amounts of water are being retained as a result of a renal disorder: a traditional preparation consists of 30g of fresh chopped horseradish root, 15g of bruised mustard seed and 550ml of boiling water. The herbs should be left immersed in the water in a covered pot for four hours, then strained off. Three tbsp of the liquid should be taken three times daily.

A herb tea is recommended for the types of kidney and urinary problems associated with old age—in the present context, these are likely to include benign enlargement of the prostate gland, ATHEROMA affecting the renal arteries, and ascending infection resulting in attacks of pyelonephritis. The tea consists of a brew of the following ingredients: buchu leaves, bearberry, cubeb berries and althea or marshmallow root. Other herbs, such as hydrangea leaves, anise and liquorice, can be added for balance and flavour.

Aromatherapy

For uraemia and abnormal protein in the urine: four drops of juniper essence on a little brown sugar after every meal.

Homoeopathy

For burning pains in the bladder (present in infection of the bladder, leading to pyelonephritis): *Cantharis*.

Acupuncture

This can be used to lower raised blood pressure (see under Hypertension, III/5). Success has also been claimed for the use of acupuncture in the treatment of pyelonephritis and renal insufficiency.

Manipulative therapy

Reflexology The kidneys, ureters and bladder can be induced to relax in a healthy fashion if reflex pressure is applied to the correct area on each foot. Because the kidneys, ureters and bladder are regarded as a single functional unit, each is worked on, one after the other, without a pause.

Relaxation techniques

Autogenics, autosuggestion and hypnotherapy can all help the patient achieve inner harmony and contribute to an improved state of well-being.

Exercise therapy

Gentle exercise for physically unfit patients (for instance, yoga, t'ai chi, simple dance therapy) can help re-educate the muscles in healthy bending and stretching postures, at the same time relieving inner tension and preparing the way for suitable aerobic exercise later.

IV/3 KIDNEY CANCER

CARCINOMA of the kidney, the commonest type of kidney TUMOUR, accounts for less than 2 per cent of all adult malignant disease. Blood in the urine is usually the first symptom to occur, and can be accompanied by non-specific ABDOMINAL PAIN, fever, or attacks of renal colic due to blood clots obstructing one of the ureters. Removal of the kidney offers the best hope of cure.

Vitamin C has been shown in a trial involving hamsters (reported in the *Journal of Alternative Medicine*) to offer significant protection against deliberate attempts to induce renal carcinoma.[59]

Wilm's tumour is a type of kidney cancer found in young children. Surgery is usually combined with radiotherapy and drug therapy.

See also Cancer (**XIII**).

IV/4 RENAL STONES

Renal STONES (calculi) can be found in the kidney, ureters or bladder. The stones vary in composition and there is no single explanation for their formation, although many theories exist. Their size varies from tiny particles to relatively huge 'staghorn' calculi, so-called because they fill the entire renal pelvis and branch out into the calcies. A number of situations are associated with renal-stone formation. These include the stagnation of infected urine (e.g. when the bladder does not empty properly); a raised level of calcium excreted in the urine, tending to produce stones composed of calcium phosphate and oxalate (several causes exist, one being overactivity of the parathyroid glands); a raised level of uric acid excreted in the urine, as occurs in GOUT; inadequate fluid intake in relation to body fluid lost in perspiration; and an extraordinarily high consumption of milk.

Conditions in which renal stones formed from oxalate crystals are particularly likely to occur include primary hyperoxaluria, a rare congenital abnormality in which more oxalic acid or oxalate than usual is present in the urine; and certain types of MALABSORPTION,[60] especially when dietary fat is poorly absorbed—e.g. COELIAC DISEASE, chronic pancreatitis.

The commonest symptoms of a stone in the kidney are dull loin pain which is made worse by movement, and perhaps pus or red-blood cells in the urine. Renal COLIC develops when a stone formed in the kidney passes down into the ureter and gets stuck; the muscular contractions of the walls of the ureter trying to free the obstruction produce pain in the loin which soon spreads down the patient's side and into the groin, and often extends into the testicle or outer lips of the vagina. The pain can reach agonizing limits, and is often accompanied by a degree of shock, with pallor, sweating, vomiting and a fast pulse. The attack, if left untreated, may disappear after 2–3 hours or continue for several days.

ORTHODOX TREATMENT

An attack of renal COLIC is treated with injected painkillers, bed-rest and anti-spasmodic drugs to control the muscular contractions of the affected ureter. Stones that reach the ureter are frequently passed of their own accord but, if they are not, a fine tube (ureteric catheter) can be inserted under anaesthetic to induce them to pass. Stones can be removed surgically from the ureter, but this is carried out only as a last resort, since surgery in this region often causes narrowing of the ureter afterwards. Stones in the bladder or kidney pelvis may likewise have to be removed surgically.

Patients with renal stones are usually advised to drink plenty of water in order to ensure that throughout the renal tract the substances capable of forming stones are kept in as dilute a solution as is possible. Attempts might also be made to keep the patient's urine alkaline or acidic, depending upon the type of stones he or she tends to form. For example, stones with a high phosphate content are found only in alkaline urine, so a possible preventative measure might be to acidify the patient's urine with a daily dose of ammonium chloride.

Dietary advice might also be given with respect to the avoidance of foods with a high oxalate or purine content: these substances encourage the formation of oxalate and uric-acid (or urate) stones, respectively.

ALTERNATIVE THERAPIES

Natural medicine

Certain eating and drinking habits are believed to increase the likelihood of renal-stone formation, and, besides a wholefood diet rich in natural fibre, fresh fruit and vegetables, pulses, whole grains, etc., advice would be given to avoid certain items of food and drink. All advice would be directed to the needs of the individual patient.

Patients forming stones with a high oxalate content would be advised to avoid the following, since they are oxalate-rich: rhubarb, spinach, peanuts, oranges, chocolate, beetroot, strawberries and tea.[60]

Patients with the malabsorptive states mentioned above would of course have additional advice with respect to their underlying malabsorptive problem. Coeliac patients would be given gluten-free diets to follow, and people with chronic pancreatitis would be given supplementary pancreatic enzymes. Both these measures would reduce DIARRHOEA and malabsorption, and in this way discourage the formation of oxalate stones.

The research paper cited above[60] also suggests a low-fat diet for patients suffering from CROHN'S DISEASE of the final part of the small bowel (the ilium), as the most important dietary restriction, since this 'will normalize oxalate excretion (normally too high) and 'stop the diarrhoea'.

Patients forming uric acid or urate stones would be advised to avoid the following purine-rich items: offal, sardines and fish roe.

Naturopathic doctors—like orthodox ones—would advise most renal-stone patients to drink as much water daily as possible. But there is evidence that tap-water can actually contribute to stone formation if it has a high calcium content. The calcium content of the patient's normal water supply should be questioned, and the patient if necessary advised to substitute bottled mineral water with a low calcium content or to boil his or her tap-water, to precipitate out the calcium salts, before drinking it.

Specific dietary supplements Pyridoxine (Vitamin B_6) helps to reduce the concentration of oxalic acid and oxalate salt in the urine by helping to limit the body's production of oxalic acid (only a certain percentage of the oxalic acid excreted in the urine is derived from food—the rest we manufacture ourselves). The dose can either be tailored to individual requirements, judged by measuring the reduction in the concentration of oxalate in the urine, or up to 100mg can be taken per day as a dose which is likely to help.

Magnesium is also suggested as useful, in the form of its amino-acid chelate (dose about 300mg daily). Its effect is to make urine more solvent with respect to oxalates.

An abnormally high level of calcium in the urine (a condition known as hypercalcuria or hypercalcinuria) and renal stones have been found to respond to a dietary supplement of defatted rice bran;[61] the dose used was 20g daily. Processed rice bran was found to be less effective.

Raw juice therapy Beetroot, carrot and cucumber juice mixed in equal volumes, about 0.5–1 litre taken daily, are claimed to dissolve renal stones.

Biochemic tissue salts For patients with pain on passing urine, together with gravel (a fine deposit) in the urine: *Natr. Sulph.*, *Magnes. Phos.*

Herbal medicine

For kidney stones, an infusion of a half-handful of each of the following herbs: dog's tooth roots, borage flowers and burdock leaves, plus one handful of maize tassels. Drink three cupfuls per day. Also, a compress on the kidneys and foot and hand baths of the same ingredients as above, plus a half-handful of celandine leaves. Or, if these herbs are unavailable, an infusion of four pinches of the inner bark (or new wood) of the lime tree and a pinch of mint to one cupful of water. Drink three cupfuls daily.

Aromatherapy

For kidney stones: three drops of essence of hyssop on a little brown sugar three times daily.

Homoeopathy

When the stone is causing renal colic: *Berberis* (10 drops every 15 minutes of the tincture). Severe cramping pains and vomiting, improved by local application of heat: *Calcanea Carb.*

Acupuncture

This is said to be able to help relieve the pain of renal colic in some patients.

Manipulative therapy

Reflexology   Massage of the reflexes of the kidneys, pituitary, thyroid and parathyroid glands.

Exercise therapy/relaxation techniques

Insofar as stress and too little physical exercise may play a part in the production of kidney and urinary-tract disorders, both gentle exercise and relaxation are likely to help individual patients overcome personal problems and deal with stress more effectively.

IV/5 CYSTITIS AND URETHRITIS

Cystitis refers to INFLAMMATION of the bladder lining, and does not necessarily imply a bacterial infection of that organ. It is very much commoner in women, and the reason usually given is that the urethra is much shorter in the female and thus the bladder interior that much more easily reached by bacteria from the perineal region. This is true, so far as bladder infection goes. But it is also relevant to other causes of cystitis, such as chemical and mechanical irritation (see below).

Urethritis is inflammation of the lining of the urethra, or bladder outlet, and can, for the most part, be considered together with cystitis, the only exception being non-specific URETHRITIS in a man.

Some women suffer one attack of cystitis which is never repeated; others get repeated attacks without any underlying cause being immediately apparent. The symptoms can be mild or severe, transient or extending over several days or weeks. They include a burning sensation on passing urine, a sense of urgency to reach the bathroom on time, low-down abdominal pain or backache, and the passage of possibly cloudy, bloodstained and/or foul-smelling URINE. 'Frequency' also occurs, and often necessitates numerous visits to the bathroom, day and night, to pass small quantities of urine. The pain is due to the inflammatory process affecting both bladder and urethra, and is often aggravated by acidic urine. The blood is due to small cracks within either or both of these areas which open up like wounds and bleed when inflammation is present; they close up between attacks, and get torn open again with the next bout of inflammation, with repeated bleeding.

Women who suffer repeated attacks of cystitis and urethritis may be more susceptible than others both to bouts of infection and to other types of irritants. Some of the non-infective causes include ALLERGY (possible allergens include gluten, starch, lactose and the proteins present in onions, beans and cereals), severe changes of temperature (e.g. sitting on icy ground, or on top of a radiator), and constant vibration, such as occurs when driving a tractor or heavy motorbike for long periods. Others are physical irritants, such as dirt, sand or dust particles; too little liquid, making the urine very concentrated (see under Renal stones, IV/4); too many irritant drinks such as tea, strong coffee, cola-type drinks; food additives such as artificial chemicals used to colour, flavour and preserve; and food irritants, such as large quantities of hot, spicy dishes. Spermicidal cream, internal sanitary tampons and use of the sheath, cap or diaphragm can spark off attacks in susceptible women. Perfumed vaginal deodorants can also cause urethral irritation and pain on passing water, and other chemical possibilities include a residue of biological washing powder on under-clothes, the use of scented talcum powder and soap, and the chlorine in swimming baths. Further suspects are the use of bubblebath liquid and bath salts, shampooing your hair in the bath, and even the addition to bath water of a few drops of antiseptic.

In addition to women's anatomic tendency to develop cystitis and urethritis, bacteria may be aided in their entry into the female lower urinary tract by contamination of the urethral area with toilet paper used for the anus, poor personal hygiene, and sexual intercourse, which almost inevitably involves some transfer of anal and perineal bacteria forwards to the urethral opening.

ORTHODOX TREATMENT

Bed-rest and plenty of non-irritant fluids are advised. Potassium citrate solution (or a more palatable equivalent) is sometimes prescribed, and antibiotics are nearly always given. Women who suffer repeated attacks of cystitis are sometimes given a 'urethral stretch' under anaesthetic, since dilatation of the urethra sometimes treats symptoms successfully.

ALTERNATIVE THERAPIES

Natural medicine

The following is a mixture of (a) the type of advice a naturopath would give to a cystitis patient and (b) self-help guidance.

Besides advising the cystitis patient to change to a wholefood diet, the naturopath would try to discover whether any dietary items might be causing allergic reactions or irritation; for instance, it is possible to follow a perfect wholefood diet, excluding all processed foods and artificial additives, only to find that you are allergic to the organically grown beans or wheat that you eat! It is equally possible to eat a nutritionally sound diet and yet cause bladder and urethral inflammation because you add too much chilli pepper or some other strong spice to which you are sensitive. Tea, coffee (even decaffeinated) and certainly cola drinks would be banned—and possibly alcohol during the 'test' period when likely irritants were being sought.

Advice would also be given about matters of personal hygiene, emphasizing the greater need cystitis patients have for meticulous cleanliness. Angela Kilmartin, in her excellent book *Cystitis—A Complete Self-Help Guide*, advises passing urine straight after making love and washing the perineal area immediately while still sitting on the toilet. This, the author suggests, is best done by pouring cool boiled water over the perineum from a bottle, leaning back slightly and allowing the water to drench the vaginal and urethral openings and to flow down over the anus.

The safe way to use toilet paper is to wipe from front to back and then to wash the anus with warm soapy water and dry it with clean cotton wool.

It is also a sound idea to wear cotton underwear rather than nylon panties, and to choose skirts, loose-fitting trousers and open-crotch tights in preference to tight jeans, ordinary nylon tights and tight trousers which do not allow air to reach the perineal area. Unscented hand-soap is better for washing underclothes than biological washing powders—all garments should still be rinsed very thoroughly. Scented soap, talcum powder, vaginal deodorants, etc., should also be avoided to see whether symptoms improve.

The best way to deal with an attack of cystitis is to take a specimen of urine in a clean container to your doctor for bacteriological examination, and to rest at home, drinking at least 300ml of water every half-hour for the first day. Avoid drugs, drink chamomile tea for a change from the water when you wish, and try alkalinizing your urine by taking a mixture of 1 tsp sodium bicarbonate with sufficient water or runny honey.

Two other points worth noting in relation to cystitis are, firstly, that recurrent bladder infection in a small child is often associated with chronic constipation, caused by the loaded rectum weighing down on the neck of the bladder. Small children are especially prone to this cause for retention of URINE as the space within their pelvis is small. Bacteria, having reached the bladder from the perineum, are very likely to multiply in stagnant urine (Recurrent attacks in children suggest an underlying pathology.) Adults with chronic constipation are also more liable than others to have cystitis attacks.

Secondly, another habit which leads to bacterial cystitis is 'holding' one's urine for a long time rather than passing it as soon as the desire is present.

Raw juice therapy A mixture of equal volumes of freshly squeezed apple and carrot juice is said to aid cystitis. Try 600ml daily.

Specific dietary supplements Dolomite tablets have been found to relieve cystitis symptoms—the dose is six tablets with plenty of water, three times daily.

Vitamin C acidifies the urine and, while pain-relief will doubtless be far greater with an alkalizing agent (such as the bicarbonate mentioned above), making the urine more acid can put an end to the attack. The dose of Vitamin C should be 3g daily for four days, or longer if required.

Cases of cystitis have been greatly improved by taking one propolis capsule three times daily.

Biochemic tissue salts For the early stage of cystitis, when urination is frequent and burning and there is a constant urge to pass small quantities: *Ferrum Phos*. For blood in the urine: *Kali Mur*. For cystitis with prostration and scalding urine, producing a cutting pain: *Kali Phos*. For ineffectual, painful straining, producing only a few drops of urine, plus a constant urge to urinate: *Magnesia Phos*. Dosage: during acute attack, four tablets of the appropriate tissue salt half-hourly, less frequently after relief is obtained.

Herbal medicine

An infusion of a handful of each of the following to one litre of water: maize tassels, cherry stalks and bilberries, plus a half-handful of poppy. Drink 2–3 cupfuls daily. *Or* a decoction of two pinches of heather flowers to one cupful of water (2–3 cupfuls daily).

Aromatherapy

For cystitis: inhale essence of cajeput and take five drops of the essence on a little brown sugar three times daily.

Bach flower remedies

Homoeopathy

For burning pains in the bladder and painful urination: *Cantharis*. For a constant urge to urinate, especially after drinking cold water: *Cantharis*.

Acupuncture

This is claimed to help bladder irritation and cystitis.

Manipulative therapy

Reflexology.

IV/6 BLADDER CANCER

Blood in the urine is always a sign to seek professional opinion. When it occurs in cystitis, the accompanying symptoms usually make the diagnosis clear; but a growth in the bladder rarely produces pain or any other problems at first and so the only sign is occasional blood in the urine. A cystoscopy and biopsy need to be carried out in order to identify the nature of the growth (if any).

Small benign TUMOURS are the commonest type of growth inside the bladder but need to be distinguished from CARCINOMA, known to be an occupational hazard in those who work with certain chemicals, as in the rubber and dye industries. Smoking is a further risk factor.

See also Cancer (**XIII**).

V   Disorders of the Reproductive Organs

The *female breast** (mammary or milk-gland) is situated on the outside of the chest wall, on top of the chest muscles. It lies immediately below the skin and is surrounded and infiltrated by the subcutaneous (i.e. 'below-the-skin') fat in that region. Each breast consists of between 12–20 lobes, separated from one another by bands of fibrous tissue, and radiating out, starfish fashion, from the centrally placed nipple. The glandular tissue inside each lobe develops during pregnancy, and is able to produce milk when the appropriate chemical stimuli are present after birth. The milk drains into numerous small collecting ducts, which all eventually meet up with the main duct carrying the milk from them to the nipple. Before opening onto the surface, the main duct expands to form a collection-place for the milk when the baby is suckling. When the baby is held to the breast, the sucking action and pressure upon the areola (the darker area surrounding the nipple) send a stimulus to the pituitary gland, which releases a harmone called oxytocin. This signals the release of milk from the collecting ducts, and stimulates the production of further supplies. The stimuli to the pituitary gland cease to be sent when the baby is weaned onto solid food, and the supply of milk dries up.

The other main function of the female breast is as an organ of sexual attractiveness and erotic stimulation.

The *ovaries* are a pair of almond-shaped glands, situated one on either side of the womb (uterus) just below the opening of the Fallopian tube. Instead of being covered with a layer of peritoneum like the rest of the pelvic and abdominal organs, the ovary of a newborn girl has an outside layer of germinal cells and a large number of unripe follicles, each consisting of a future ovum (egg) sorrounded by a membrane.

The *womb* (*uterus*) is hollow, thick-walled and muscular, and lies deep within the pelvis behind the bladder and in front of the rectum. Positioned like a pear with the stalk pointing downwards, its wider, upper portion (or 'body') opens into the Fallopian, or uterine, tubes on

---

* Although the breast is not a reproductive organ in the usual meaning of the term, it seems logical to discuss it in this section due to its functional association.

Reproductive Organs

Structure of the Vagina

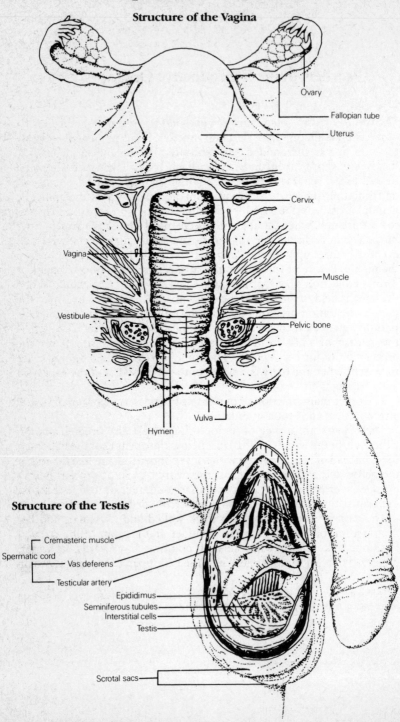

Ovary

Fallopian tube

Uterus

Cervix

Vagina

Muscle

Vestibule

Pelvic bone

Hymen

Vulva

Structure of the Testis

Cremasteric muscle

Spermatic cord

Vas deferens

Testicular artery

Epididimus

Seminiferous tubules

Interstitial cells

Testis

Scrotal sacs

each side. The womb (except during pregnancy) is typically about 7.5cm long, 5cm broad at its widest point, and about 2.5cm thick. It tapers at its lower end into the neck, or cervix, which projects and opens into the vagina. The cervix is a mainly fibrous ring which opens up during the early stages of labour.

The *vagina*, lined with mucus-secreting glands, is the passage-way between the cervix and the vulva. In the majority of girls prior to sexual intercourse or the first use of tampons, the vagina's outer opening is partially protected by a thick, fibrous membrane, the hymen. The vagina comprises the external female genitals, and includes the pair of small inner lips (the labia minora) which shelter the clitoris and the opening of the bladder (urethra).

All these structures are bounded by the pair of larger outer lips, the labia majora.

The ovary is the woman's sex gland, and its function, once the stage of puberty has been reached, is to produce a ripe ovum or egg every 28 days which is then collected by the end of the Fallopian tube. This process, ovulation, is controlled by the pituitary gland at the base of the brain. The pituitary secretes the hormone FSH (follicle-stimulating hormone) which ripens one of the immature follicles in the ovary and makes it shed a mature ovum. The ovum is encourged to fall into the open end of the Fallopian tube by finger-like processes (fimbria) at the tube's end, and travels down the length of the tube towards the hollow body of the womb. If sexual intercourse occurs around the time of ovulation the ovum may meet live sperms on its journey down the tube and be fertilized by one of them. Fertilized or unfertilized, the ovum descends to the uterus where, if unfertilized, it shrivels up and dies (atrophies). If fertilized, however, it becomes embedded in the lining of the womb wall and develops into an embryo.

While the follicle is ripening it is also secreting the hormone oes-trogen, which thickens up the thin, post-menstrual womb lining and prepares it against the eventuality of receiving a fertilized egg. When the oestrogen reaches a particular level in the blood, this is the signal for the egg inside the follicle to rupture outwards and fall into the Fallopian tube—at which point the pituitary gland ceases to secrete FSH and starts to manufacture LH (luteinising hormone) instead.

After the egg is shed, the ripe follicle from which it came develops under the influence of LH into a tiny glandular structure called the corpus luteum. At this point it produces only a little oestrogen but starts to secrete progesterone. This has the effect of thickening the lining of the womb in preparation for a developing embryo, should fertilization be successful. If the ovum is indeed fertilized the corpus luteum continues

273

to thrive and secretes hormones important to the developing baby. If the egg is unfertilized and finally discarded the corpus luteum starts to shrivel and the level of progesterone in the blood drops correspondingly. This coincides with about day 22 of the menstrual cycle (taking day one as the day on which the previous period began). The womb lining and egg are shed together as the next period, starting around day 28.

Aside from its role in the birth process, the function of the vagina clearly is to harbour the man's erect penis during intercourse, and accept the ejaculated sperms. These swim up through the cervix, and some manage to complete the journey through the womb into the Fallopian tubes.

The two *testicles* are contained within the scrotal sac. Each consists of masses of tiny coiled tubes (seminiferous tubules) enclosed in a thick fibrous protective jacket. Ultimately all the minute tubules end in the 'waiting area' or 'epididymis', a small smooth lump on the side of the testis from which the sperm tube (vas deferens) leaves on its way through the groin to the penis and the urethral opening. The vas deferens is accompanied on its course by blood vessels, and collectively these structures are known as the 'spermatic cord'. If this becomes twisted the blood supply to the testis and the flow of blood away from it are obstructed. The condition is known as torsion of the TESTIS and is a surgical emergency.

Before reaching the urethra, the vas deferens passes behind the bladder and through the substance of the prostate gland. This is about the size of a walnut, and somewhat similar in shape. It surrounds the neck of the bladder and first part of the urethra, and consists of glandular and muscular tissue.

The testicle (testis) is the organ in which the sperms (spermatozoa) and male sex hormones (androgens) are made.

There is an excellent reason why the testis is situated outside rather than inside the pelvis. Sperm production requires a temperature below body-heat to take place satisfactorily; and, when the testis fails to descend into the scrotum from the position within the abdomen it occupies during the baby's development in the womb, it is very unlikely to produce live sperm. (The production of androgens, however, is unaffected.) About 1 in 10 baby boys are born with one or both testes incompletely descended. Some need surgical correction at a later date, but in the majority of cases the missing testis will be found to have completed its journey into the scrotum within a month or two of birth.

About 200 million sperms are produced per ejaculation.

V/1 BREAST CANCER AND BENIGN BREAST DISORDERS

Benign (non-cancerous) breast disease and CARCINOMA of the breast are the two main types of breast disorder, the first being a greater deal more common than the second. There are several overlapping varieties of benign breast disease—breast pain and swelling, which can be irregular, or occur only during the days leading up to a period (see PREMENSTRUAL SYNDROME); fibrocystic disease, consisting of INFLAMMATION of fibrous tissue and the development of cysts (this can also be more severe before a period starts); benign breast TUMOURS; and breast cysts.

Benign disorders of the breast are common among women whose diet includes a high proportion of saturated animal fat and rare among those who eat little saturated animal fat but take in a high proportion of essential fatty acids (e.g. those present in cold-pressed vegetable oils). Because the hormone prolactin, secreted by the pituitary, stimulates breast development, it was thought for some time that high levels of it were responsible for benign breast disease. High prolactin levels are found in a few women with this complaint, but the majority of women with benign breast disease have normal levels of prolactin. Consequently it has been suggested that the underlying cause is unusual sensitivity to the influence of normal levels of prolactin. Essential fatty acids, and a class of prostaglandins (hormone-like substances) derived from them, can inhibit the effect of prolactin in certain body tissues, including breast tissue, and since benign breast complaints are associated with a low intake of essential fatty acids a partial deficiency of them and the relevant prostaglandins was suggested as the underlying cause.

BREAST LUMPS

It is vital to distinguish between harmless tumours and early malignant ones. If you discover any kind of a lump you should get your doctor to examine you as soon as possible.

You should examine your breasts once a month (to be on the safe side). Do this by inspecting them first of all to note any changes in shape, position, nipple appearance or skin colour or texture. Carry this out by viewing them in a large mirror in a good light, first with your arms by your sides and then with them raised above your head. Squeeze each nipple to test for a discharge, and then examine each breast with the flat of the fingers and the fingertips of the opposite hand. Go over the entire area in a clockwise direction, including the armpit area (where the lymph glands might be enlarged) and the area of skin up to the top of your ribs. Some women carry out this part of the examination in the bath. If you do this, make sure you carry out the fingertip examination when you are standing upright as well, as the breasts should be felt when you are both horizontal and vertical.

Mastitis is INFLAMMATION of a breast lobe, generally occurring during breast-feeding and due to a blocked main milk duct followed by bacterial infection. The condition normally responds rapidly to antibiotics. Breast-feeding should then be continued.

BREAST CANCER

CARCINOMA of the breast is (with the possible exception of lung cancer) the commonest malignant disease in women, most cases occurring in the age group 45–59. Oestrogen is suspected to play a large part in malignant breast disease, both the natural hormone secreted by the ovaries and the synthetic product given in the Pill, etc. In fact, much controversy has surrounded the link between the Pill and breast cancer. Some studies have failed to show any connection; but others have found a definite link.

In some countries breast cancer is a rarity—these include the underdeveloped countries and Japan. Among the reasons suggested for this are that, in underdeveloped countries, women tend to have babies shortly after puberty, to breast-feed them as long as possible, and to have a far greater number of pregnancies than is usual in the West. The effect of this is that ovulation and the secretion of oestrogen are suppressed for long periods, and oestrogen has less opportunity to have a harmful effect.

Also, in many places in the developing world women eat a great deal less animal fat and sugar than we do in the West. This is true also of Japanese women, and evidence is accumulating to link this type of cancer with dietary factors. A likely explanation seems to be that obesity and a high fat intake effect the way the body deals chemically with and stores oestrogen.

The *Journal of Alternative Medicine* (November 1984) quoted the results of a trial[62] that had been carried out to test the hypothesis that carbohydrates (specifically sugar) may play a role in causing cancer of the breast. Rats were used to test the effects of three dietary carbohydrates: sucrose, lactose and cornstarch. The rats fed on lactose had the lowest incidence of chemically induced TUMOURS, whereas those fed on sucrose and cornstarch developed a significantly greater number of cancerous tumours. This result suggested that dietary carbohydrates have a significant effect in promoting breast cancer.

A further report in the same journal (August 1984) quoted a review[63] citing evidence suggesting that a high intake of total fat (i.e. the total intake of fat, whatever the source) increases our susceptibility to cancer, particularly of the breast and the colon.

ORTHODOX TREATMENT

Painful, lumpy breasts due to non-malignant conditions are treated with painkillers, sometimes with diuretic drugs to relieve swelling, and sometimes with the drugs danazol (Danol) and bromocriptine (Parlodel). The orthodox treatment of breast cancer depends upon the size of the TUMOUR and on whether it has spread to adjoining lymph nodes and other places in the body (see SECONDARIES); it also takes into account whether 'oestrogen-receptor protein' can be detected. The usual surgery is either a mastectomy to remove the whole breast and affected lymph glands or, increasingly, removal of the cancerous tumour only, following radiation treatment. (See also Cancer, **XIII**.)

ALTERNATIVE THERAPIES

The following account refers only to benign breast disease unless breast cancer is specifically mentioned; the alternative approaches to cancer treatment are treated in **XIII**.

Natural medicine

The best diet to follow for healthy breasts is unquestionably a wholefood one. This eliminates all artificial additives and includes plenty of natural fibre, very little sugar and animal fat, and utilizes even cold-pressed vegetable oils and polyunsaturated margarines sparingly. Chemical substances named methylxanthines (e.g. caffeine, theophylline) present in tea, coffee and cola drinks increase the effect of prolactin on breast tissue. Diets for benign breast disease should therefore exclude these items. A naturopathic practitioner would certainly attempt to correct the patient's body-weight by overall calorie reduction, if she were obese or inclined that way. Moreover, fruit and vegetables, in particular the cruciferous vegetables, show a protective effect against cancer in various areas of the body, and their inclusion in the diet is therefore an excellent idea for overall protection.[62] (The cruciferous vegetables are those with cross-shaped flowers; e.g. turnips, cabbage and cress.)

The naturopathic doctor would also review the patient's lifestyle and advise on the elimination of certain stress factors, as well as the avoidance wherever feasible of pollutants and toxins—e.g. petrol and diesel fumes, tobacco, large quantities of alcohol. Adequate exercise would be advised. Useful for well shaped youthful breasts is 'windmilling' the arms round and round, making circles as large as possible—say 20 forward windmills and 20 backward ones daily.

Hydrotherapy   This is often held to contribute to healthy breast tissue. Cold water can be splashed onto the breasts for two minutes daily, after showering in warm water. Alternatively, a special device called Aquamaid, which you attach to a cold-water tap, can be used to massage and stimulate the breasts, thereby improving the circulation and toning up the supportive connective tissue. It is said to improve the shape, and help correct 'sag'. (Aquamaid is available from the Cantassium Company, 225 Putney Bridge Road, London SW15 2PY.)

A positive correlation has been established between the patient's attitude and the prognosis of breast cancer. This was discovered by the Society for Psychosomatic Research and reported in *Doctor* (3 May, 1984), but in general naturopathic doctors are more likely than orthodox ones to be aware of the benefits of a positive mental attitude.

Raw juice therapy   For healthy breast tissue, 300ml daily carrot juice, 150ml cabbage juice and 150ml cress or turnip juice.

Specific dietary supplements   For overall breast protection, those nutrients believed to offer protection against cancerous changes in the body, namely Vitamins C, A and E, and selenium. Vitamin E was reported years ago as valuable in benign breast disease, and a more recent study carried out at the Johns Hopkins hospital confirmed this: the suggested dose is 600mg daily.

Evening primrose oil (Efamol) has been tested in a double-centre (Universities of Wales and Dundee), placebo-controlled, double-blind crossover study in women with breast pain and fibrocystic breast disease. It was found to produce 'highly significant improvement in breast pain, breast lumpiness and general well-being'.[64] The recommended dose is three 500mg capsules twice daily.

Pollen has been reported to increase the size, firmness and shape of breasts, from which one might perhaps deduce an improvement in the health of the breast tissue itself.

Biochemic tissue salts   Sore, tender breasts may be helped by *Calc. Phos.*, four tablets every half-hour and then less frequently as condition begins to respond.

Aromatherapy

For painful breasts: bathe with pure, fresh water containing 2g essence of geranium (*Pelargonium odorantissimum* or *Geranium robertianum*). Alternatively, apply the following cream on retiring: 1,000g sweet almond oil, 250g white wax, 50g essence of geranium, 600ml distilled water.

Bach flower remedies

Homoeopathy

For benign, painful breast conditions: *Calcarea Ostrearum*. Painful breasts during pregnancy: *Conium Maculatum*.

Acupuncture

It is claimed that mastitis has been helped by acupuncture, although whether this refers to true mastitis or benign breast disease is not clear.

Manipulative therapies

Reflexology For cysts, swellings and lumps which have been reliably diagnosed as benign, massage is applied to the top of the feet, from the fifth through to the second zone.

Relaxation techniques Biofeedback may be of help to anxious, over-stressed women; hypnotherapy; autosuggestion; self-hypnosis.

Exercise therapy

Yoga exercises known to aid the breast and its development include Bow, Cobra, Head of a Cow. Other exercise therapies as may be applicable for the release of tension and the establishment of fitness and weight loss—e.g. dance therapy.

V/2 OVARIAN TUMOURS AND CARCINOMA OF THE OVARY

Ovarian tumours are a common problem, and include both true cysts and solid structures. They are often referred to as 'cysts' regardless of their make-up. They may cause no symptoms, or merely vague attacks of ABDOMINAL PAIN. On the other hand they can produce long periods of irregular bleeding; an absence of periods; or PERITONITIS if they bleed into the abdominal cavity.

Some cysts arise from the retention of a Graafian follicle (a mature follicle just prior to ovulation) or a corpus luteum; these are known as *retention cysts* and do not become malignant. Others arise as 'new growths' from the ovarian cells, and 15 per cent of these are cancerous. Besides malignancy, they are also affected by the following complications. *Torsion* involves twisting of the 'stalk' by which an ovarian tumour is attached, causing, when the blood supply is obstructed altogether, severe abdominal pain, nausea, vomiting, pallor and sweatiness. *Haemorrhage* into the centre of a cyst produces similar symptoms. *Rupture* can produce peritonitis. *Infection* of an ovarian cyst occurs by spread from a nearby organ, such as an infected, inflamed appendix, and produces pain, fever and a fast pulse.

Although this can occur at any age, it is most commonly found between the ages of 40 and 60. The cancer can be cystic from a cyst or solid in consistency; the first symptom is usually enlargement of the abdomen. Periods remain regular, but the patient may complain of vague ABDOMINAL PAIN and INDIGESTION.

The November 1984 issue of the *Journal of Alternative Medicine* mentioned two studies which had detected links between ovarian cancer and the diet. The first of these,[65] carried out in New England, revealed an association with high animal-fat consumption; the second report,[66] from Milan, indicated that drinking coffee probably increased the risk of ovarian cancer. The contraceptive Pill, incidentally, may help to protect against it.

TREATMENT

Many retention cysts regress spontaneously. Often a laparoscopy (diagnostic operation) is carried out if the diagnosis is in doubt. A bleeding corpus luteal cyst may well be misdiagnosed as an ectopic pregnancy (pregnancy situated in the Fallopian tube instead of the womb). If this is found on operation, the bleeding is stopped and the abdominal cavity mopped out.

Other varieties of ovarian cysts are treated as though malignant change were present, and a laparotomy is carried out. The possible operation then decided upon depends on the sort of cyst found. Either the cyst is removed and the rest of the ovary reconstituted (this is for benign cysts in girls and women still of reproductive age), or the whole ovary is removed—this would be the case with large cysts leaving little normal ovarian tissue, or when torsion of haemorrhage into the cyst had occurred. Both ovaries are generally removed if CARCINOMA is present. Radiotherapy and cytotoxic drugs might also be used.

For the alternative approach to malignant tumours, see **XIII**.

V/3 PELVIC INFLAMMATORY DISEASE

This can be an imprecise term, referring in many cases to infection of the Fallopian tubes (salpingitis—see **V/4**). The term can also be used of any condition giving rise to lower ABDOMINAL PAIN, tenderness on movement of the cervix and inside the fornix, and often to fever as well. However, the term is a very useful one, because it recognizes that the infection often involves much of the pelvic region, not just a single organ or area.

In this book, for the sake of convenience, we will take the term to include the most important conditions involving inflammation of the pelvic organs; i.e. salpingitis, pelvic abscess (**V/5**), endometritis (**V/6**), cervicitis (**V/7**) and vaginitis (**V/8**). Alternative therapies for these are discussed under **V/8**. Atrophic vaginitis, thinning of the vaginal lining membrane in post-menopausal women, is discussed under Menopause (**V/14**).

V/4 SALPINGITIS

One or both Fallopian tubes can become inflamed as a result of infection, the organism most usually responsible being the gonococcus (which causes gonorrhoea). Other bacteria which can be responsible include streptococci and staphylococci; infection by them was a common complication of illegal abortions when the operation was not performed under sterile conditions. *Chlamydia* is another likely cause, and salpingitis can also follow acute appendicitis (see **I/16**).

The symptoms of *acute salpingitis* are lower ABDOMINAL PAIN, irregular bleeding, malaise, fever and pain when the cervix is moved on internal examination.

Chronic salpingitis is a common condition, producing pain on intercourse and heavy, painful periods. The ovary on the affected side is usually inflamed as well. The bacteria frequently involved include intestinal ones—*Escherichia coli* and *Streptococcus faecalis*; the gonococcus is involved when the condition results from gonorrhoea. Fertility is often adversely affected, and ectopic pregnancy may become more likely. The seriousness of pelvic inflammatory disease should not be underestimated.

ORTHODOX TREATMENT

For the acute condition bed-rest is prescribed, together with pain-killers and antibiotics. A chronically infected and damaged Fallopian tube might be incised and drained, or removed surgically.

The chronic form is harder to treat. Antibiotics are generally prescribed only when the symptoms periodically become acute, when bed-rest is also indicated. The operation salpingostomy is sometimes performed for infertility: it involves opening up the Fallopian tube.

V/5 PELVIC ABSCESS

The symptoms and treatment are similar to those of salpingitis (**V/4**). See also ABSCESS.

V/6 ENDOMETRITIS

The cause of an inflamed womb lining is usually bacterial infection. This was a common complication of 'back-street' abortions, and is still seen following serious pelvic injury allowing the entry of bacteria. The symptoms include low ABDOMINAL PAIN, low BACKACHE, and sometimes heavy loss of blood during periods.

ORTHODOX TREATMENT

Bed-rest, antibiotics, pain-killers.

V/7 CERVICITIS

Chronic cervicitis and cervical erosions cause a vaginal discharge which may be white or bloodstained, or contain pus if infection is present. Itching and irritation are uncommon, but the discharge is invariably worse in the days before a period starts. Vaginal bleeding between periods may occur: this is a symptom about which you should always consult your doctor.

The commonest organism to cause infective cervicitis is the gonococcus; such cases are due to the venereal infection, gonorrhoea. The *Chlamydia* organism too can cause cervicitis. Herpes simplex (see **XII/3**) can also be the cause; the genital-herpes virus (HSV-2) produces painful blisters and ulcers on the cervix, and in the vaginal lining and the vulva (the penis tip and shaft are affected in the man). Lesions can spread to the perineum, thighs and buttocks. Genital herpes is being recognized more and more often now; more than 10,000 new cases are reported annually in the UK. The widely publicized association of cervical cancer with genital herpes remains unproven.[67]

THRUSH can also cause cervicitis.

ORTHODOX TREATMENT

Antibiotics are prescribed when a cervical swab shows evidence of bacterial infection. It is usually a good idea to include the woman's sexual partner in the treatment.

Herpes infections of the cervix, vagina and vulva are treated with acyclovir (Zovirax). This can be given by intravenous injection, by mouth, or applied to the lesions. It is said to be virtually nontoxic, but some doubt exists.

Candida infection is treated with the anti-fungal drug nystatin (Nystan).

V/8 VAGINITIS

Inflammation of the vagina is generally accompanied by irritation of the area and a vaginal discharge. The most usual infectious causes are THRUSH, due to *Candida albicans*; trichomoniasis, due to *Trichomonas vaginalis*; and gonorrhoea.

Thrush causes a cheesy white discharge, and can be intolerably itchy. Trichomoniasis, generally acquired during sexual intercourse, produces a copious, bubbly, greenish discharge with a fishy smell, and is accompanied by soreness and irritation. Intercourse is often painful. Conococcal vaginitis typically inflames the urethra (bladder outlet) as well, and often accompanies cervicitis. Discharge is present in the urethra as well as the vagina.

Another possible cause of vaginitis is the presence of a foreign body in the vagina—for instance, a variety of objects are inserted for sexual gratification, and tampons can be forgotten about and get lost.

ORTHODOX TREATMENT

This consists of the appropriate antibiotic (anti-fungal in the case of *Candida* infection). Metronidazole (Flagyl) is given by mouth for trichomoniasis; and intramuscular penicillin is given for gonorrhoea. Foreign bodies are removed if present.

ALTERNATIVE THERAPIES

Natural medicine

For pelvic inflammatory disease generally (see exceptions below), a wholefood diet with particular emphasis upon the reproductive parts of plants and animals, including raw, leafy and root vegetables, nuts and seeds, a little fresh milk and fish roe. Sufferers from genital herpes are advised to avoid activities known to stimulate viral activity; e.g. smoking, excessive alcohol, and drugs such as aspirin, diuretics and antidepressants. Emotional and physical stress should also be avoided. Women should blot well after urination and wipe from front to back. Twice-daily vaginal douching with water is advised, as is douching after intercourse. Loose cotton underclothes are recommended.[68]

Recurrent infections—including thrush and herpes—are regarded by holistic practitioners as a sign that the body's defence mechanism is out of order. In particular, repeated courses of antibiotics, steroid drugs and the contraceptive Pill are regarded as contributory factors.

For dietary advice specific to thrush infection, see THRUSH. For the alternative treatment of herpes, see herpes simplex (**XIII/3**).

Hydrotherapy Immersion of the bottom and pelvis up to the navel in cold water for half a minute once or twice daily, keeping the rest of the body warmly clothed.

Specific dietary supplements Raw garlic has natural bactericidal properties, and four large cloves of it should be eaten daily. The amino acid arginine enhances the function of the thymus gland, thus assisting the body's defence mechanism. Dose: 1–2g daily on an empty stomach. (NB: arginine should not be taken by people who suffer from herpes or schizophrenia.)

For infection of the sexual organs, take 3g propolis daily for the first three days, and 2g daily for the next eight days.

Pollen is said to increase vigour and speed recovery following illness, which may well be helpful in cases of pelvic inflammatory disease.

Raw juice therapy For decreased resistance to infection, carrot juice, 170ml, and celery juice, 170ml.

Biochemic tissue salts For profuse white vaginal discharge: *Kali Mur*. For yellow-green, slimy (i.e. pus-containing) discharge: *Kali Sulph*. Dose: four tablets every 15 minutes, reducing as the condition improves.

Herbal medicine

For vaginal discharge, 2–3 douches daily of the following ingredients (one handful of each to 2 litres water): elecampane leaves, bramble leaves, rose petals, sage. *Aloe vera* gel has been found useful for THRUSH infection of the vagina, PRURITUS VULVAE and venereal sores.

Aromatherapy

For heavy vaginal discharge: 4–5 drops of essence of rosemary on a little brown sugar after each meal.

Homoeopathy

For pelvic inflammatory disease when pus is being produced: *Hepar Sulphur*.

Acupuncture

This is claimed to help pelvic pain, vaginal discharge, heavy menstrual bleeding, vaginal pain, itching, and ovarian pain.

Relaxation techniques

These are of great general benefit, perhaps especially so for sufferers from genital herpes, as herpetic infections are known to break out under conditions of mental fatigue, repressed emotions and stress. Biofeedback, autogenics, hypnotherapy and autohypnosis all have something to offer.

Exercise therapy

Dance therapy, T'ai chi and yoga can improve overall fitness. Asanas (yoga postures) recommended for uterine disorders and vaginal discharge are Shoulderstand, Headstand, and Locust.

V/9 CANCER OF THE CERVIX

Much has been written about cervical cancer in recent years, and much of this about the inadequate screening facilities and instances of inexcusable failure to inform women of positive cervical smears. It is one of the commonest forms of cancer in women but is curable if detected early by a smear test. This test was introduced in the 1950s, since when deaths due to the disorder had—until recently—dropped dramatically wherever the smear was used.

Cervical cancer is now regarded as developing through two separate mechanisms, the familiar one affecting older women and a new one affecting younger women and previously low-risk groups such as the non-promiscuous and the higher social classes. The first of these typically occurs in the ages 45–55, and a predisposing factor is believed to be early promiscuity. The second variety is believed to be due to the human papilloma virus (HPV), present in genital warts (see V/17). One study revealed that 9 out of 25 women whose partners had penile warts had precancerous smears. When a particular variety of HPV was present (type 16) 80 per cent of women had precancerous changes. In some cases, the man's occupation is associated with an increased or decreased risk of inducing cervical cancer in their partners. Fishermen and lorry drivers carry a high risk, clergymen a low risk.

It has also been found that second wives run six times the normal risk of contracting cervical cancer if first wives have had it.

The new variety of cancer is harder to treat than the older type. It progresses more rapidly, and the survival chances are considerably lower—especially since its rapid progress means that screening may very well be far too late.

TREATMENT

Surgery and radiotherapy are the mainstay of treatment. Attempts are being made to grow the virus believed to be responsible for the new type of cervical cancer, and thereby ultimately to develop a vaccine to it.

For alternative approaches see XIII.

V/10 FIBROIDS

These are benign growths in the wall of the womb (uterus), composed of smooth muscle fibres and fibrous connective tissue. Their most important symptom is abnormal bleeding, in particular a very heavy flow of

blood during periods (MENORRHAGIA). Fibroids produce this by projecting into the uterine cavity and increasing the total bleeding area, and
by preventing the blood vessels from clamping down properly at the end
of the period. Their cause is not known. The symptoms they can
produce (besides heavy periods) include: ABDOMINAL PAIN due to the
torsion of a fibroid's stalk (pedicle; some, just below the outer surface of
the womb, grow outwards on a stalk into the abdominal cavity); a lump
in the abdomen; a desire to pass water often (due to pressure on the
bladder); bleeding between periods (metrorrhagia); and infertility.

ORTHODOX TREATMENT

Small fibroids can safely be left alone. Large ones are removed either by
a myomectomy, in which the fibroids are removed from the wall of the
womb, or by a hysterectomy. The latter is usually performed only when
the fibroids are both large and multiple.

V/11 ENDOMETRIOSIS

A condition in the tissue normally lining the womb (the endometrium)
is also located elsewhere, such as in the wall of the womb, the wall of the
bladder, or in other pelvic organs, most commonly the ovary. The tissue
clumps, which appear as small, mauve-black spots in the pelvic cavity,
bleed inwards in sympathy with the womb lining itself, in response to
the menstrual-cycle hormones. In areas permitting the clumps to expand, such as the ovary, cysts (known as chocolate cysts) full of altered
blood form. Symptoms include MENORRHAGIA, painful periods (see
V/12), pain on intercourse (DYSPAREUNIA) and infertility.

ORTHODOX TREATMENT

This includes surgery to destroy the abnormal clumps of womb lining.
Sometimes drugs are used to suppress cyclical activity in the clumps.
Pregnancy also often alleviates the symptoms, both for the duration
(because menstruation ceases) and thereafter.

ALTERNATIVE THERAPIES

Natural medicine

A diet which has been successfully recommended for heavy or prolonged periods, and sometimes successfully for fibroids and endometriosis, eliminates sugar and includes protein at a rate of 1g/kg bodyweight, plus supplements. The aims of the diet and supplements are to counteract the injurious effect of oestrogen in the body and to speed the liver's conversion of naturally produced oestrogen into the harmless form, oestriol. Naturopathic doctors would recommend also that the diet followed should be wholefood.

Specific dietary supplements

- Vitamin-B complex, 100mg, twice daily
- Vitamin B_6 (pyridoxine), total of 50mg, three times daily
- lecithin granules or capsules, sufficient to supply 244mg each of choline and inositol
- dessicated liver tablets, go by manufacturer's instructions
- yeast tablets (not when *Candida* infection is/might be present), go by manufacturer's instructions
- Vitamin E, build up to 400iu daily over a course of one month. Selenium, 50mcg daily

Raw juice therapy   The following is recommended for TUMOURS and may perhaps contribute to the shrinking of fibroids: a combination of watercress, spinach, carrot and turnip leaves in equal parts, 1.2 litres of the combination to be drunk daily.

Biochemic tissue salts   For dysmenorrhoea and congestion of the pelvic organs, starting several days before the period: *Ferrum Phos.* alternating with *Magnesia Phos.* during the attack. Dose: four tablets every 15 minutes, less frequently when symptoms start to respond.

Herbal medicine

For metrorrhagia (bleeding between periods), vaginal douches, foot and hand baths using one handful each of the following ingredients to 2 litres of water: hawthorn flowers, celandine, mallow, bramble and sage plus one crushed head of garlic.

Aromatherapy

For pain during menstruation: three drops of essence of cypress on a little brown sugar three times daily.

Homoeopathy

Caulophyllum 3× taken every 15 minutes when periods are heavy and when bleeding occurs between periods. Note that an orthodox medical practitioner should *always* be consulted when bleeding is irregular.

Acupuncture

This is said to help pelvic pain, irregular periods and 'flooding'.

V/12 PAINFUL PERIODS (DYSMENORRHOEA)

There are two main varieties of dysmenorrhoea. The first (*primary dysmenorrhoea*) is not associated with pelvic disease. It typically affects teenagers and young women, and is likely to disappear after the birth of a child. Period pain is associated with menstrual cycles in which ovulation takes place. Generally a girl's first few periods are not ovulatory ones, which is why periods are often trouble-free when they start but become difficult after a year or so. The mechanism for the pain in primary dysmenorrhoea is believed to be due to the womb manufacturing an excess of hormone-like substances named prostaglandins. These can be helpful or injurious to us, depending upon their type. Those made by the uterus during a period cause the womb to clamp down in a cramp-like fashion, causing low BACKACHE and ABDOMINAL PAIN. They also escape into the bloodstream, where they are thought to affect organs elsewhere in the body, producing other symptoms associated with difficult menstruation. These include headache, nausea, vomiting, intestinal upsets and FAINTING spells.

The second type of painful period (*secondary dysmenorrhoea*) is far commoner in older women. There is usually an underlying cause of this variety in the form of a pelvic disorder: possibilities include fibroids (V/10), endometriosis (V/11) and chronic pelvic inflammatory disease (V/3 *et seq.*). In a small number of women an IUCD (intra-uterine contraceptive device) can cause very severe period pain.

ORTHODOX TREATMENT

Many women rely on home remedies for painful periods, including bed-rest, a hot-water bottle applied to the stomach or low back, and mild pain-killers such as aspirin or paracetamol.

Drugs prescribed for primary dysmenorrhoea include prostaglandin-synthetase inhibitors (i.e. drugs which suppress the formation of the prostaglandins, examples being mefanamic acid [Ponstan] and indomethacin [Indocid]); the combined oestrogen/progestogen contraceptive Pill, which suppresses ovulation; and progestogen hormones (e.g. dydrogesterone [Duphaston], norethisterone [Primolut N]).

Treatment for secondary dysmenorrhoea is related to its underlying cause.

ALTERNATIVE THERAPIES

Natural medicine

The menstrual blood-flow is regarded by many alternative practitioners as the body's periodic elimination of toxic waste matter (although exactly what is meant by 'toxic' in this context is open to doubt). Painful periods, associated headaches, nausea, etc., are seen as representing an underlying disharmony within the body rather than a chemically mediated effect. This includes secondary dysmenorrhoea, in which the underlying chronic inflammation of the pelvis or the fibroids (V/10) are seen more as the agent by which troublesome menstruation is brought about, rather than the basic reason for its occurrence.

A naturopathic practitioner would advise a wholefood diet and possibly periodic fruit or fruit-juice fasts as a means of cleansing the body of accumulated wastes. A routine of gentle exercise would be advised, building up to sessions of aerobic exercise carried out several times weekly. The learning of relaxation would be advised as well.

Specific dietary supplements

- Magnesium orotate, 500mg daily
- Vitamin-B complex, 50mg twice daily (see that your total intake of Vitamin B_6 is 100–150mg daily, including what you get in the B-complex preparation)
- Vitamin E, chewable tablets, 100iu, twice daily
- Vitamin C, 1,000mg daily
- ferrous gluconate
- folic acid, 25mcg daily
- Vitamin B_{12}, 5mcg daily
- Pollen, taken with royal jelly, has been tested in a Yugoslavian gynaecology clinic and found to relieve severe primary dysmenorrhoea in a large number of cases

Raw juice therapy   A 600ml glass of blueberry and huckleberry juice, daily.

Biochemic tissue salts   For painful periods in girls shortly after puberty, still having a scanty show of blood: *Calcarea Phos*. Chief remedy for cramping labour-like pain during periods: *Magnesia Phos*.

Herbal medicine

For painful periods, vaginal douches using each of the following to 2 litres of water: yarrow, mint leaves, parsley and sage. Also for painful periods, foot and hand baths made from two handfuls of fresh nettle leaves in 1 litre of water. To reduce heavy periods, an infusion of two handfuls of fresh nettle leaves in a small cup of water; take three cupfuls daily.

Bach flower Remedies

Aromatherapy

For irregular periods: two drops of cumin essence on a little brown sugar twice daily between meals. To treat painful or irregular periods: five drops of tarragon essence on a little brown sugar between meals.

Homoeopathy

For irregular periods, too early and maybe too heavy: *Calcium Phosphate*. Periods delayed, scanty yet protracted, in fair-haired, blue-eyed women: *Pulsatilla*. Periods delayed, in dark-haired women: *Sepia*. For heavy periods in young girls: *Calcium Carbonate*.

Acupuncture

This is suitable for painful and irregular periods.

Relaxation techniques

Tension and stress tend to make painful periods more painful. Yoga is often recommended for women suffering from period pains, especially helpful positions being Uddiyana, Cobra, Posterior Stretch, Fish and Plough.

Exercise therapy

Dance therapy, to get the physically unfit girl or woman used to 'moving again', followed at a later date by some type of aerobic exercise. Exercise should not be relinquished because the period is due. T'ai chi is very useful.

V/13 PROSTATE-GLAND ENLARGEMENT

In humans the prostate gland tends to enlarge in middle or old age due to the excessive growth of the glandular cells it contains. This increased growth is in no sense malignant, and the only ill-effects in mild to moderate cases are the desire to empty the bladder more often than before and often some difficulty in the subsequent emptying. This difficulty may increase to the point that the bladder is never emptied entirely, and the residual urine can become infected. Unless the condition is treated the infection can damage the lining of the bladder and ascend to the kidneys via the ureters, causing further damage to these organs.

ORTHODOX TREATMENT

The prostate is examined by feeling it through the front wall of the rectum, by means of an internal examination in that area. The doctor is able to feel if the gland is enlarged and if its consistency is normal (i.e. firm but soft or hard and 'shotty', which would imply a malignant growth). The usual way of dealing with benign enlargement is by surgical removal of a part of the gland. Early surgery, before any serious damage has been done to bladder or kidneys, is nearly always advised; another reason is that a small number of cases of enlarged prostate gland are due not to benign enlargement but to malignant change. The treatment of choice in most cases of cancer of the prostate (see XIII) is surgical removal as soon as possible after diagnosis.

ALTERNATIVE THERAPIES

Natural medicine

The prostate gland contains zinc in 10 times the concentration found in most other bodily organs. There is some evidence that zinc-rich foods and zinc supplements help benign prostatic enlargement so, in addition to the patient's diet being wholefood and high in raw vegetables and fruit, he or she would be advised to eat some or all of: lean lamb chops, brewers' yeast, wheatgerm, eggs (in moderation), pumpkin seeds, non-fat dry milk powder and powdered mustard. Coffee, cola drinks and chocolate would be proscribed since the active chemicals in their caffeine content (methylxanthines) can aggravate benign enlargement of the prostate.

Specific dietary supplement Zinc gluconate, 50–100mg daily. Courses of pollen have been reported (in clinical trials in both Sweden and Japan) to relieve the symptoms of prostatic enlargement.

Raw juice therapy Half a litre to a litre daily of the following three juices in roughly equal volumes: carrot, cucumber, beetroot.

Biochemic tissue salts When the condition becomes acute, with irritation in that region and difficulty in passing urine (perhaps fever): *Ferrum Phos*. For enlargement of the prostate gland, perhaps with a little swelling of the testicles and the muscles flabby and relaxed: *Calcarea Fluor*. When there is dribbling of the prostatic fluid and a generally run-down condition: *Calcarea Phos*. Dose: four tablets every two hours.

Herbal medicine

Herbs useful in the treatment of prostatic problems include damiana, saw palmetto, couch-grass and horsetail. These should be administered by a qualified practitioner. The inclusion of raw onion in the daily diet is said to be very useful.

Aromatherapy

A soupspoonful of the alcohol preparation taken at the start of every meal is recommended: macerate 500g raw chopped onion in 500g 60° alcohol for two weeks. Strain. The flavour may be improved by the addition of lemon juice and sugar.

Homoeopathy

Sabal Serrulata often produces a rapid and dramatic improvement in prostatic-enlargement problems. Treatment from a qualified practitioner is to be preferred to attempts at self-treatment. Any attendant bladder weakness may very well benefit from *Causticum*.

Acupuncture

This has been known to help benign enlargement of the prostate and its problems in the early stages.

V/14 MENOPAUSE

The menopause is the last menstrual period. Varying terms (e.g. 'the change', the 'climacteric') are used to refer to the 2–3 year period during which a woman's periods come to an end, and are also often used to refer to the symptoms that affect some, although by no means all, women at that time. In the UK the average age for women's periods to cease is 51.4 years, although they can come to an end before the age of 40 (due to autoimmune disease [see ALLERGY] or to the surgical removal of the ovaries). Some women continue to have regular periods long into their 50s, although this is not very common.

Signs to look out for (and consult your doctor or gynaecologist about without delay) are irregular bleeding, with periods coming at 2–3 week intervals, and episodes of prolonged bleeding. The average age at which the menopause occurs is also the age at which cancer of the womb (see **XIII**) occurs most commonly, and all abnormal bleeding should be investigated at the earliest opportunity on this account.

The normal menopause can come about in one of three ways: the periods can suddenly stop; the menstrual loss, though still regular, may become less and less until it dies away altogether; or the intervals between periods may get longer and longer—instead of arriving every 28 days, the periods arrive at two- then at three-monthly intervals (this may even extend to six months).

The symptoms that can occur during the menopause are of three main types, and in most cases can be related directly to the falling level of oestrogen as the active life of the ovaries draws to a close. Osteoporosis (see below and **VI/8**) is another common symptom.

Hot flushes, night sweats and palpitations   These are due to faulty control of the state of constriction and dilation of the blood vessels, probably due in turn to a response error within the hypothalamus area of the brain. There is an increased flow of blood to the skin, resulting in a rise in skin temperature and an increase in heart rate of about 20 beats per minute.[70] The associated flushes and sweats can cause much discomfort and embarrassment, and during the night occur for no apparent reason. During the day, they seem to be brought on by warm rooms and hot baths, coffee or tea, alcohol, spicy foods and stress.

Vaginal and urinary problems The urethra and the vagina are both derived from the same tube in the developing embryo, and so their surface linings are affected in much the same way when the blood-levels of oestrogen start to fall. A common result is degeneration of the cells and consequent urethral irritation and vaginal dryness. The symptoms are having to pass water more frequently than usual, soreness on doing so, and perhaps blood in the urine. A mistaken diagnosis of cystitis (see **IV/5**) due to infection is commonly made at this time. The vaginal symptoms are pain on intercourse, due to failure to lubricate and to shrinkage of the lining membrane, and an increased tendency to contract vaginal infections (see THRUSH).

Psychological symptoms Depression, anxiety and pronounced lack of self-confidence are liable to arise at this time in women with a tendency towards these complaints. Not all of these problems are due to the falling oestrogen level: in many cases they can be related to concern about the ageing process and reluctance to enter the change of life. Relief of the urinary and vaginal symptoms frequently relieves also many of the emotional problems; where this does not happen straightforward treatment for depression (**XIV/3**) and anxiety (**XIV/4**) obtains better results than attempts to treat them with oestrogen supplements.

Osteoporosis Another outcome of diminishing oestrogen levels— indeed, the most important long-term effect—is accelerated loss of substance from the bones of the skeleton. All our bones start to lose some of their density from the age of 20 onwards, but men are far less affected by this process than women, and the final outcome of abnormal bone-substance loss—osteoporosis—is a great deal more common in elderly women than it is in men in this age group.

The bones become more porous and thereby weaker and brittler, and more inclined to fracture. The most serious fracture likely to be sustained by elderly women is that involving the neck of the femur (the upper end of the long thigh-bone as it enters the hip-joint): 15 per cent of elderly patients with this injury die within three months, and the condition costs the NHS more than £100 million annually.[70] (See also **VI/8**.)

ORTHODOX TREATMENT

The standard treatment for menopausal symptoms, and as a preventive measure against post-menopausal osteoporosis, is supplementation with oestrogen, nowadays in combination with progestogen (synthetic progesterone). This combination greatly reduces the risk of cancer of the uterus associated with the administration of synthetic oestrogen, but many women prefer to do without the therapy and seek alternative methods of treatment.

It is well worth quoting in this context the opinion of a leading medical expert, Dr A. Fowler, stated in a letter to the *British Medical Journal* (vol. 287, p. 286): 'If the post-menopausal woman is an active exerciser, does not smoke, and eats oily fish or has moderate exposure to sunlight, she is unlikely to suffer from appreciable osteoporosis.'

Antidepressants and tranquillizers are also given for emotional and psychological problems arising during the menopause; and KY jelly is recommended as a lubricant to assist the problem of vaginal soreness (which is treated also with oestrogen cream).

ALTERNATIVE THERAPIES

Natural medicine

Leon Chaitow[71] recommends a wholefood diet with the elimination of all sugar, tea, coffee and cola drinks and the reduction of alcohol intake to no more than two glasses of wine daily (or equivalent). He suggests a daily breakfast, ideally consisting of yoghourt, fruit, seeds and nuts; one main meal daily of mixed raw salad, with cottage cheese, wholemeal bread or jacket potato; and, for the other main meal, lots of lightly cooked fresh vegetables with fish, lean meat, poultry or a vegetarian savoury. Desserts and snacks should consist of fresh fruit and drinks of juices, herb teas and mineral water. Chaitow also recommends a brisk 10–20 minute walk daily, and the learning and practice daily of a form of meditation or relaxation. And he suggests the following dietary supplements:

- 6–10 brewers' yeast tablets
- 2 kelp tablets
- 1 multivitamin/mineral tablet
- 2 garlic capsules

For hot flushes:

- 400iu Vitamin E, twice daily; this should contain at least 50mcg of selenium (if not, then take it separately, although not in excess of 100mcg daily)
- Vitamin C, 1g twice daily, in combination with bioflavonoids (stated on the package)

- 1 high potency Vitamin-B tablet daily, containing at least 50mg of each of the chief B vitamins

Also:

- calcium pantothenate (Vitamin B_5), 500mg daily
- 1g B_{13} calcium and 500mg B_{13} magnesium at bedtime to help sleep problems
- 500mg evening primrose oil (Efamol)

Pollen has been found in controlled clinical trials to decrease the tendency to put on weight during the menopause, and substantially to reduce the score of the 'climacteric index' (a numerical scale on which menopausal symptoms were graduated) in 35 out of 38 women.[72] With post-menopausal women still suffering menopausal symptoms (age-group 40–65 years) similar results were obtained.

Regarding a sore, dry vagina, there is evidence that continued and frequent sexual activity before, throughout and after the menopause helps to prevent the vaginal changes that cause this. When masturbation frequency was taken into account in addition to the frequency of sexual activity, even more striking evidence was found suggesting that masturbation may be helpful in lieu of intercourse.

Raw juice therapy The famous potassium broth recommended by John B. Lust: 200ml carrot juice, 110ml celery juice, 55ml parsley juice and 85ml spinach juice. He suggests 600ml daily and the above formula provides only 450ml, so for the sake of convenience I recommend an extra 55ml each of celery and carrot; or an extra 30ml each of all four.

Biochemic tissue salts

For nervous tension and irritability arising during the menopause: *Kali Phos.*, four tablets every two hours until symptoms abate.

Herbal medicine

Passiflora tablets, 1–3 daily, especially if tense and anxious. Sarsaparilla (liquid form) and ginseng tea are reputed to help hot flushes.

Aromatherapy

Three drops of essence of clary sage on a little brown sugar after each meal.

Homoeopathy

For a very heavy menstrual flow (associated symptoms often include headache, flushes, cold hands and feet, tightness in chest and fatigue): *Lachesis*. For a heavy flow associated with bearing-down pains and backache, improved by violent quick movements and in the middle of the day and the afternoon: *Sepia*. For hot flushes with intense congestion of the face and a throbbing in the head, aggravated by heat in any form; attacks sudden, violent and unexpected: *Glonoine*.

Acupuncture

Leon Chaitow states that there is strong evidence that acupuncture can prove very helpful to menopausal women, and that improved well-being and vitality can often result. He especially advocates combining acupuncture with a nutritional plan such as the above (pages 296–7) and a relaxation programme.

Relaxation techniques

Biofeedback, yoga and meditation can all help, as can autogenics and autohypnosis.

Exercise therapy

Dance therapy can prove very useful for re-establishing flexibility and suppleness prior to the reintroduction of more strenuous activities.

V/15 INFERTILITY

The failure of intercourse to result in a pregnancy can be due to the man's inability to father a child, to the woman's inability to conceive/retain a fertilized egg within her womb, or to both. Possible causes include imcompatibility between the woman's vaginal mucus and the man's sperm; a low (or absent) sperm count; poor-quality sperm (e.g. when a factor or series of factors interferes with their production —varicose veins [III/6] in the sperm tubes can do this); failure on behalf of the woman to ovulate; failure of the sperm to meet with and fertilize an ovum in the Fallopian tubes (e.g. when one or both tubes are blocked by scarring due to previous infection or endometrial deposits). Of healthy couples, 90 per cent achieve conception within a year of trying to, and infertility is considered only after this time has passed without success.

ORTHODOX TREATMENT

Treatment with surgery or medication helps about 35 per cent of couples diagnosed as suffering from infertility. A similar number of untreated couples as well as 41 per cent of unsuccessfully treated couples, also achieve pregnancy later on—which does not say a great deal for the treatment (or perhaps for the diagnosis).

For couples who cannot conceive—in particular, those in whom no apparent cause of the problem can be found—the organization Foresight, the Association for the Promotion of Preconceptual Care, can be of great help and encouragement; Belinda Barnes, chairperson, believes that in many cases the problem can be put right. Diet is a highly important factor, as are lifestyle and ability to handle stress, and Foresight feel that more couples should learn about these essentials before trying to conceive, not wait until they may have become frustrated and strained by the inability to conceive. (It is also true that, the better the couple's health, the better the health of the intended offspring.)

Couples are counselled on diet, smoking and drinking habits, and investigated for allergy problems, toxic metals (by hair analysis) and mineral deficiencies. Doctors in private practice in many parts of the UK hold Foresight clinics, and the address of the nearest in any given area can be obtained by writing to Foresight.

ALTERNATIVE THERAPIES

Natural medicine

Expert Leon Chaitow recommends the following diet[73]: wholefood only, eaten as three meals a day, and never taken when stressed or angry; no alcohol, and a minimum of fat. Breakfast should be yoghourt and fruit or sugar-free muesli; an egg and wholemeal bread and honey or sugarless jam and a herb tea; or porridge, fruit and yoghourt. One major meal should contain 85g of protein, such as low-fat cheese, fish, poultry, lean meat, with a raw salad or lightly cooked vegetables. The other should be based on salad with brown rice, wholemeal bread or baked potato, low-fat cheese or cereal/pulse mixture (e.g. lentils and millet, or chickpeas and rice). Desserts should be yoghourt and fruit. Drink spring water, fresh juices and herb teas. Snacks should be of nuts and seeds, or fresh fruit. In addition, neither partner should smoke.

Hydrotherapy   For men with poor sperm production, a cold hipbath (sit in cold water in the bath) for 1½–3 minutes at least once daily, but not in the few hours prior to lovemaking. Also, avoid hot baths, saunas, tight underwear and jeans, and electric blankets: the rationale here is that sperms are best produced at lower than body temperature.

Exercise   At least on alternate days and for not less than 30 minutes, preferably outdoors. Walking is especially good. Aerobics only when a fitness check has been passed.

Relaxation   This is especially recommended—not less than one and preferably two 15-minute sessions daily.

Specific dietary supplements

- Inadequate sperm production can be aided by the amino acid arginine: try 8g daily for a month. Take under the supervision of a nutritional expert.
- Carnitine (an amino acid found in large amounts in the testicles): 200mg thrice daily is recommended.
- Vitamin C: 1g daily (essential if carnitine is taken).
- Zinc (for both partners): 100mg zinc orotate is recommended daily; important for potency and for conception.

These supplements should be taken as part of the daily recommended dietary supplements.

When ovulation is sporadic rather than regular, but inflammation is not present, liquid extract of the herb *Agnus castus* (marketed under the name of Agnolyt) can be very helpful. It contains no hormones, and should be taken continuously for at least six months.

When nutritional improvement does not restore fertility, a fertility drug can help, but for many reasons it is better to try natural methods first. The following supplements—again taken as part of a dietary supplement programme—can help restore fertility in the temporary decline that frequently follows the use of contraceptive measures such as the Pill or an IUCD (intrauterine contraceptive device):

- potent B-complex supplement: at least 50mg strength of major vitamins and at least 400mcg of folic acid
- Vitamin C: 1g
- zinc: 100mg as B_{13} zinc or as zinc orotate
- selenium and Vitamin E combined, 50mcg selenium and 200iu Vitamin E

Other important minerals, such as calcium and magnesium, are included in the recommended daily supplement. Stress, anxiety and depression can be aided by a daily dose of pollen.

Herbal medicine

See information about *Agnus castus* above. Also used by doctors of herbal medicine in the treatment of infertility are helonias root, blue cohosh and dong quai for women; and damiana, saw palmetto, oats and sarsaparilla for men. *Aloe vera* gel is a good lubricant with excellent healing properties for sore, damaged membranes, and can be used instead of KY jelly if discomfort on penile penetration of a dry vagina suggests that a moisturizing agent is required.

Homoeopathy

When associated with scanty periods and painful breasts: *Conium*. When there is associated leukorrhoea ('whites'—see VAGINAL DISCHARGE): *Borax*. Another useful remedy: Silicea.

Acupuncture

This has been used to treat sterility.

Exercise therapy

Dance therapy can be helpful in relieving stress and toning up muscles unaccustomed to exercise. Yoga can also be useful.

Relaxation techniques

Yoga, meditation, autogenics; hypnotherapy, especially when patient finds relaxation difficult and suffers anxiety and tension.

V/16 IMPOTENCE

The inability to obtain, or to sustain, an erection suitable for penetration and ejaculation can be due to an underlying physical disorder. This is termed *organic impotence*: examples of possible causes include disorders of the heart and blood vessels; diabetes; renal failure and liver disease; anaemia; injuries (e.g. pelvic fracture, brain or spinal cord injury); the effects of a surgical operation upon, e.g. the bladder or pelvic blood vessels; the effects of the ageing process; neurological problems such as spina bifida and multiple sclerosis; DRUG DEPEND-ENCE; and hormonal abnormalities. Organic impotence usually comes on slowly over a period of time.

In the majority of cases, however, the underlying cause is of a psychological nature. Such impotence is called *psychogenic impotence*, and its onset is usually sudden. The fading of an erection at the moment of penetration is the hallmark of psychogenic impotence. Causes include guilt, aggression and feelings of inadequacy. Usually, a past or present unsatisfactory sexual/emotional relationship is at least partly responsible, and this may go back to childhood and stem from the child being scolded, smacked or otherwise punished for playing with his own genitals or exploring another child's.

A man's ability to obtain an erection with masturbation or with another partner but not with his usual sexual partner suggests that counselling is needed, as does the presence of normal waking erections coupled with the inability to sustain an erection during intended intercourse.

Psychogenic impotence can also feature in depression (see **XIV/3**) and in anxiety neurosis (see **XIV/4**), or be a side-effect of any of a number of drugs. The latter include among them alcohol; some anti-hypertensives (e.g. methyldopa [Aldomet], clonidine [Catapres]); some diuretics (e.g. bendrofluazide [Neo Naclex, Aprinox]); barbiturates (e.g. phenobarbitone, as in Epanutin with phenobarbitone, and Luminal); antidepressants (e.g. lithium [Camcolit], phenelzine [Nardil]); antianginal drugs (e.g. perhexilene); appetite-suppressants (e.g. fenfluramine [Ponderax]); anticholinergic drugs (e.g. propan-theline [Pro-banthine]); peptic-ulcer drugs (e.g. cimetidine [Tagamet]).

ORTHODOX TREATMENT

Any suggestion in the case history or physical examination of a so far undiagnosed underlying physical disorder is likely to lead to further investigations. Impotence which seems to be or clearly is of psychogenic origin may result in referral of the patient for psychiatric or sexual counselling.

ALTERNATIVE THERAPIES

Natural medicine

The approach adopted by most naturopaths to impotence may well be eclectic—as it is in the case of many other disorders. The naturopathic treatment as such would take an extensive case history, with special reference to past and present general health, past and present lifestyle including alcohol consumption and regular medication taken, and, most of all, to stress factors of recent origin and/or encountered on a regular basis. Advice would embrace diet (wholefood, high-raw percentage), regular exercise according to the individual's age and health, the possibility of stopping certain drugs (in cooperation with the patient's GP), and coping with stress factors. Relaxation sessions would indubitably be recommended on a daily or twice-daily basis, and possibly psychotherapy if this were considered necessary. In addition, homoeopathic or herbal remedies might be found desirable as adjuncts (see below).

Pollen is said to have a rejuvenatory effect and to increase stamina by combating fatigue.

Raw juice therapy   Twice daily, 140ml red cabbage juice, 85ml celery juice and 55ml lettuce juice.

Biochemic tissue salts   As a treatment for debility, including weightloss, being generally run down, and anaemia: *Calcarea Phos.* Where the nervous system is involved; and where depression is in evidence: *Kali Phos.* alternating with *Calcarea Phos.*; dose: four tablets every three hours.

Herbal medicine

For psychogenic impotence: damiana, Asiatic ginseng and saw palmetto may well be useful.

Aromatherapy

Five drops of essence of ylang-ylang on a little brown sugar after each meal.

Homoeopathy

As a useful remedy in more persistent cases: *Lycopodium*. For temporary impotence, not psychogenic in origin but following injury and bruising: *Arnica*. Of value in the earliest stages of the problem: *Agnus Castus*. When there is marked anxiety and fear of intercourse: *Argent. Nit.* For impotence in the elderly and associated with debility: *Sabal Serrulata*.

Acupuncture

This has been used successfully for impotence, usually psychogenic and when due to debility, nervous stress and strain and exhaustion.

Relaxation techniques

Any of these may be very useful: yoga and meditation; autogenics; biofeedback (in helping individual to recognize and control stress); autohypnosis.

Psychotherapy

Psychotherapy, in particular hypnotherapy, during which the arts of relaxation and autohypnosis are taught, can be very beneficial.

V/17 GENITAL WARTS

These have been mentioned in the discussion of cancer of the cervix (**V/9**) since they are now considered to be a risk factor in the development of that condition. Although of the several different varieties of HPV (human papillomata virus) which can cause genital warts only type 16 has been associated with an increased risk of cervical cancer, caution must be taken wherever genital warts are involved in either partner. It is not yet possible to isolate which variety of HPV a person is infected with, and doctors at the Whittington Hospital (where much of the work in this connection is being done) advise all partners of men with genital warts to be screened yearly for signs of cervical cancer. Even if the women has no signs of genital warts herself, she is still at risk if her partner suffers from them. It is possible to have a subclinical infection which can be recognized only on colposcopy (internal examination of the vagina using an instrument called a colposcope). The infection can even pass unnoticed in the male partner, who may have no clinically apparent warts yet still carry type 16 HPV and pass it on to his partner.

The number of cases of genital HPV infection is increasing annually, as is cervical cancer—especially in young women; in the past decade reported cases from VD clinics have more than doubled, and many other patients are probably reporting directly to their GPs. At present, no attempt is being made to follow up the female partners of men with genital warts, but a spokesman from the research unit at the Whittington Hospital feels that this situation ought to alter. Meanwhile, the safest approach a woman can adopt is to have a yearly cervical examination and to keep a look-out for any signs of genital warts in both herself and her partner.

ORTHODOX TREATMENT

Genital warts are treated by the carbon-dioxide laser technique, or by the application of podophyllin, sometimes reinforced by the addition of inosine pranobex (Imunovir), the dose of which is six 500mg tablets daily for 14–28 days.

ALTERNATIVE THERAPIES

Natural medicine

A wholefood diet with a high daily percentage of raw fruit and vegetables will help to reinvigorate the body's immune system, which will then be better able to fight infection. Consumption of saturated animal fats should as usual be minimal, and cold-pressed vegetable oils and their products should be used instead of butter. Of particular help to the immune system are certain vitamins and minerals; the following daily regimen is especially suitable: Vitamin A, 25,000iu; a mega-B complex; Vitamin C, 3g; zinc, 10mg daily in its orotate or chelate form. Vitamin-E oil squeezed from a capsule onto the warts can help get rid of them.

Herbal medicine

Paint the heads of the warts with fresh garlic or lemon juice daily.

Aromatherapy

Dab the warts each evening with essence of lemon.

Psychotherapy

Warts can be 'charmed' away, success depending upon the person concerned being convinced that his or her warts are going to disappear. Also visualization, either combined with a relaxation technique such as yoga or incorporated into a session of autohypnosis can in many people help warts (and other conditions) to clear up, provided it is practised daily or even twice daily, again with conviction.

VI   Disorders of Bones, Tendons and Muscles

Bone (together with cartilage) is the building material of the skeleton. Each individual bone has a specific role to play, and its structure is designed accordingly. Nevertheless, it is possible to name two major functions which all the skeleton's composite bones share to a greater or lesser extent. The first of these is support for the soft tissues of the body. Without a firm supporting structure to which muscles can be attached movement of any part of the body would be impossible. The second is the protection the skeleton affords to the delicate organs.

At a microscopic level, bones consist of a ground substance, or matrix, in which are arranged living cells. The matrix is inert and hard, and consists of fibres of protein impregnated with insoluble salts, mostly calcium phosphate. Bones have an outer, ivory-like layer of compact bone, arranged as fine channels named Haversian canals, and an inner core containing the soft marrow situated in gaps and spaces in relatively spongy bone. The bone is enclosed in an outer, tough, fibrous membrane, the periosteum.

The function of muscles is closely associated with that of bones. There are in fact three different types of muscle, and together they account for just under half our total body-weight. The three are (a) skeletal or voluntary, (b) involuntary and (c) cardiac muscles; the latter two are discussed on pages 310–11.

Skeletal muscle, attached to various parts of our skeleton, is known also as 'voluntary' because for most of the time its action is controlled by our will. Skeletal muscle clothes the shafts of the long limb bones and of the digits; and forms two massive columns on either side of the spine. It helps to support and mobilize the head on the neck; runs in short

Skeleton

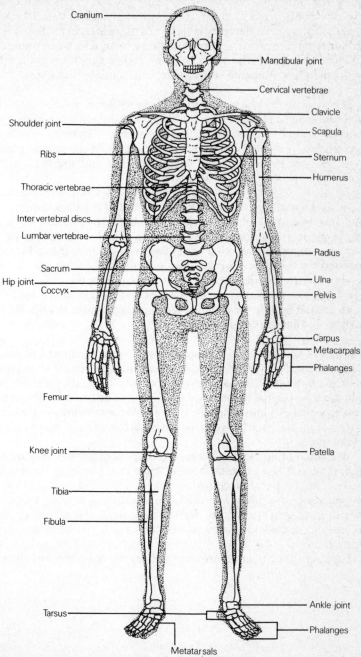

Cranium

Mandibular joint

Cervical vertebrae

Clavicle

Shoulder joint

Scapula

Ribs

Sternum

Thoracic vertebrae

Humerus

Inter vertebral discs

Lumbar vertebrae

Radius

Sacrum

Ulna

Hip joint

Coccyx

Pelvis

Carpus

Metacarpals

Phalanges

Femur

Knee joint

Patella

Tibia

Fibula

Tarsus

Ankle joint

Phalanges

Metatarsals

strips between the curving ribs, where it plays a part in breathing; and forms the front wall of the abdomen.

The structural unit of skeletal muscle is the fibre. This is made up of elongated cells tapering (like the whole muscle) at each end. It is specially constructed to contract (i.e. shorten) in response to signals received from motor nerves originating in the spinal cord. These nerves receive two types of 'instructions', the net sum of which determines the outcome in terms of how much muscular contraction takes place. Some of the messages stimulate contraction, others inhibit these stimuli and dampen their effect.

Tendons are the connecting ropes of the skeleton. Except in specialized cases, skeletal muscles have a belly, or main portion, which tapers to a point at either end in a roughly lozenge shape. Attached to each end is a tendon, the outer connective-tissue sheath of the muscle passing imperceptibly into the sheath of the tendon, and the tendon then binding the muscle firmly to a bone.

Tendons are immensely strong. One well known example is the Achilles tendon, running from the lower end of the back calf muscles and inserting itself in the back of the heel-bone. When we walk, messages pass from our brain down the spinal cord and along the nerves, causing (among other complementary actions) the calf muscles to contract. As they shorten, they pull upwards upon the Achilles tendon, which lifts the back of the foot by raising the heel. When we place that foot on the ground the muscles on the outer side of our calves contract and pull the front of the foot upwards while, in turn, the calf muscles behind relax and lengthen.

The *skull* consists of 20–30 named bones, some composed of several parts and all closely interlocked with one another. For the most part, it is easiest to think of the skull as one complete bone, the cranium, with which are associated three movable joints. The first two of these are the two mandibular joints, one on either side of the cranium, and the third is the joint at the back between the lower surface of the skull and the top of the spine.

The cranium houses the brain. Its component parts—frontal, parietal, temporal and occipital bones—have small holes in them which permit blood vessels and cranial nerves to pass to and from the brain to surrounding structures. The chief construction of nervous tissue, the spinal cord, passes up into the brain through the widest of these apertures, the foramen magnum, after leaving the shelter of the spine's bony arch.

Looking into the cranium from above, the floor consists of three tiered compartments, the anterior (front), middle and posterior (back) fossae. The first of these is the highest, like the 'gods' row of seats in the theatre; it both supports the frontal lobes of the brain and forms the roof of the nose and eye orbits. The middle fossa, comparable to the balcony stalls, houses the brain's temporal lobes. Lastly, the posterior fossa (the expensive stall seats) supports the back of the brain, the cerebellum. On the undersurface of the posterior fossa are the areas of attachment for the powerful neck muscles.

The facial bones open to form the passageways and hollows for the eyes, nose and mouth. The maxilla, containing one of the air sinuses, supplies the floor of the eye orbit, the upper jaw and part of the structure of the nose.

The *spine* or backbone runs from the underside of the skull down to the tip of the coccyx or vestigial tail, a remnant of our evolutionary history. It contains 33 separate units, or vertebrae, arranged as follows: 7 cervical in the neck; 12 thoracic in the chest; 5 lumbar in the lower back; 5 sacral fused together to form the sacrum (back of the pelvis); and 4 coccygial, representing the coccyx. Tough discs are sandwiched between the bodies of adjacent vertabrae, which arch to provide a passageway for the spinal cord. Each vertebra also has a number of bony prominences to which muscle and connective tissues are attached.

There are 12 pairs of *ribs* in both men and women. The 'floating' ribs are the last two pairs, and are so-called because they 'float'; i.e. are connected to muscle in front rather than joining with the cartilaginous ends of the ribs above. All the ribs are connected behind with the vertebral column. The upper seven join onto the breastbone (sternum) via the 'costal cartilages'. The front ends of the next three pairs (false ribs) are joined by means of the cartilage to the rib immediately above.

The scapulae (shoulderblades), the clavicles (collarbones) and the upper end of the breastbone together constitute the *pectoral girdle*. The upper end of the arm-bone (humerus) on each side articulates at the shoulder joint with the pectoral girdle and at the lower end with the two forearm bones, the radius and the ulna, to form the elbow joint. The ulna is the longer of these two, projecting beyond the lower end of the humerus to form the elbow point. At the wrist the lower end of the ulna articulates with the lower part of the radial shaft; unlike the radius, it plays no part in the wrist joint. The lower end of the radius articulates with a group of small bones collectively called the carpus. The carpus in turn forms joints with the long bones of the hand (metacarpals), which finally articulate at their further ends with the finger bones (phalanges).

At the wrist joint, the tendons of the forearm muscles pass to their insertion points on the hand-bones. Those on the inner surface of the joint pass below strong bands of fibrous tissue running between the lower ends of the radius and ulna, together with the median nerve. The hollow space below the bands is known as the carpal tunnel; the tendons move smoothly here because they are enclosed in specially lubricated sheaths.

Unlike the pectoral girdle, which is composed of mobile parts, the *pelvic girdle* is fixed. Its two largest constituents are the large, heavy hip bones which unite with one another in the midline in front. Their meeting point can be felt as the first hard structure you feel when you run the tips of your fingers down the front of your abdomen in the midline.

The hip bones do not meet one another behind, but are attached one on either side of the sacrum at the sacroiliac joints. On the outer aspect of each hip bone is situated a deep cavity or cup into which the head of the femur (thigh bone) fits. You are far less likely to suffer from a dislocated hip joint than a shoulder joint simply because the cup into which the humerus fits on the outer part of the scapula is, comparatively speaking, very shallow.

The femur runs from hip to knee joint, where its lower end articulates with the upper end of the tibia, the larger of the two calf bones. The other calf bone is the fibula, situated on the outer aspect of the tibia. The lower ends of both bones help to make up the ankle joint by articulating with the upper surface of the talus, one of the ankle bones collectively called the tarsus.

The bony lump on the inner surface of your ankle is the inner malleolus, at the lower end of the tibia; the lump on the outer surface, the outer malleolus, is the lower end of the fibula. Together, these two knobs hold the talus tightly in a kind of mortice device.

There are seven tarsal bones in all. The calcaneum, the largest, projects backwards to form the heel bone. Into its outer surface is inserted the lower end of the Achilles tendon, and it is this bone which can develop a small, painful spur of bone (see CALCANEAL SPUR). The tarsals articulate in front with the metatarsals. The little bones making up the toes (phalanges) are attached in rows to the spherical heads of the metatarsals. The bone configuration in both fingers and toes is the same: two phalangeal bones in the first digit (i.e. thumb, big toe), and three in each of the other four digits.

The basic unit of *muscle*, the fibre, has been described above. In voluntary muscle the fibres are arranged in bundles with all the fibres pointing the same way so that muscular contraction is the sum total of a united effort on behalf of all the component fibres. In smooth muscle (e.g. the muscle of the large and small bowel) the fibres are arranged with some bundles lying parallel to the length of the organ or tube, and others situated in rings around it. Thus in a transverse section of, say, the duodenum, looked at under the microscope, two different muscle layers can be identified: the longitudinal and the transverse. This arrangement of the contractile units permits the characteristic peristalsis (squeezing movement) of the bowel to take place. This type of muscle has a dual nerve supply, receiving separate stimuli to contract and to relax.

Cardiac muscle consists of a highly specialized type of cellular arrangement, lacking individual functioning units like the fibres of the other two muscle types. Instead, the whole heart is really a mass of cells that do not begin or end as discrete entities, but run into one another in an arrangement known as a syncytium. The most important inherent property of cardiac muscle is rhythmic contraction. This is controlled at the physiological rate of around 70 beats per minute by the intervention of the sinu-atrial node in the heart's left atrium (see page 227).

Tendons (known also as sinews or leaders) bind muscles to bones, and consist of very strong fibrous connective tissue. *Ligaments*, on the other hand, bind bone to bone; they are fibrous bands, and help to strengthen joints.

Joints between bones are mobile or fixed. The former, notably the *synovial joints*, are lined with cartilage covered with moist slippery (synovial) membrane. The membrane secretes synovial fluid, whose purposes may include lubricating the opposing bone surfaces. Examples are the ankle, the hip, the shoulder and the mandibular joints. *Fixed joints*, such as those formed by the two hip bones in front, the interconnecting skull bones, the bodies of adjoining vertebrae, and the sacrum and hip bones (sacro-iliac joints), are united by fibrous connective tissue and permit little or no movement.

VI/1 ARTHRITIS

Arthritis is INFLAMMATION of a joint. It is a feature of many different diseases, such as rheumatic fever and psoriasis, and its main symptoms are pain and stiffness. Three commonly occurring varieties of arthritis are osteoarthritis (VI/2), rheumatoid arthritis (VI/3) and gout (VI/4). Therapies for all three are discussed under VI/4.

VI/2 OSTEOARTHRITIS

This is the biggest single cause of joint pain and malfunction: it affects 5–10 million people in the UK. Traditionally, osteoarthritis has been regarded as a progressive disorder of weight-bearing joints in the elderly, but this is nowadays widely doubted. The joints benefit from being used, and everyday wear and tear do not generally predispose to premature joint disease. Other possible explanations include age changes in synovial joints; the existence of one or several different disease processes; and gradual deterioration of the joints' function due to numerous possible causes, including injury.

Inside the joint the cartilage gets worn away, and the exposed bone thickens, producing cysts and small bony projections called osteophytes. The synovial membrane thickens, and the joint may fill with fluid (a joint effusion). The joint becomes swollen, crackles when used, and its range of movement is reduced. The patient notices pain, and difficulty in walking (typical joints to be affected are the knees and hip joints). Symptoms often occur intermittently or may be entirely absent. They appear to coincide with episodes of inflammation of the damaged synovial membrane, injury to the affected joint (to which osteoarthritis predisposes it) and certain seasons of the year, namely late spring and late autumn.

Some patients with this disease improve spontaneously, others remain much the same, and yet others deteriorate, with severe pain, loss of movement, joint deformity, nerve-trapping and muscle-wasting.

VI/3 RHEUMATOID ARTHRITIS

This is chronic inflammation of connective tissue, most often the fibrous connective tissue around joints, and its cause is not known. The joint cartilage and synovial membrane can also become inflamed and damaged, and the muscles over the affected joints become tight and tense. Autoimmunity has been cited as a major contributory factor (see ALLERGY); and a viral cause has been suggested.

Pain, swelling, heat and stiffness in the knuckles, wrist and elbow joints are typical symptoms, although the shoulder, hip, knee, ankle and intervetebral joints can also be affected. Accompanying problems can include weight-loss and tiredness, ABDOMINAL PAIN, headaches, generally feeling under the weather, enlarged tender lymph nodes, and small painful nodules appearing below the skin.

There is a slight hereditory factor in rheumatoid arthritis, and women are more predisposed to the illness than men. Untreated patients, or patients who fail to respond to treatment, develop distorted and ultimately useless joints and severe muscle-wasting.

VI/4 GOUT

Gout is the name for those diseases in which arthritis occurs due to uric-acid crystals. Uric acid is a waste product normally excreted in the urine, but gout sufferers have defective body chemistry which causes them to deposit the substance as crystals in their joints, as small lumps beneath the skin (tophi), and inside the kidney where they can form renal stones (see **IV/4**). Gout is sufficiently common in Europe today to account for 5 per cent of all arthritis cases.

Men are more often affected than women. One of the commonest joints to be affected is the first (metacarpo-phalangeal) joint of the big toe. Others are the instep joints, ankle, heel, knee, wrist, finger and elbow. Both alcohol and unaccustomed exercise can bring on an attack, and the affected joint becomes intensely painful, red, hot and swollen.

Untreated gout patients can suffer from progressive kidney damage leading to kidney failure (see **IV/1**, **IV/2**). In addition, the tophi can become very large, and the skin overlying them can ulcerate due to interference with its blood supply.

ORTHODOX TREATMENT

Osteoarthritis is treated with pain-killers and drugs in the NSAID (non-steroidal anti-inflammatory drug) group; examples are in-domethacin (Indocid), piroxicam (Feldene) and phenylbutazone (Buta-zolidin). Aspirin is often very effective, as is weight reduction in very heavy patients. Replacement of the joint with an artificial one can be highly successful.

Patients with rheumatoid arthritis are prescribed bed-rest and a combination of immobilization alternating with gentle exercise for the affected joints and associated muscles. Drugs include aspirin, NSAIDs, gold salts, penicillamine, and, where unavoidable, steroids, Surgery can help a number of patients.

Gout too is treated with NSAIDs and attempts are made to prevent further attacks by the use of allopurinol (Zyloprim), which reduces the amount of uric acid produced by the body.

Various forms of physiotherapy are recommended for arthritic patients, depending upon their conditon and requirements.

ALTERNATIVE THERAPIES

In addition to the approaches discussed below, the reader is referred to those treated under PAIN.

Natural medicine

Dietary correction is considered very important in the control of most types of arthritis. Besides diet, the patient's lifestyle, past medical history including physical injuries and allergies, and stress exposure and response are also carefully examined. The Schroth cure is often recommended for arthritis, especially the rheumatoid variety.

Weight reduction is advised where this is applicable, and osteopathy is recommended for most joint problems in the early stages. Manipulation can do less for joints affected by advanced arthritis, so the sooner osteopathic (or chiropractic) help is sought the better for the patient.

Incorrect diet is known to aggravate many aspects of arthritis; alternatively, the correct diet and supplements can do much to control or cure it. A mainly vegetarian diet is recommended for both osteo-arthritic and rheumatoid-arthritic patients, and great care should be taken to identify and eliminate all possible allergens. The health of the bowel flora (bacteria) and of the digestive processes should be considered.

Food substances rich in sulphur are recommended, including garlic and live yoghourt. All red meat should be avoided, as should salt, sugar and white-flour products, cows' milk and its products (use goats' milk and goats' yoghourt), acid fruit such as citrus fruit and strawberries, and alcohol—this last is especially important to gout patients. A lightly cooked egg is permitted twice weekly, and 50–75g poultry or fish on alternate days if vegetarian foods are not liked. Basically, the diet is wholefood with the above exceptions, and the patient is encouraged to eat large raw salads and lightly steamed vegetables daily. It is recommended that one day per week raw food only be eaten.

Poultices Large poultices of cold green clay can be applied to acutely inflamed joints (mix with water and apply as a paste). Frequent hot applications can be used for chronic arthritic conditions. Both types should be left on for 2–4 hours. (Leon Chaitow quotes from Raymond Dextreit's *Our Earth Our Cure*, in his article.[74] (Green clay is marketed in the UK by the Cantassium Company.)

Bee-sting therapy Some therapists keep bees which they cause to sting arthritis sufferers. This has been found to be highly effective in a number of patients, although it has no effect in others.

Copper bracelets   Many people find great relief from arthritis through wearing a copper bracelet. This may be due to the absorption of trace elements.

Raw juice therapy   During the acute inflammatory stage: 600–1,200ml celery juice daily. Also 170ml carrot juice, 140ml beetroot juice, and 140ml cucumber juice, twice daily.

Specific dietary supplements   Green clay (see above) taken internally. Leon Chaitow recommends this, again quoting Dextreit, as a means of detoxifying the system. Either stir ½tsp of green clay into half a tumbler of water and drink every morning on an empty stomach before breakfast, or mix the clay with water to make a paste, roll little bits up into small balls, and bake these in the oven; drink down several of these small pillules with water on an empty stomach, several times daily.

Green-lipped muscle extract is a short-term aid. Take it according to the supplier's instructions.

Leon Chaitow also suggests hair mineral analysis to determine mineral deficiencies—possible ones are zinc and copper—and he recommends the following supplements:

- Garlic capsules. A possible dose would be one perle (capsule) four times daily.
- Zinc, if required. Many people in this country are zinc-deficient. A helpful dose might be 100mg chelated zinc daily.
- Calcium, 6–9 bone-meal tablets daily have helped arthritis greatly.[75] Perhaps even better are dolomite tablets, which supply calcium and magnesium in balanced amounts. Try five dolomite tablets daily (supplying 750mg calcium and half as much magnesium); if partial relief is gained, try twice this quantity. Alternatively, a chelated calcium and magnesium supplement can be taken daily in the orotate form.
- Vitamin C, 1,000mg daily in 1–3 doses. If orthodox drugs are combined with alternative therapies and aspirin is being taken, much Vitamin C is lost due to this drug.
- Vitamin E, 200iu, twice daily.
- Vitamin-B complex, 100mg, three times daily.
- Vitamin B_{12}, up to 2,000mcg daily.
- Vitamin A, 10,000iu, Vitamin D, 400iu, 1–3 capsules, three times

daily (take for five days, stop for two). *As an alternative* in the case of rheumatoid arthritis patients: five Max-EPA capsules, twice daily.
- Evening primrose oil (Efamol), three 500mg capsules, twice daily.

Pollen B tablets have been found very useful in numerous patients; e.g. a three-month course has been reported to help severe arthritis in the knee and arm in October (see discussion of seasonal variations of osteo-arthritis, VI/2).

Honey is claimed by many to help arthritis.

Cider vinegar: Maurice Hanssen quotes Dr Jarvis's recommendation for rheumatoid arthritis, osteoarthritis, BURSITIS and gout:[76] (a) 2tsp cider vinegar and 2tsp honey in a glass of water taken at each meal, or between meals if preferred; (b) on Monday, Wednesday and Friday, at one meal add one drop of iodine to the mixture; (c) one kelp tablet at breakfast or at all three meals; (d) avoid wheat foods and cereals, white sugar, citrus fruit and muscle meats such as beef, lamb and pork, as these produce an adverse reaction. Hanssen's own recommendation is for the addition of molasses, as follows: (a) on rising, 2tsp cider vinegar in a tumbler of water; (b) with each meal, 2tsp each of cider vinegar and molasses with one of honey, sipped during the meal in a tumbler of water; (c) a natural vitamin and mineral supplement, daily; (d) a diet very low in sugar and refined flour.

Biochemic tissue salts For gout, to treat the fever and other signs of inflammation: *Ferrum Phos*. Chief remedy in this disorder: *Natrum Sulph*. In acute attacks, alternate this with *Ferrum Phos*.

Herbal medicine

Tablets of Devil's claw (*Herpagophytum procumbens*). Alfalfa: as tablets or as a tea made from simmering (not boiling) 30g untreated seeds (such as are used for sprouting) in 700ml of water in a glass or enamel pan for half an hour. Strain and squeeze out seeds, cool and refrigerate, but do not keep for longer than a day. To use, mix a cupful with an equal volume of water (or to taste), and add honey if you wish. Drink 6–7 cups daily. Persist for at least 2 weeks.[77]

According to one source cherries apparently help arthritis, especially gout. (The source does not give a quantity.)[77] It is worth also trying sour cherries—0.25–0.5kg daily.[77]

Specifically for gout, an infusion, taken four cupfuls daily, made of the following in a litre of water: four slices of lemon, a pinch of lavender and a pinch of dog's tooth.

Aromatherapy

For gout and other types of arthritis: four drops of essence of juniper on a little brown sugar after every meal. For gout alone: rub afflicted joint with olive oil containing 10 per cent essence of juniper.

Bach flower remedies

Homoeopathy

The basic remedy for large single joints or for small multiple joints of the hands or feet: *Rhus toxicodendron*. For very painful joints, worsened by slight movement: *Bryonia*. A useful general remedy is *Ruta*.

Acupuncture

Arthritis can be helped by use of this.

Manipulative therapy

Osteopathy (including manipulation, exercise, neuromuscular and other soft-tissue techniques) can be useful, as can chiropractic. The Alexander technique has helped patients with osteoarthritis, and remedial massage may be useful.

Reflexology   Massage applied to the reflexes of the affected organs, as well as to the reflexes of the bronchial tubes, lungs, adrenals and ileocaecal valve.

Exercise therapy

Yoga and T'ai chi both help when gentle remedial exercises are recommended, as does dance therapy. All these gently exercise the body, convey inner balance and combat stress.

Psychotherapy

This is useful to combat anxiety and depression. Also useful are hypnotherapy and autosuggestion.

Relaxation techniques

These can be used to combat tension. Autogenics and biofeedback may be especially useful.

Spiritual therapy

Electrocrystal therapy can be very useful in relieving pain in arthritis. Also recommended are art, music and colour therapy, and Aurasoma.

VI/5 RHEUMATISM

This is a loose term for painful joints and muscles, excluding disorders due to infection or injury. Aside from arthritis (VI/1–VI/4) other 'rheumatic' complaints include fibrositis VI/6, RHEUMATIC FEVER, polymyalgia rheumatica (VI/7) and other disorders of soft tissues such as TENDINITIS, BURSITIS and SYNOVITIS. General treatments are discussed under VI/7.

VI/6 FIBROSITIS

Sometimes called muscular rheumatism, fibrositis is a vague term referring to painful muscles. The affected areas are usually located in the upper back, one of the commonest sites being between the upper part of the shoulderblade and the backbone (thoracic vertebrae). The pain can be intense, and sufferers sometimes liken it to a 'toothache in the muscle'. It can be present for several days or weeks at a time, and then disappear for months, for no apparent reason. One factor that has been observed to precipitate an attack is sweating, followed by rapid atmospheric cooling of a fibrositic area. Thus, if a sufferer plays sports or becomes overheated by wearing too heavy a garment in warm weather, and reduces his body heat by removing the garment and allowing the air to cool the skin directly, an attack of fibrositis frequently follows.

The underlying cause is thought to have something to do with nerve compression due to localized muscle SPASM or to minor abnormalities of the vertebrae. Another idea is that small areas of muscle herniate out through weak spots in the muscle's outer fibrous coating.

VI/7 POLYMYALGIA RHEUMATICA

Elderly patients are most often affected by this condition, which typically starts with pains and stiffness in the neck and shoulders and sometimes in the lower back, buttocks and thighs. Signs of fever are sometimes present, and this condition is associated with temporal ARTERITIS in a high proportion of patients.

ORTHODOX TREATMENT

The treatment for fibrositis includes simple pain-killers (such as aspirin), the application of heat and massage. Polymyalgia rheumatica is usually treated by a short course of steroids.

ALTERNATIVE THERAPIES

Natural medicine

The approach taken to the rheumatic complaints above is much the same as that taken to arthritis (see under VI/4). Tension is believed to play a part in generating fibrositis, as is poor posture, and both of these factors are considered and corrected if necessary.

Treatment may well start with the Guelpa fast. Subsequently, a similar diet to that recommended for arthritis sufferers would be likely to help generalized rheumatic aches and pains. Hydrotherapy, in terms of immersion in warm baths, could well be useful, and it is possible that green-clay packs on fibrositic 'trigger points' and polymyalgic muscles might also be of benefit. Toxin excretion would be encouraged, also, by deep breathing.

Raw juice therapy   Carrot juice (350ml) and spinach juice (110ml), twice daily.

Specific dietary supplements

- Calcium pantothenate (a B vitamin) may be helpful in the following regimen: 500mg daily for two days; 1,000mg for three days; 1,500mg for four days; and 2,000mg daily thereafter for two months or until relief is obtained. Daily intake should then be the minimum required for relief to be maintained (see also below).
- Vitamin C, 4,000mg daily in divided doses.
- Nicotinamide, 3g daily.

- To prevent recurrence, 100mg calcium pantothenate, 500mg Vitamin C and 100mg nicotinamide daily.
- As with arthritis (see under VI/4), a three-month trial of daily pollen is said to be very effective in many cases.

Cider vinegar   A dose of 55ml cider vinegar is said to work wonders for arthritic cows. This should be subjected to clinical trials in humans!

Biochemic tissue salts   For pain in the back muscles: *Ferrum Phos*. For fibrositic pain: *Magnesia Phos*. Dose: four tablets every hour in acute stage, less frequently when relief is obtained.

Herbal medicine

An infusion of one pinch each of camomile and lavender, and two pinches each of violet, sage and rosemary to a litre of water; take four cupfuls daily. At the same time, foot baths and hand baths of a handful of each of the following plus a chopped onion to 2 litres of water: camomile, heather, burdock, celandine, dog's tooth roots, broom flowers and lavender.

Also advisable are a bed of fern, and a hot cabbage poultice on the affected parts.

Aromatherapy

Massage in the following: oil made from 1,000ml olive oil plus 50g essence of origanum (wild marjoram). Also, three drops of origanum essence on a little brown sugar after every meal.

Homoeopathy

Rhus toxicodendron is the most important single remedy. When aggravated by motion and warmth: *Bryonia*. When worse for a change in the weather or an impending storm: *Rhododendron*. When jaw and neck areas are troublesome: *Causticom*.

Acupuncture

Can be very helpful.

Manipulative therapy

The Alexander technique for posture correction (useful in some fibrositis cases), osteopathy, chiropractic; remedial massage. Reflexology, too, can be very helpful.

Relaxation techniques

Yoga, autohypnosis, biofeedback.

Exercise therapy

Yoga and T'ai chi could help. Particular yoga postures for rheumatism include Mountain, Shoulder Sand, Knee to Chest, Twist and Posterior Stretch.

VI/8 OSTEOPOROSIS

Osteoporosis is an advanced stage of the bone-thinning process that affects everyone (especially women) from the age of 20 onwards. Factors that accelerate the process include, most notably, a declining level of oestrogens in the blood (during the menopause); Cushing's syndrome (overactivity of the adrenal glands); rheumatoid arthritis (see VI/3); and overactivity of the thyroid gland (see X/1). Because of the close association of osteoporosis with the menopause, detailed discussion of this disorder is to be found under V/14. The same dietary and exercise advice should be followed by non-menopausal sufferers.

VI/9 SARCOMA

Sarcoma is cancer of bone, connective tissue or muscles. It is far less common than CARCINOMA. The most commonly seen sarcomas are those involving bone; osteogenic sarcoma is one of these, and is especially common in childhood. Orthodox treatment includes radiotherapy, anticancer drugs and surgery. For further discussion see XIII.

VII   Disorders of the Skin, Hair and Nails

The skin consists essentially of two layers, the epidermis (outer) and the dermis below it. The epidermis consists of an external covering of dry, tough cells (keratin) which frequently flake off and are renewed from live cells below. Immediately below these are the cells which produce the skin pigment melanin. Hairs emerge from their follicles (roots) and push through the epidermis, and the pores of sweat glands open onto it. Both hair follicles and sweat glands originate in the developing baby in the epidermis layer and grow down into the dermal layer below. Besides sweat glands and hair follicles, the dermis consists of muscle fibres, strong, stretchy connective tissue, sensory organs and nerves (transmitting sensation), and capillary blood vessels. Sebaceous glands are found in association with the hair follicles.

Hairs, like the outer horny layer of dead epidermal cells, consist of keratin. Finger and toenails are made of a dense variety of keratin.

The skin serves many purposes. It provides protection for the underlying soft tissues. It also acts as a water-tight covering for these structures and prevents the loss from them of blood and tissue fluid. It helps to guard the body against the entry of invading bacteria and viruses; it is an important organ of sexual attractiveness and stimulation; and its blood vessels help to regulate the temperature of the body by dilating and bringing blood nearer to the surface when heat needs to be lost and by constricting when heat needs to be conserved. The skin is also an important organ of excretion.

VII/1   ACNE

This is an inflammatory skin condition especially prevalent in teenagers. It particularly affects the skin of the face, upper chest and upper back, and is due to the sebaceous glands at the base of the hair follicles producing larger amounts of skin grease (sebum) than usual. The sebum blocks up the gland openings on the skin and, as it continues to be produced, pimples, lumps and spots (whiteheads and blackheads)

Structure of the skin

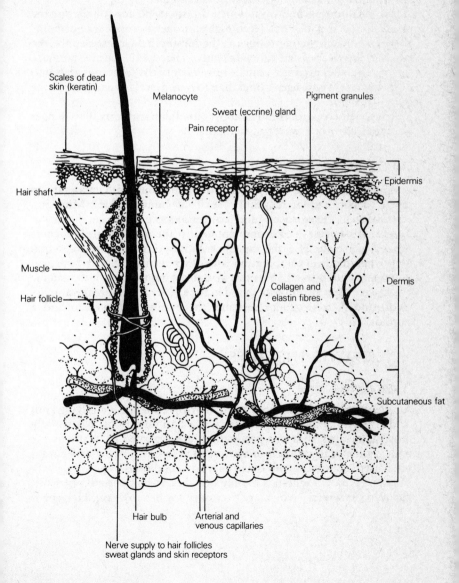

Scales of dead
skin (keratin)

Melanocyte

Pigment granules

Sweat (eccrine) gland

Pain receptor

Epidermis

Hair shaft

Muscle

Hair follicle

Collagen and
elastin fibres.

Dermis

Subcutaneous fat

Hair bulb

Arterial and
venous capillaries

Nerve supply to hair follicles
sweat glands and skin receptors

occur. Red spots, with a yellow centre of pus, show that the sebaceous ducts are getting inflamed.

Acne can cause a great deal of distress at an age when young adults are especially sensitive about their appearance. One in five boys and one in three girls need medical treatment for it. An expert on acne, dermatology consultant Dr W. J. Cunliffe does not ask girls with acne to do without cosmetics, 'since a girl with bad acne needs (at least for the first few months) some make-up to boost her morale'.[78]

It is the hormone androgen which is responsible for stimulating the production of extra sebum. (Although androgen is a male sex hormone, both males and females produce it, the former in their testicles and the latter in their ovaries and adrenal glands.) The actual causative mechanism of acne is believed to be undue sensitivity of the sebaceous glands to normal levels of androgen rather than to raised levels of androgen in the bloodstream.

Acne can leave permanently lumpy, pitted skin and scars. This danger is minimized by not squeezing the spots.

ORTHODOX TREATMENT

Long-term antibiotics are prescribed for patients with moderate to severe acne; e.g. tetracyclines such as minocycline (Minocin), erythromycin (Erythrocin) and co-trimoxazole (Bactrim, Septrim). Topical treatments (treatments applied to the affected area) include benzoyl peroxide as a gel, cream or lotion (Acnegel, Acetoxyl) and benzoyl peroxide in combination with other agents, e.g. with hydroxyquinoline (Quinoderm). (Retinoic acid is less used in the UK than in the USA.) Two topical antibiotics used in the UK are Actinac (chloramphenicol) and Neo-Medrone (contains the antibiotic neomycin and a steroid).

ALTERNATIVE THERAPIES

Natural medicine

Alternative therapists are interested in discovering the underlying fault in the body's homoeostatic mechanism. Skin eruptions, particularly those associated with pus production, are regarded by many as the body's attempt to rid itself of accumulated toxins. The Schroth cure is often used in the treatment of chronic skin conditions.

Leon Chaitow suggests a mainly raw diet, rich in natural nutrients, including enzymes[79] which are necessary for healthy skin. Hygiene is vital: unperfumed soap should be used, and the area swabbed dry with a clean towel and then with clean cotton wool soaked in surgical spirit (this may need to be repeated up to five times daily). Mr Chaitow also suggests that scarring can be treated with a cream containing both RNA and Vitamin E. He recommends also an overall improvement in nutrition, and detoxification. The following diet and supplements are based on his advice:

- Foods to avoid: white sugar and products, refined flour and products, fried and oily food, stale nuts, chocolate (substitute carob), iodine and kelp, animal fats and full-fat milk.
- Breakfast should be based on a mixture of natural grains, millet, oat flakes, wheatgerm, seeds, natural yoghourt, fresh fruit, or oatmeal porridge with fresh fruit and seeds. Twenty minutes before breakfast (unless you have thrush): 1tsp active bakers' yeast in a little warm water.
- Main meal: one main meal should be a large mixed salad with wholemeal bread, jacket potato, or rice dressed with lemon juice and olive oil, and seeds if liked. The other main meal should include fish, free-range eggs, poultry, lean meat or vegetarian savoury, and lightly cooked vegetables.
- Desserts: fresh fruit, yoghourt; once a week a raw-food day to help detoxify the system.
- Drinks: herb tea, mineral water, yeast (unless you have THRUSH).

Raw juice therapy   600ml of mixed carrot, grapefruit and celery juice, taken twice daily.

Specific dietary supplements

- Vitamin A (emulsified), 25–50,000iu daily
- B complex, 50mg strength
- B_2, 5–15mg daily
- B_3, 100–300mg daily
- B_5 (calcium pantothenate), 100–300mg daily
- B_6, 150mg daily
- choline, 50–100mg daily
- Vitamin C, 1g daily
- Vitamin D, 200mg daily
- Vitamin E, 200iu daily
- garlic capsules, four daily; also garlic rubbed on the spots
- zinc, as orotate, 200mg daily

Continue the above regimen for three months. If there is a vast improvement, maintain with same diet and daily supplements of Vitamin A (10,000iu), Vitamin-B complex (as before), Vitamin C (1g), Vitamin E (as before), zinc 100mg. Keep this up for six months; the diet should then be adequate to the individual's needs. Also advised are regular outdoor exercise; vigorous skin friction with a loofah; a three-month course of pollen tablets; and propolis tincture or ointment (a small dab on spots, several times daily, can sometimes improve acne dramatically).

Biochemic tissue salts   For pimples and pustules occurring in adolescence: *Calcarea Sulph*. Four tablets an hour, reducing as acne starts to clear.

Herbal medicine

Foot and hand baths of the following ingredients (a handful of each in 2 litres of water): burdock leaves, artichoke leaves, celandine leaves, sage flowers, mallow flowers and roots. (Two baths a day if associated with an upset liver.)

Aromatherapy

Bathe with lavender water (distilled water with 2 per cent essence); then apply lavender cream (1,000g sweet almond oil, 250g white wax, 750ml distilled water, 20g essence of lavender, 5g aspic).

Bach flower remedies

Homoeopathy

For chronic acne: *Kali Bichromicum*. For red, sore infected spots, circular and raised: *Sulphur*. For severely infected acne, with itching: *Psorinum*.

Acupuncture

This can help acne sufferers.

Manipulative therapy

Reflexology   Massage reflexes to liver, pituitary, thyroid and adrenals.

Exercise therapy

Regular dance therapy or yoga for toning body and improving circulation.

Psychotherapy

Hypnotherapy and autosuggestion can both be helpful.

VII/2 ECZEMA

This is a skin disorder involving INFLAMMATION and severe itchiness as well as the formation of blisters, weeping sores, scabs and loss of dry skin scales. (The terms dermatitis and eczema are often used synonymously.) Several varieties exist and all represent a skin reaction to one or several irritant factors. Emotional disturbances frequently make eczema worse, especially in children. Common types of eczema include: (a) varicose eczema, present in people with varicose veins (see III/6) and sometimes preceding ULCER formation; (b) contact eczema, due to contact with some chemical substance in the home or at work; and (c) atopic eczema, which mainly affects babies and small children and is associated with asthma (II/15) and hay fever (II/4).

ORTHODOX TREATMENT

Efforts are made to identify irritant substances which may be responsible. Steroid creams, lotions and ointments are given to reduce the inflammatory reaction, and itchiness is treated with steroids or antihistamine creams and tablets.

ALTERNATIVE THERAPIES

Natural medicine

The Schroth cure may be recommended. A natural wholefood diet free of any food items suspected of producing the eczema would follow. Since eczema attacks can be brought on by emotional factors, the patient's lifestyle would be discussed, and any stress factors brought to light. Adequate exercise would be advised, as well as psychotherapy for excessive anxiety, and daily relaxation sessions. Applied kinesiology might be used to identify food sensitivities and possibly to correct them.

327

Raw juice therapy

Carrot juice (170ml), beetroot juice (140ml) and cucumber juice (140ml), daily. *Or* carrot juice (230ml) and celery juice (230ml).

Specific dietary supplements

- 1 multivitamin supplement
- Vitamin E, 400iu, once or twice daily
- Vitamin A, 25,000iu, once daily, six days a week
- chelated zinc, 50mg, three times daily with food
- acidophilus capsules or tablets, 3–6, three times daily
- evening primrose oil (Efamol), 500mg capsules, three capsules twice daily, and the contents of one or several capsules applied to the rash
- many eczema sufferers have benefited from a course of pollen tablets
- the application of propolis cream once daily can have an outstanding effect on *dry* eczema, plus propolis capsules for a few days at the commencement of the treatment (propolis is not recommended for wet [weeping] eczema)
- honey can be useful for eczema patients who suffer from nervous tension; its tranquillizing properties are obtained from 1tsp taken six times daily

Biochemic tissue salts　In the first stage, for the inflammation: *Ferrum Phos*. For small, white dry scales on the skin and a white-coated tongue: *Kali Mur*. For scabs with offensive irritating secretions causing rawness and soreness of the affected areas, and for eczema in nervous persons: *Kali Phos*. Dose: four tablets every hour in acute condition, 3–4 times daily in chronic eczema.

Herbal medicine

Foot and hand baths (two daily) of a handful of each of the following ingredients to 2 litres of water: elecampane leaves and flowers, artichoke leaves, celandine leaves and cabbage leaves.

Aromatherapy

Dab areas with cotton wool soaked in this blend of oils: olive or sweet almond oil enriched with essence of chamomile (100g per litre) and of Borneo camphor (50–100g).

Bach flower remedies

Homoeopathy

Skin cracked and weeping: *Graphites*. At the borders of hair: *Natrum muriaticum*. Much itching, uncontrollable desire to scratch which then results in burning and smarting: *Sulphur*.

Acupuncture

This can be helpful to eczema.

Manipulative techniques

Reflexology   Massage to the reflexes of the liver, pituitary, thyroid and adrenals.

Psychotherapy

This can be useful when there is a strong emotional and nervous element in the production of the eczema. Sometimes rashes can be removed entirely (at least for a time) by hypnotherapy and autosuggestion, but nevertheless the underlying cause for imbalance needs to be identified.

Relaxation therapy

Relaxation through yoga and/or meditation is likely to be of considerable benefit. Of special use is the Sun Salutation posture.

VII/3 PSORIASIS

A psoriasis rash can take a variety of forms, but a typical one is a bright red raised area shedding silver-coloured flakes of dead cells. Its real cause is not understood, but it is thought to be associated with disordered skin biochemistry. Attacks come and go, and can be precipitated by worry, accidents and injury, but occur only in people predisposed to the complaint. Psoriasis is not contagious, and the problem is one of renewal of dead epidermal cells at a faster rate than necessary, with consequent thickening of the underlying skin. Itching rarely occurs: the worst thing about psoriasis is its appearance. It most commonly affects the arms and hands, the back and the scalp.

ORTHODOX TREATMENT

This includes steroid drugs by mouth for very severe cases; otherwise the encrusted scales and plaques can be removed by peeling agents, UV light and tar baths. Skin preparations containing steroids are sometimes prescribed.

ALTERNATIVE THERAPIES

Natural medicine

A wholefood diet with a fair proportion of the protein provided by animal sources (e.g. rabbit, poultry, fish, kidneys and liver). Adequate exercise and stress reduction. Treatment may start with the Schroth cure.

Specific dietary supplements

- Vitamin A, 10,000iu, three times daily for six days a week
- B complex, 100mg time release, morning and evening
- rose-hip Vitamin C, 1g twice daily
- Vitamin E, 400iu, three times daily
- evening primrose oil capsules, 500mg strength, two three times daily
- zinc, 15–30mg daily
- pollen promotes the health of skin
- propolis (see advice for eczema, VII/2)

Raw juice therapy   Apple and carrot juice, 600ml of each daily.

Herbal medicine

An infusion of two pinches of each of the following to a cup of water (take 3 cups per day): sage, camomile, lavender, thyme and lime flowers. Also, bath with hot and then cold water, dry the skin and apply calendula ointment into the patches (if this stings, try comfrey ointment).

Aromatherapy

A general remedy for skin diseases: dab affected part with sweet almond oil and 5 per cent essence of cajeput.

Bach flower remedies

Acupuncture

This can help psoriasis sufferers.

Manipulative therapies

Reflexology as for eczema (**VII/2**).

Spiritual therapies

Aurasoma; electrocrystal therapy. Also likely to help are psychotherapy (hypnotherapy, autosuggestion) and yoga for relaxation and reintroduction of exercise.

VII/4 IMPETIGO

This is an extremely infectious skin condition found more frequently in children than in adults and caused by invasion of the epidermal skin layers by staphylococcal or streptococcal bacteria. The lesions, which especially likely to occur on the face and around the mouth, are disfiguring to look at. They itch and the blisters form scabs which weep and ooze yellow fluid and pus. The condition can be serious in newborn babies and chronically sick children.

ORTHODOX TREATMENT

The lesions are soaked with warm water and disinfectant and gently rubbed to remove dried secretions and scabs. Antibiotics are prescribed, both as ointment and by mouth.

ALTERNATIVE THERAPIES

Natural medicine

The body's defence system requires a boost, and this may start with a 2—3 day fruit-juice fast followed by a strictly wholefood diet of which a large proportion of the foods are eaten raw. Fresh air and exercise would be recommended, and relaxation taught and prescribed for daily practice.

Raw juice therapy   Grape juice is especially good for spots and skin eruptions: take 600ml twice daily. Also, 1.2 litres daily of mixed carrot, spinach, cucumber and garlic juices (for boils, abscesses and septic spots).

Specific dietary supplements

- Vitamin A and D capsules (10,000iu and 400iu), 1–3 times daily (lower dose for a child) for five days out of seven
- Vitamin E, 100–400iu, once daily
- rose-hip Vitamin C, 500mg, twice daily
- propolis tincture can be applied to the infected lesions

Biochemic tissue salts   For the early stages, the following in alternation: *Ferrum Phos.* and *Kali Mur.* When the swelling has become soft and pus has started to form: *Silicea.*

Aromatherapy

Bathe lesions with boiled water and 2 per cent sassafras essence. Smear on the following compound: 1,000ml sweet almond oil, 250g white wax, 750ml distilled water and 25g essence of sassafras.

Homoeopathy

For septic lesions in unhealthy skin which is highly sensitive: *Hepar Sulphur.* When suppuration has taken place and is slow to clear: *Silicea.*

Acupuncture

Acupuncture helps ABSCESSES so may also help impetigo.

VII/5 LOSS OF HAIR

Possible causes for hair-loss include a deficiency of the thyroid hormone thyroxine (see X/1), anaemia (see VIII/1), a lengthy and debilitating illness, and taking of the Pill, steroid drugs, antibiotics and barbiturates. If no underlying cause can be found by conventional methods, a specialist in hair (trichologist) ought to be consulted. Too much Vitamin A can also cause hair to fall out.

ORTHODOX TREATMENT

Possible underlying causes (including skin conditions) are investigated and treated if present. A vitamin supplement or tonic might be prescribed if no apparent cause could be found.

ALTERNATIVE TREATMENT

Natural medicine

A wholefood diet would be recommended, with a relatively high protein content—e.g. liver, wheatgerm, beans and pulses, tofu, low-fat cheese, skimmed milk, eggs, lean meat and poultry, and fish. Stress elements would be identified and discussed, and the patient counselled to counteract these either by a change in lifestyle or by learning and practising relaxation, or both. Many commercial oils and other preparations are available for improving the strength, growth and general condition of the hair. Those containing jojoba extract are often very effective. Also beneficial is warmed pure almond oil massaged gently into the scalp and very gently into the hair, and leaving it in place for an hour before shampooing with a pure, unscented shampoo of the correct formulation for the individual's hair type.

Specific dietary supplements

- brewers' yeast tablets: six daily
- a potent B-complex supplement, one twice daily
- choline and inositol, 1g each, daily
- a multimineral formula containing 1g calcium and 500mg magnesium, one daily
- Vitamin C, 1g, twice daily, together with bioflavonoids
- kelp, one tablet, twice daily
- zinc orotate, 100mg, once daily
- desiccated liver: follow maker's instructions and take the maximum dose
- pollen is reputed by a number of users to both invigorate the elderly and help restore hair in areas which have been bald for years.

Raw juice therapy   Lettuce juice, 140g, twice daily.

Herbal medicine

A remedy reputed to be excellent consists of a hair tonic made from equal volumes of the following ingredients: best brandy, 4711 Eau de Cologne, coconut oil.

Aromatherapy

Massage the scalp with 40° alcohol containing 3 per cent essence of herb sage.

Homoeopathy

Lycopodium and *Vinc. Minor* are said to be helpful in restoring hair in some cases of middle-age balding.

VII/6 RINGWORM

A very common skin infection caused by the fungus *Tinea*. Only the epidermis is attacked by this parasite, the resultant INFLAMMATION being due to irritation from the metabolic products of the fungus or to a delayed allergic response (see ALLERGY. In certain types of *Tinea* infection the involved area or areas of skin form a disc-like shape, with the centre healing before the periphery to produce a ring effect.

Common areas of the body to be affected include: the scalp, with scaly patches and hair-loss; the hands; the groin (dhobie itch); the trunk, limbs and face; the beard; the feet (athlete's foot); and the nails. Itching is a common feature wherever the infection occurs. When the nails are involved they may crumble, become deformed and eventually separate from the underlying nail-bed.

ORTHODOX TREATMENT

Local treatment (i.e. substances applied to the rash areas) is reserved for minor skin infections. The more recent imidazole preparations have largely superseded the time-honoured preparations such as tolnaftate and compound benzoic acid ointment (Whitfield's ointment BNF), and are normally applied once a day. Examples are sulconazole nitrate 1 per cent cream (Exelderm) and econazole nitrate 1 per cent cream (Ecostatin). Griseofulvin in tablet form is given for ringworm of the scalp and nails and for widespread or chronic infections of the skin that have failed to respond to local treatment. Griseofulvin's brand names are Fulcin and Grisovin.

ALTERNATIVE THERAPIES

Natural medicine

A wholefood high-raw diet would be advised to help boost the strength of the patient's immune system, which is then in a better position to combat infections itself. Stress factors would be looked into and relaxation advised, and outdoor exercise recommended several times a week. It is very probable that a naturopathic doctor would approve of herbal or perhaps dietary-supplement remedies for ringworm infection as an adjunct to his or her longer-term management. He or she would also suggest that the infected area be exposed to the air as much as possible. If athlete's foot were the problem the patient would be advised to go barefoot whenever this was possible. Dabbing the affected areas morning and night with cider vinegar is useful.

Specific dietary supplements The following nutrients are especially important to the health of the skin:

- Vitamin A, 25,000iu daily for three weeks
- a potent B complex containing at least 50mg each of the major B vitamins, one, twice daily
- Vitamin C with bioflavonoids, 1g, twice daily
- Vitamin E, 400iu in chewable-tablet form, once a day for a week, then twice daily for two weeks
- essential fatty acids: take evening primrose oil (Efamol) capsules, 500mg strength, two, twice daily
- Earl Mindell suggests in his *Vitamin Bible* that Vitamin-C powder or crystals applied directly to affected areas seem to help ringworm infection

Other supplements and applications A little raw honey applied to the ringworm areas and left in place for as long as possible has proved effective in at least one recorded case. Propolis ointment may well be effective, applied daily and left in contact with the infected areas. Pollen taken by mouth is said to boost the body's natural resistance and encourage it to overcome infections.

Raw juice therapy Strawberry and date juice (use fresh dates) are recommended by Dr John Lust as one of the best skin-cleansing foods known; he specifically mentions ringworm in this context. I would recommend pulping raw fresh dates, making strawberry juice with a juicing machine, and then liquidizing the date-pulp together with the strawberry juice (as the dates contain little moisture). No quantities are given by Lust and the strawberry juice would be expensive, but I suggest a daily consumption of, say, 170g fresh dates and 340ml strawberry juice.

Herbal medicine

Make a strong tea with golden seal root, bathe the area, dry thoroughly and dust area with powdered golden seal root.

Aromatherapy

Take four drops of lavender essence on a little brown sugar half an hour before each meal; also dab the areas daily with lavender alcohol and 40 per cent of essence.

Manipulative therapies

Reflexology Massaging the reflexes to the liver, pituitary, thyroid and adrenal glands can stimulate the natural healing processes of the skin.

VIII Disorders of the Blood

Our blood is composed of fluid—plasma—in which three different types of solid particle are suspended (see below). The body of an adult man contains about 4.5–5 litres of blood.

The plasma is clear, slightly sticky and yellowish in colour, and accounts for about 55 per cent of the total volume of the blood. It contains proteins in solution as well as the breakdown products of digestion: amino acids, fat, and glucose, derived respectively from the protein, fat, and carbohydrates we consume in food. Plasma contains also dissolved gases as well as waste products resulting from the metabolic processes of the cells. These waste materials (e.g. urea, uric acid) are given off by the active tissue cells and pass with ease through the capillary walls, where they enter into temporary solution in the plasma. They are eventually removed by the kidneys and lungs and excreted. Plasma in this way acts as a transport medium for waste material, for a certain amount of our oxygen and carbon dioxide, and for the nutrients required by the tissues.

The plasma proteins are large molecules mainly manufactured in the liver. One of their chief functions is to keep what is known as the osmotic pressure of the plasma at a desirable level. They are unable to pass through the capillary walls, and their effect on the plasma is to combat the loss of large amounts of fluid out into the surrounding tissues. The tendency of fluid to flow outwards is increased by the pressure of blood within the capillaries, and the plasma proteins (especially albumin and globulin) resist this outward flow by drawing fluid into the capillaries again. In certain liver diseases, the manufacture of plasma proteins is adversely affected, and some of the osmotic pressure of the plasma is lost. The outward flow of plasma fluid is then insufficiently opposed and the fluid tends to collect in the tissues, waterlogging them and producing OEDEMA. Renal diseases also result in plasma loss.

Globulin has an additional important function. There are several different classes of globulin in the plasma, and the one known as gamma-globulin, made in the lymph nodes and spleen, provides immunity to infectious illnesses.

Other types of plasma protein exist, including fibrinogen, which is responsible under the right conditions for producing the fine fibrous threads that are an essential part of clot-formation.

There are two different types of blood cells: red cells (erythrocytes) and white cells (leukocytes); also there are the cell-like platelets (see below). The first of these differs from most other body cells in lacking a nucleus. The nucleus is actually present in the immature red cell, but simply fragments and is absorbed by the time the cell has matured.

There are approximately five million red cells in every millilitre of blood; their lifespan is about 120 days. Old red cells are broken down in the spleen and their number is constantly being replenished from primitive cells in the marrow of the long bones. This production is controlled by a hormone (erythropoietin) associated with the kidneys.

Red cells have the extremely important function of carrying oxygen around the bloodstream from the lungs to the tissues of the body, whose need for it is constant. This is done by the oxygen passing through the red-cell membrane and becoming attached to the red oxygen-carrying

337

pigment inside, haemoglobin. The oxygen circulates in the bloodstream until it reaches the capillaries and tissues, whereupon it is released. The amount of haemoglobin in a normal blood sample is in the region of 14.5g per 100ml. Iron and a variety of other factors, including Vitamin B_{12} (cyanocobalamin) and folic acid (another B vitamin), are necessary for the manufacture of haemoglobin.

The white cells too are derived from cells in the bone marrow; they do have nuclei. They are larger than the red cells, although fewer in number, an average count in an adult being in the region of 8–9,000 per millilitre of blood. There are three different types of white cell, the most prolific (70 per cent) being the granulocytes. Three types of granulocytes exist: neutrophils, basophils and eosinopils, named for their slightly different staining properties when examined in the laboratory. Their function is to surround and destroy bacteria, and their number increases greatly under the stimulus of an acute bacterial infection.

The other two types of white cell are the lymphocytes and the monocytes. Lymphocytes are present in the lymph nodes and spleen as well as in the bloodstream, and manufacture gamma-globulin. Their number tends to be raised in the presence of chronic infection and when the invader is a virus.

The remaining particle at large in the plasma is the thrombocyte, or platelet. This is not a true cell but is formed (again in the bone marrow) by the fragmentation of a cell. Platelets play an important part in the clotting mechanism owing to their ability to adhere to one another when a blood vessel is torn: They stick to the injured site in a clump and prevent blood escaping by plugging the hole. At the same time they secrete a factor that is essential to the formation of fibrin threads from fibrinogen. An adequate supply of platelets in the blood is essential for clotting to occur normally. The normal platelet count is around 250,000 per millilitre of blood.

VIII/1 ANAEMIA

Anaemia is a reduction in the quantity of haemoglobin in the blood. This limits the blood's ability to carry oxygen around the body and produces the commonest symptoms of anaemia, including exhaustion, breathlessness and/or dizziness after minimal exertion; and an unnaturally pale complexion, fingernail beds and eyelid-linings.

Slight degrees of anaemia are very common. Women are prone to develop iron-deficiency anaemia due to their monthly blood-loss, and adults of either sex can become anaemic due to the chronic loss of small amounts of blood over a long period. This can happen in cases of a bleeding peptic ulcer (see I/9) or bowel TUMOUR, in the presence of severe piles, or when varicose veins exist in the foodpipe (see OESOPHAGEAL VARICES).

Two basic mechanisms are capable of producing anaemia: the first is inadequate production of red cells, and the second is heavier than normal loss of them.

Inadequate production can be caused by a deficiency of iron, usually as a result of blood-loss; this is often aggravated by insufficient dietary iron and/or insufficient iron in storage to meet the extra demands of periods, pregnancy and lactation. Other factors affecting the production of red cells include cancer, long-standing infectious illnesses, and a failure by the kidneys to secrete the essential hormone erythropoietin. Also important is vitamin deficiency, especially of cyanocobalamin (Vitamin B_{12}) and of folic acid: abnormally small numbers of red cells are formed, and some of these are of poor quality and soon destroyed. A shortage of folic acid can result from an insufficient dietary intake of fresh vegetables. A shortage of Vitamin B_{12}, though, is most likely to be caused by the absence of a substance known as intrinsic factor, normally produced in the stomach. Anaemia results because, in order to be absorbed, Vitamin B_{12} has to combine with intrinsic factor. This variety of anaemia is called *pernicious anaemia*: until 1926 it was a terminal disease.

A heavier than normal loss of red cells means that larger numbers are either lost (due to haemorrhage) or broken down than is usually the case. In health, the only red cells to be 'lost' are those that reach the end of their natural lifespan; these are broken down by a process called haemolysis, and their iron is carefully stored in the liver, their number being replaced by newly mature red cells from the bone marrow.

Frequent small blood-losses deplete the body of red cells and of its total iron complement (in the form of the red cells whose iron content would have been stored). Some of the circumstances in which this is likely to occur were noted above. This type of blood-loss may lead to *iron-deficiency anaemia*, as is HAEMORRHAGE resulting from an injury. When a litre or two of blood is lost thanks to an accident the blood still (initially) contains the same amount of red cells and haemoglobin per millilitre, even though the total blood volume has been severely depleted. The blood volume is made up either by means of a transfusion or by the body itself, since fluid from the tissues will enter the blood circulation with the object of maintaining the blood pressure. When this takes place, the blood becomes progressively more dilute and severe anaemia is present until the body has managed to restore the circulating number of red cells to normal.

More than the usual numbers of red cells are destroyed (haemolysed) when cells are unusually delicate (examples include sickle-cell anaemia). Other causes of *haemolytic anaemia* include certain toxins such as lead, sensitivity to a drug, incompatible blood transfusion and autoimmune disease.

ORTHODOX TREATMENT

The orthodox approach to anaemia is to discover the mechanism responsible and to direct treatment at that. Pernicious anaemia, for instance, is treated with injections of Vitamin B_{12} (patients are unable to absorb this vitamin by mouth). Iron-deficiency anaemia, due for example to heavy periods, would be treated with supplementary iron, and the periods themselves treated too if necessary.

Haemolytic anaemia due to blood-group incompatibility can occur in a newborn baby when his or her blood group is incompatible with that of the mother. Severe examples would be treated by exchange transfusion, the damaged blood cells and the plasma of the baby being gradually withdrawn and replaced by fresh donor blood of a compatible group.

ALTERNATIVE THERAPIES

Natural medicine

Treatment would depend to a certain extent upon the cause. In life-threatening situations it is likely that the orthodox approach would be used, and the patient referred for immediate treatment to a medical doctor. After the emergency treatment had been given, though, a naturopathic doctor would advise the patient on diet, lifestyle and stress-reduction in order to speed up convalescence as much as possible.

For a state of chronic anaemia, perhaps resulting from an inadequate body-store of iron or the production of fragile red cells (for instance, due to a lengthy infection), advice would be given along similar lines.

A good diet for the treatment of iron-deficiency anaemia would include some of the following iron-rich foods: pork-liver, beef-kidney, heart and liver, egg yolks, oysters and raw clams, nuts, beans, asparagus, molasses, oatmeal and dried peaches. A suitable diet for someone with pernicious anaemia (due to dietary deficiency, not lack of intrinsic factor) would include liver, kidney, eggs, milk and cheese, since all these are sources of Vitamin B_{12}.

Specific dietary supplements For iron-deficiency anaemia chelated iron is most readily absorbed. Organic iron exists in the following compounds: ferrous gluconate, ferrous fumerate, ferrous citrate and ferrous peptonate, none of which neutralize Vitamin E (avoid the inorganic iron preparation ferrous sulphate which can destroy Vitamin E). Take about 300mg three times a day. Also take 1g of Vitamin C, twice daily.

Sickle-cell anaemia sometimes responds to Vitamin E, 400iu daily.

Raw juice therapy Fresh spinach juice, mixed with carrot, nettle and a little horseradish juice—four cups per day. Molasses as a supplement may be helpful, as it contains riboflavin, pyridoxine and iron, all of which are important in the manufacture of healthy red cells. Take a dessertspoonful twice daily. Also, pollen taken in a high-potency form is reported to help anaemia.

Biochemic tissue salts *Calcarea Phos.* is the chief biochemic tissue salt remedy for iron-deficiency anaemia. When this has helped to form healthy red cells, to help replenish their supply of haemoglobin: *Ferrum Phos.* For simple anaemia in young girls, when the blood takes a long time to clot: *Natrum Mur.* For when skin eruptions coexist with the anaemia: *Kali Phos.* alternating with *Calcarea Phos.* Dose: four tablets of the appropriate remedy every two hours.

Herbal medicine

An infusion of three pinches of rosemary in a cupful of water. For pernicious anaemia, comfrey tablets, taken as the manufacturer suggests.

Aromatherapy

Five drops of essence of lemon on a little brown sugar half an hour before each meal.

Homoeopathy

For iron deficiency anaemia: *Ferrum Metallicum.* Helpful for pernicious anaemia: *Arsenicum.* For tall, pale, weak sensitive people, overactive and breathless: *Phosphorus.*

Acupuncture

This is reported to help anaemia.

Spiritual therapy

Electrocrystal therapy may help.

VIII/2 GLANDULAR FEVER

This is an infectious illness caused by a virus of the same group as that which causes herpes (see **XII/3**). The medical name of this disorder is infectious mononucleosis, referring to the change which occurs in the microscopic appearance of the blood. The white-cell count (total number per millilitre) increases to 10–30,000, and lymphocytes instead of granulocytes become the predominant type. The most notable of these lymphocytes are some—around 10 per cent of the total number of white cells present—which assume an atypical appearance: these are the mononucleocytes of the disorder's medical name.

Glandular fever is commoner in children, adolescents and people in their 20s than in older age groups. It seems to be passed from one person to another in saliva. It starts insidiously with a slight temperature rise after an incubation period of 4–8 weeks. The patient feels very under the weather and develops a sore throat, enlarged tender lymph glands, and muscular aches and pains. Occasional accompaniments to these symptoms include jaundice and a rash.

ORTHODOX TREATMENT

The patient is advised to go to bed, keep warm and drink plenty of fluids. Occasionally tetracycline as prescribed, as well as aspirin and throat lozenges.

ALTERNATIVE THERAPIES

Natural medicine

A wholefood diet, with plenty of fresh fruit and vegetables, as a general health measure against infection. For a patient with glandular fever (whose appetite is usually very poor), freshly squeezed vegetable and fruit juice would be excellent nutrition.

Specific dietary supplements

- Vitamin C: 500mg, three times daily
- high-potency Vitamin-B complex: try 50mg strength, three times daily
- amino acid L-lysine: 1,500mg daily
- honey: mix 2tbsp honey and 2tbsp glycerine with a pinch of powdered ginger or a little of the grated fresh root and 1tbsp fresh lemon juice; keep this mixture warm and take as needed to relieve the sore throat

Biochemic tissue salts   For swellings of the glands of the neck and the throat: *Kali Mur*. For the fever and pain in acute swelling of the glands: *Ferrum Phos*. Dose: four tablets every two hours, reducing in frequency as symptoms abate.

Herbal medicine

A gargle made by infusing one handful of each of these ingredients in 2 litres of water: cabbage leaves, elecampane flowers, dog's tooth roots, poppy flowers, mallow flowers and violet flowers.

Aromatherapy

Essence of thyme, three drops on a little brown sugar half an hour before each meal. With the following gargle this soothes the sore throat: lukewarm boiled water containing 2 per cent essence of thyme.

Homoeopathy

For fever and swollen glands: *Belladonna*. *Ailanthus glandulosa* has proved useful. Of value for glandular symptoms: *Baryta Carbonica*.

VIII/3 CANCER OF THE BLOOD

Leukaemia is often referred to as cancer of the blood. The term refers to a group of diseases whose common factor is the manufacture of excessively large numbers of abnormal white blood cells by the bone marrow. Immature white cells, normally kept within the bone marrow until mature, are also released into the circulation, and can be identified by means of the microscope.

The malignant cells in the bone marrow multiply to such an extent that the manufacture of red cells and production of the platelets cease. As a result, symptoms of anaemia appear, and the clotting ability of the blood is reduced due to the platelet deficiency.

There are two main classes of leukaemia, acute and chronic. The acute varieties tend to affect young children, the chronic ones to occur later in life.

Hodgkin's disease is often mentioned together with leukaemia, but this is a malignant disease of the lymphatic system rather than of the bone marrow and blood. It shares a number of symptoms with chronic leukaemia in adults, especially with the chronic lymphatic variety. Both illnesses cause fatigue, anaemia, stomach pains and enlargement of the spleen and the lymph glands.

TREATMENT

Some patients do very well with modern treatment, which consists of anticancer drugs and/or radiotherapy. For alternative treatments see under Cancer (**XIII**).

VIII/4 MALARIA

This tropical parasitic blood infection is due to a single-celled animal belonging to the genus *Plasmodium* which spends part of its lifecycle in man and the rest of it in the mosquito (both hosts are necessary to it). Transmission from human to mosquito occurs when the mosquito drinks the blood of an infected person. Later, at the right stage of its lifecycle, *Plasmodium* is transmitted in the insect's saliva to a new human host when the mosquito again sucks blood. Once in man, the parasites develop further in the liver, enter the bloodstream, and multiply inside the red blood cells. After 48–72 hours the red cells burst open, causing the characteristic symptoms of malaria—i.e. chills, fever and sweating. The parasites enter fresh red cells, and their lifecycle continues.

The parasitic invasion of man by *Plasmodium* causes also anaemia, enlargement of the spleen, jaundice, renal failure and potentially fatal blockage of blood vessels in the brain. Signs of the illness may not occur for weeks or months after infestation occurs.

ORTHODOX TREATMENT

This aims at prevention, and is done mainly with chloroquine (Avloclor).

ALTERNATIVE THERAPY

Herbal remedy

This aims at reducing the fever: either an infusion of one pinch of vervain to a cupful of water; or an infusion of eucalyptus leaves, using half a handful of broken dried leaves to a litre of water (take 3–4 cups daily).

VIII/5 AIDS (Acquired Immunodeficiency Syndrome)

This was recognized as a new illness in the spring of 1981, and is now known to be due to the HTLV virus, which can be transmitted through the blood and by sexual intercourse (especially anal). The virus interferes with the activities of specialized T-lymphocytes whose function is to repel viral and other infections.

The main features of AIDS[80] are profound fatigue, weight-loss, night sweats, persistent diarrhoea, cough and breathlessness. Spontaneous skin bruising can occur (see PURPURA) and lymph-node enlargement is common. A malignant form of sarcoma can feature (Kaposi's sarcoma): this is a form of skin cancer in which purple nodules and blotches spread generally in the skin and to the mouth and nose. Secondary infections often occur due to the poor state of the auto-immune system, which is already overburdened with the AIDS virus. THRUSH is a common secondary infection, herpes another.

There is at present no effective treatment for AIDS and the mortality rate is 100 per cent. The incubation period is from nine months to six years, with an average of two years.

AIDS is chiefly a disease of male homosexuals (75 per cent of patients). A further 20 per cent of patients are drug addicts 'mainlining' (i.e. using intravenous routes), and the remaining 5 per cent are people who have received infected blood transfusions (e.g. haemophiliacs), women partners of bisexual males or partners of intravenous drug users, and the babies of mothers with AIDS. There is no evidence that AIDS can be transmitted in any other way—e.g. by touching, kissing, breathing or eating. People who suffer from AIDS and then suffer further from being treated as pariahs are therefore victims not only of the disease but also of ignorance and prejudice.

ORTHODOX TREATMENT

The orthodox treatment of AIDS is symptomatic since there is no specific drug therapy and as yet no antiviral agent. Secondary infections are treated with antibiotics, antifungal or antiviral drugs, and pain-relief is given for malignant TUMOURS.

ALTERNATIVE TREATMENT

Not a great deal of literature on this subject at present exists, but the general aim of alternative practitioners would be to bolster and strengthen the body's immune defence system. AIDS is typically a disorder in which alternative therapists from a variety of specialities would doubtless wish to collaborate; obvious ones include naturopathy, acupuncture, herbal medicine, aromatherapy, homoeopathy and possibly reflexology. Electrocrystal therapy might be of help in strengthening the depleted energy of the body's defence mechanism.

IX Disorders of the Brain, Spinal Cord and Nerves

The brain is recognized as having three main regions—the fore-, mid- and hindbrain—but most of what you see when you look at a model of the brain is forebrain. This consists of two halves, the right and left cerebral hemispheres, which are joined deep down in the midline by a body of white nervous tissue called the corpus callosum.

In the spinal cord (see below) the grey matter is enclosed in an outer layer of white matter; but the reverse is true in the forebrain, where the two halves have their grey material (cerebral cortex) on the outside.

One of the most noticeable features of the cerebral hemispheres is their wavy surface, full of regular and symmetrical humps and dips. The functions of the cerebral hemispheres (in humans at least) are self-awareness, intellectual activity and the initiation of voluntary action. A motor area (governing movement) and a sensory area (interpreting

Brain, Spinal Cord and Nerves

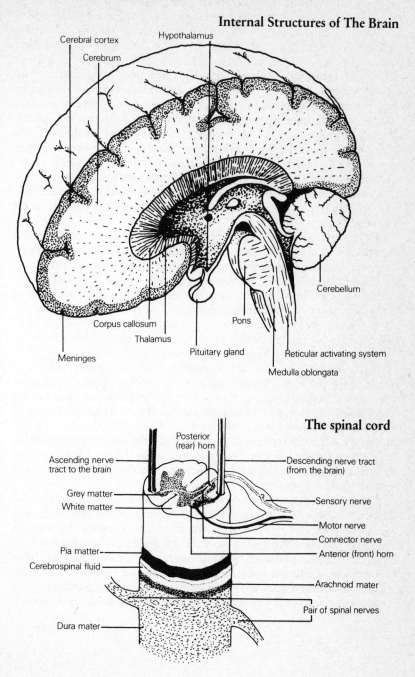

Internal Structures of The Brain

Cerebral cortex

Cerebrum

Hypothalamus

Cerebellum

Corpus callosum

Thalamus

Pons

Meninges

Pituitary gland

Reticular activating system

Medulla oblongata

The spinal cord

Posterior (rear) horn

Ascending nerve tract to the brain

Descending nerve tract (from the brain)

Grey matter

White matter

Sensory nerve

Motor nerve

Connector nerve

Pia matter

Anterior (front) horn

Cerebrospinal fluid

Arachnoid mater

Pair of spinal nerves

Dura mater

most of our sensations) have been distinguished, but some of our functions have yet to have their specific areas of operation identified.

Also in the forebrain are the thalamus and hypothalamus. The first relays sensations it receives either to reflex centres or to the higher centres where we become aware of them; it also interprets, at a basic level, the sensations of pain, crude touch and temperature. The hypothalamus, below it, controls the autonomic nervous system, in which capacity it helps to regulate heartbeat, blood-pressure and glandular secretions. Beneath the hypothalamus is the pituitary gland, the master endocrine gland in the body. Just behind where the pituitary gland arises we find the pineal body, or 'third eye'. Also deeply buried within the forebrain are the basal ganglia (referred to again under Parkinson's disease [IX/3], which can be more easily understood when it is realized that the basal ganglia are responsible for the moment-by-moment control of voluntary muscle tone—i.e. its state of contraction or relaxation).

The midbrain is far less complex than the forebrain. The two cerebral hemispheres are joined one on either side of it, and it relays messages from the eyes and ears as well as helping to coordinate movements.

The hindbrain's most important structure is a large corrugated body called the cerebellum, which governs, among other things, our sense of balance and the maintenance of posture. Just below the origin of the cerebellum is the area where spinal cord and brain actually merge. This, the medulla (or medulla oblongata), contains among other things the vital centres regulating heartbeat and respiration.

The spinal cord, like the brain, consists of grey nerve-cell bodies and white nerve-cell fibres, the arrangement of which is opposite to that in the cerebral hemispheres. A cross-section shows the arrangement of the central grey matter into a butterfly shape, with two anterior horns in front and two posterior horns behind.

The spinal cord has two main activities. It is the vital link along which messages pass to and from the brain, and is also the local headquarters at various levels for reflex activity (such as the withdrawal of a limb way from a source of pain).

The spinal nerves leave the spinal cord in 31 pairs, between each two adjacent vertebrae. They contain both sensory and motor fibres and serve the skin and muscles with sensation and movement pathways running between them and the spinal cord. Paired nerves also leave the brain. These cranial nerves, of which there are 12 pairs, originate from nerve nuclei within the substance of the brain and supply structures of the head, face, and neck with sensation and movement pathways. The 10th cranial nerve, the vagus, also sends branches down to the heart and the stomach. In the heart it has a 'braking' effect upon the rate at which that organ beats; in the stomach it helps to regulate the rate at which hydrochloric acid is secreted by the cells of the stomach lining.

The spinal cord ends in nerves descending downwards to the lumbar and sacral vertebrae. Because of its appearance, this arrangement of spinal nerves is known as the 'cauda equina', or horse's tail.

The brain and the spinal cord are enclosed in the meninges, three layers of membranes named (from the outside in) the dura mater, the arachnoid mater, and the pia mater. The first of these layers is tough, and lines the inside of the skull; it also sends a fold downwards between the right and left cerebral hemispheres, superficially separating them. The arachnoid mater is a flimsy membrane lining the inner surface of the dura mater, and is connected by strands to the innermost and very delicate pia mater, which follows the contours of the cerebral hemispheres faithfully.

IX/1 EPILEPSY

A group of diseases in which the electrical activity of the brain-cells gets temporarily out of control. Effects include (a) brief losses of conscious awareness, (b) 'fits' (convulsive seizures) and (c) transitory uncontrolled movement of certain muscle groups. The first two types are called *petit mal* and *grand mal* attacks; the third is known as a Jacksonian seizure. (Occasionally a high fever in childhood, a brain ABSCESS or a TUMOUR, injury or other damage is found to be the underlying cause of attacks, in which case epilepsy is not the culprit.) Warning symptoms of an approaching attack include headaches, spells of dizziness, and repeated yawning. These are followed by odd physical sensations (e.g., sudden tingles in the skin) and a feeling of unreality which constitute the 'aura', or first part of the attack.

While *petit mal* attacks may pass unobserved (people think that they've merely lost a few moments in daydream), *grand mal* attacks are far more dramatic and therefore considerably worse for the patients. They may realize an attack is going to begin but are usually unable to avert it: they pass out and the voluntary muscles contract very strongly, especially those of the jaw. They then convulse violently, and may vomit or pass urine or faeces. Finally, they fall asleep or enter a phase a bit like an hypnotic trance.

349

ORTHODOX TREATMENT

The barbiturate phenobarbitone was the drug of choice for many years but has now been superseded by others such as carbamazepine (Tegretol) which can control seizures efficiently.

ALTERNATIVE REMEDIES

Natural medicine

Lifestyle, diet, stress factors, exercise habits, etc., would be scrutinized by a naturopath. Some alternative practitioners claim to ease epileptic patients off their anticonvulsive drugs and maintain them in good health. Many, however, would prefer to work in cooperation with an orthodox doctor and try by lifestyle modification or a combination of therapies to help the patient reduce the need for such drugs to a minimum. A wholefood diet, high in raw foods, would be prescribed. (Food additives are suspected of causing convulsions in some instances.)

Specific dietary supplements   Some research findings have indicated that deficiency of Vitamin D or of pyridoxine (Vitamin B_6) can be associated with convulsions, and that supplements of either or both, given under professional supervision, may reduce the frequency of attacks.

Calcium and magnesium supplements very occasionally help; for example, in one reported case two dolomite tablets daily (in addition to usual anticonvulsive drugs) stopped convulsions.

Biochemic tissue salts   For muscular convulsions in any part of the body: *Magnesia Phos.* For spasms in teething babies and children: alternate *Magnesia Phos.* with *Calcarea Phos.* For feverish conditions frequently associated with spasms, especially during teething: *Ferrum Phos.* Dose: 2–4 tablets every 15 minutes during attacks, less often when relief is gained; during teething, give *Calcarea Phos.* 3–4 times daily.

Herbal medicine

A preparation of skullcap is sometimes given alongside orthodox drugs to help reduce convulsions.

Aromatherapy

Essence of chamomile, 3–4 drops, on a little brown sugar, three times daily between meals. Also, 3–4 drops essence of basil in a spoonful of lime-blossom honey, three times daily. In addition, prepare a sugar compound of 100g finely ground brown sugar to which you add essence of basil (1g) essence of lavender (1g) and essence of rosemary (1g). From it take ½ coffeespoonful to sweeten an infusion of verbena or mint after every meal (if you are not following a homoeopathic course of treatment).

Bach flower remedies

Acupuncture

Some cases of *petit mal* are reported to respond to this.

Physical manipulation

Cranial osteopathy has claimed some success in treating epilepsy.

Relaxation therapy

Stress reduction would be very likely to help, especially where tension and anxiety were particular trigger factors to attacks. Recommended are yoga, autohypnosis, autosuggestion, and meditation.

Spiritual therapies

Aurasoma; music and colour therapies.

IX/2 MIGRAINE

This disorder consists of severe recurrent headaches, usually confined to one side of the head and often accompanied by nausea, vomiting, poor appetite and acute sensitivity to light (photophobia). Three main varieties are recognized: classical, common and cluster migraine. An attack of *classical migraine* gives warning of its approach by causing disturbances in vision (blurring, loss of sight), taste, touch or speech. This warning is known as the aura, and is thought to be due to the constriction of blood vessels in one area of the brain. The pain can be very severe, and usually recurs on the same side each time. Nausea and vomiting are common accompaniments. *Common migraine* rarely gives any warning other than perhaps slight nausea. It can be very severe, and also causes nausea and vomiting. *Cluster migraine* occurs in 'clusters' of attacks lasting 2–12 weeks during which 3–4 headaches per day sometimes occur. The trouble-free periods between attacks last from several months to several years. The pain of cluster migraine is also intense and is often worst behind the eye, which may water and become red. The nose may become blocked on the affected side.

ORTHODOX TREATMENT

Mild tranquillizers are given to some patients, but the mainstay of treatment is ergotamine tartrate (Migril, Cafergot). Clonidine (Dixarit) is given as a preventive measure.

ALTERNATIVE THERAPIES

Natural medicine

Emphasis is upon dietary correction, stress-reduction and lifestyle-modification where necessary (e.g. avoidance of visits to noisy places with brightly flashing lights, such as discos, where an attack is very likely to be brought on). Also recommended are a wholefood diet, with perhaps applied kinesiology to identify any food allergies present, and possibly to correct them. Also known to precipitate attacks in some sufferers are HYPOGLYCAEMIA, sinusitis (see II/8), synthetic oestrogen (in the Pill or in hormone-replacement therapy for menopausal symptoms), and the food additives monosodium glutamate (present in many processed foods), nitrates and nitrites (present in hot dogs, bacon, ham and salami). Food triggers include milk and other dairy products, chocolate, cola, pork, onion, garlic, corn, eggs, citrus fruit, wheat, coffee, alcohol, cheese, chicken liver, pickled herrings, broad-bean pods and canned figs.

In some patients the use of a bonnet-type hair-dryer at the earliest sign of an impending migraine attack can prevent that attack.

Raw juice therapy   Where fatigue, nervous tension, a hangover and gastric upset are associated factors, the following is recommended: two parts tomato juice to one part celery juice, plus 2tsp onion juice. Take one wineglassful every two hours until the attack disappears.

Specific dietary supplements

- niacinamide (Vitamin B$_3$) can help prevent or ease the severity of migraine headaches; take 50–100mg once or twice per day in your stress-B supplement
- calcium pantothenate: 100mg, three times daily
- pyridoxine (Vitamin B$_6$): 50mg, three times daily (if regimen gives relief, reduce levels of these last two to your own maintenance level)
- pollen is reported to have helped relieve migraine attacks very effectively

Biochemic tissue salts *Ferrum Phos.*, four tablets every half-hour during acute stage, reducing as the attack lifts.

Herbal medicine

A compress on the forehead during an acute attack; or foot and hand baths (as regular treatment) of the following ingredients: five chamomile flowers and a handful each of balm and lavender to 2 litres of water. *Or* an infusion of a pinch of each of the following to a cupful of water: basil, chamomile and wild thyme.

Feverfew (a type of chrysanthemum) is renowned for its ability to help many migraine sufferers. A test devised by herbalist Simon Mills suggests a way of determining whether feverfew is likely to help a particular migraine patient: if the migraine attack is helped by applying heat to the head, feverfew (which dilates the blood vessels) could be beneficial; if cold-packs are effective, however, feverfew is unlikely to be beneficial. Mills also points out that a professional judgement with respect to suitable treatment in each case is preferable, since migraine is a complicated condition.[82] It is important, according to Mills, that the correct variety (*Tanacetum parthenium*) of feverfew is used and that the herb is freeze-dried to preserve the essential volatile oils. The correct dose is likewise vital. The traditional folk remedy suggests chewing one raw leaf of feverfew, but it seems that its content of active substance is extremely low. Hospital trials suggest that the best dose is one 200mg tablet daily for 90 days. If taken over this period, relief is often long-term. Some herbalists feel that 250mg daily should be taken.

Aromatherapy

Four drops of essence of sweet marjoram on a little brown sugar after each meal. Also, massage forehead, temples and nape of neck with marjoram alcohol (1,000ml 80° alcohol, 100g borneol and 60g essence of sweet marjoram).

Bach flower remedies

Homoeopathy

Feverfew in liquid or tablet form. Also, for migraine preceded by misty vision or zigzag lights: *Natrum Muriaticum*. For migraine that begins in the nape of the neck, comes over the head and settles in one eye: *Silicea*. For headache usually over right eye, nausea, dizziness: *Lycopodium*. For migraine preceded by blurred vision: *Kali Bichromicum*. Left-sided headache, with faintness and palpitations: *Spigelia*. Right-sided headache, with variable symptoms (worse for heat): *Pulsatilla*.

Acupuncture

This is helpful in migraine cases.

Manipulative therapy

Reflexology   Helpful in migraine cases, massage being applied to the reflexes to the solar plexus, the tip of the big toe and the cervial reflexes on the edge of the big toe. Massage also applied to the reflex to the colon if it is tender, and the reflex to the coccyx.

Cranial osteopathy   This helps some cases.

Relaxation techniques

Definitely suitable, as tension triggers migraine attacks in many sufferers. Yoga, meditation, autohypnosis and autosuggestion would be appropriate. Yoga postures recommended for the treatment of all types of headache include Corpse Posture, Neck and Eye exercises, and the Shoulder Roll.

Exercise therapy

This might be suggested if the naturopath felt it relevant. Dance therapy and yoga sessions could also be helpful.

Psychotherapy

This may be needed to get to the root of inner tension and anxiety.

Spiritual therapy

Electrocrystal therapy may prove helpful. Also, art, music and colour therapies.

IX/3 PARKINSON'S DISEASE

Parkinson's disease results from degeneration of cells in the basal ganglia and the brain stem. The chief effects are upon the control of voluntary muscle; posture, voluntary movement of the skeletal muscles, speech and facial expression can all be affected. The disorder can be a product of the side-effects of certain drugs (e.g. those used to treat schizophrenia), or result from a number of poisons, one (named MPTP) being sometimes present as a by-product in the illegal home production of narcotic drugs (e.g. pethidine, morphine). These substances damage the basal ganglia, but Parkinson's disease proper (the drug/poison-induced version is usually called Parkinsonism to distinguish it), arising for no apparent cause, seems to be an exaggerated aspect of 'normal' ageing processes. Certain cells, called dopaminergic neurones, from within the basal ganglia are lost, and a deficiency of dopamine occurs —dopamine being an essential chemical messenger carrying electrical stimuli from one neurone cell to another.

Symptoms of Parkinson's disease include an uncontrollable tremor (shaking) of the hands, arms and head, a shuffling walk, slow stiff awkward movements in general, and in some patients degeneration in condition until the patient is completely helpless. Because the patient's facial muscles are immobile many people believe Parkinson's disease patients to be mentally affected. They do not, in fact, lack intelligence, but sometimes serious mental and emotional changes can occur.

ORTHODOX TREATMENT

Levodopa (Brocadopa, Madopar, Sinemet) is the most important drug in the treatment of Parkinson's disease. It is changed within the brain cells to dopamine, and this goes part of the way to relieving the symptoms and signs of the disease in many patients. Another very useful drug used at present in conjunction with levodopa is selegiline hydrochloride (Eldepryl). This acts by inhibiting the effect of a substance called monoamine oxidase, which breaks down dopamine in the brain cells.

ALTERNATIVE THERAPIES

Natural medicine

It is likely that a naturopathic doctor would work in cooperation with an orthodox physician since no satisfactory natural treatment has yet been found to surpass or even equal the effectiveness of levodopa therapy. The naturopathic aim would be to improve the general health of the patient, as far as possible, with wholefood diet, suggested supplements, gentle daily exercise and stress-reduction. Most diseases —in particular those involving the brain and spinal cord—are aggravated by nervous tension and severe mental and physical stress.

Raw juice therapy   These combinations are recommended by John B. Lust for maintaining the general health of the nervous system:

- carrot juice (340ml) and spinach juice (115ml), daily
- carrot juice (170ml), beetroot juice (140ml) and cucumber juice (140ml), daily

Specific dietary supplements   The normal vitamin and mineral daily supplementation should *not* include any pyridoxine (Vitamin B_6) because this neutralizes the effects of the levodopa treatment. The side-effects of the levodopa, on the other hand (e.g. emotional and mental disturbance and 'freezing' attacks in which all movement is temporarily suspended), can be partly or totally counteracted by the daily 1g Vitamin C in the supplementation.

The amino acid methionine was found in an Alabama hospital trial involving 15 patients to relieve the following symptoms of Parkinson's disease: low level of activity; difficulty in moving; rigidity; poor mood and sleeping patterns; poor concentration and attention-span; inaudible, incoherent voice; and weak muscular strength. Symptoms that did not improve were drooling and tremor. The improvements occurred in 10 of the 15. The dose of methionine started at 1g a day and was increased over a period of three weeks to 5g daily. Levodopa therapy was maintained throughout the trial; the full methionine dose was maintained for 2 months.[83]

Aromatherapy

Trembling may be reduced by four drops of lavender essence on a little brown sugar half an hour before each meal.

Bach flower remedies

Acupuncture

This may help relieve the trembling.

Relaxation techniques

Much might be gained if the patient started to follow relaxation techniques as soon as the complaint were diagnosed—autohypnosis, yoga and autosuggestion might retard the development of symptoms for a certain period. Yoga could be usefully pursued for as long as possible.

IX/4 CANCER OF THE BRAIN

The brain contains two main types of cell, neurones which are nerve cells and cannot become cancerous because they cannot reduplicate themselves, and neuroglial cells, which form connective tissue and are capable of multiplying. It is the latter which can become malignant and form one type of brain TUMOUR, called a glioma. Symptoms of a brain tumour, which are largely due to the resulting increase in pressure within the brain (intracranial pressure), may include vomiting, blurred vision and head pain. Orthodox treatment usually aims at surgery, wherever possible, and/or radiotherapy. For discussion of alternative approaches to cancer see **XIII**.

IX/5 MULTIPLE SCLEROSIS (MS; DISSEMINATED SCLEROSIS)

This disease attacks the myelin sheaths that protect and insulate the nerve cells throughout the brain and spinal cord. Evidence of its effects occur in patches of destroyed myelin, which are then replaced by thickened tissue or 'plaques'. The condition's cause is not known. Symptoms in the early stages vary. The earliest sign might be, for example, lack of feeling in an area of skin; weakness of a particular muscle-group, perhaps giving rise to a limp; or blurred vision in one or both eyes. Although the disease is progressive, long periods of partial or complete remission occur. After a variable number of years, though, the patient may become increasingly handicapped physically as well as more difficult to deal with on an emotional level. On the other hand, a remission may last for years, or the disease may fail to progress and thereafter cause little real problem.

ORTHODOX TREATMENT

There is no specific treatment for MS. Usually the patient's health is maintained in as good a state as possible with an adequate diet and vitamin and mineral supplements. Physiotherapy may be recommended to enable the patient to keep as mobile as possible for as long as possible.

ALTERNATIVE THERAPIES

Natural medicine

The emphasis would be on a strictly wholefood diet, supplements, gentle remedial exercise and regular relaxation and visualization. Some success has resulted from adopting macrobiotic diet and the philosophy behind it. A diet formulated by Dr R. L. Swank has been successful in that it has seemed to stabilize the disorder at the point it had reached when the diet was started.[84] Anyone deciding to follow this diet ought to start upon it as soon as the diagnosis is confirmed. (See also below.)

Specific dietary supplements   The health of the nervous system depends upon—among other factors—an adequate intake of Vitamin-B complex and Vitamin E. The following are recommended: stress-B complex, 100mg strength, one twice daily; 200iu Vitamin E twice daily, building up to 400iu twice daily.

Herbal medicine

Clinical trials of the use of evening primrose oil in MS[85] have shown significant relief resulting in cases where treatment started shortly after diagnosis; it has not been effective in long-established cases. The recommended dose is three 500mg Efamol capsules twice daily. Action for Research on Multiple Sclerosis (ARMS) in Britain recommends that its members take evening primrose oil in this dosage immediately on diagnosis.

As with Dr Swank's diet, few patients actually improve on supplementation, but the regimen seems to stabilize the condition and stop its progression. In a few fortunate patients, there may be substantial improvement.

Aromatherapy

Muscular paralysis resulting from either injury or disease is said to be helped by smearing the affected part with oil and essence of juniper (olive oil with 10 per cent of essence).

Bach flower remedies

Acupuncture

MS may respond in the early stages to this.

Manipulative therapy

Remedial massage is useful.

Relaxation techniques

Since it now seems that a definite link exists between MS and prolonged stress, relaxation techniques are likely to be highly beneficial. For example, hypnotherapy and visualization; autohypnosis; autosuggestion; yoga combined with meditation.

Psychotherapy

This might be of use where past trauma still affects the patient and produces tension symptoms.

Exercise therapy

Therapeutic, mentally and physically, as long as they can be carried out gently and without strain: yoga, dance therapy, T'ai chi.

IX/6 SHINGLES (HERPES ZOSTER)

This disorder is due to the infection of the sensory root of one (or several) spinal nerves. These nerves are a mixture of sensory and motor fibres, but the two different types of fibre issue separately from the spinal cord before uniting to make a 'mixed nerve'. The infecting agent is the herpes zoster virus, responsible also for chickenpox (see XII/1). The rash is typically preceded by pain in the area supplied by the relevant nerve. This can be severe and also puzzling—until the rash breaks out, whereupon the diagnosis is obvious because the spots are characteristic. They follow the course of the sensory fibres as a band travelling around the body from back to front. (Sometimes a pair of spinal nerve roots are infected so that two bands encircle the body, meeting in front in the midline. (It is a myth that if this happens you die!) The spots appear first as red blotches which soon break down into vesicles (or blisters) containing fluid. The spots are both itchy and painful, and can be dangerous when the virus infects the ophthalmic nerve (one of the cranial nerves), so that the spots involve the eye.

Pain can continue for a long time after the rash has disappeared. Shingles is sometimes connected with a period of stress or debilitating illness when the natural defences of the body are depleted.

ORTHODOX TREATMENT

The usual treatment consists of oily calamine lotion, to apply to the rash, and pain-killers for the pain, although antiviral drugs are indicated when the rash involves the eye. Acyclovir (Zovirax) is virtually nontoxic, and in severe cases is given by intravenous injection. Acyclovir and trifluorothymidine are also applied to the rash on the eye itself.

For pain that continues after an attack (post-herpetic neuralgia) a new treatment has recently been tried with promising results. Intramuscular injections were given of adenosine monophosphate (AMP), a naturally occurring purine compound. After four weeks 88 per cent of patients who received it were pain-free in contrast to 43 per cent of the placebo patients. No recurrence of the pain occurred in the 18 months following the trial, and AMP was found not only to relieve the pain but also to accelerate the healing of the rash. Research is currently being carried out into the effects of AMP upon other tissues of the body.

ALTERNATIVE THERAPIES

Natural medicine

Wholefood diet, gentle exercise when patient sufficiently fit, lifestyle-improvement wherever necessary, special attention to stress-reduction and relaxation.

Raw juice therapy   The following should help to speed recovery from ophthalmic herpes: two cups carrot juice, one cup celery juice and 1tbsp parsley juice: take three cups daily.

Specific dietary supplements

- Vitamin A: 10–25,000iu, 1–3 times daily for five consecutive days out of seven
- Vitamin-B complex: 100mg, morning and night.
- rose-hip Vitamin C with bioflavonoids: 1–2g, morning and night)
- Vitamin D: 1,000iu, 1–3 times daily for five consecutive days out of seven
- cider vinegar, dabbed neat on the rash, has been found to give better pain relief than medication; the treatment needs to be repeated every couple of hours
- propolis: a trial in Yugoslavia in 1978 showed a 5 per cent solution of propolis tincture, applied daily, relieved pain within 48 hours; the pain did not reappear and itching continued for a long time in only three of the 21 patients in the trial.

Biochemic tissue salts   *Kali Mur*. and *Kali Phos*. alternately, four tablets of each every half-hour during the acute stages, reducing the dose as symptoms abate.

Herbal medicine

A compress, foot and hand baths of a handful of each of the following to 2 litres of water: poppy flowers and seed capsules, meadowsweet and lime flowers. At the same time, an infusion of a pinch of each of the following in a cup of water: thyme, rosemary, lavender, chervil and lime flowers.

Aromatherapy

Dab rash and blisters with cotton wool soaked in water containing 2 per cent essence of lemon.

Homoeopathy

Patient feels better for warmth and movement, worse in bed: *Rhus toxicodendron*. For much swelling and large blisters: *Urtica*. For burning, stinging pain, restless, no thirst: *Apis*.

Acupuncture

This may be of help in accelerating recovery.

Relaxation techniques

This is especially likely to be of value to patients in whom stress has precipitated the attack of shingles.

IX/7 STROKE

Stopping of the circulation of the blood to an area of the brain. This usually happens without warning and generally causes permanent damage to the cells in the affected area. The damage is due to the absence of oxygen and glucose, of which the brain-cells normally receive a constant supply. PARALYSIS is often experienced by the patient following a stroke because the area of the brain which controls voluntary movement (the 'motor' area in the cortex) is frequently the one affected by the sudden stoppage. Speech, too, is often impaired. On the other hand, some minor strokes fail to produce symptoms; other, major, strokes are fatal.

There are three chief ways in which a stroke can come about. A cerebral HAEMORRHAGE may occur, in which a weak artery in the brain ruptures and bleeds. A cerebral EMBOLISM may occur. Alternatively, a thrombus may form (see THROMBOSIS), obstructing the blood flow more gradually as it develops within a diseased artery (see hardening of the ARTERIES).

There is frequently a considerable degree of improved function during the weeks following a stroke. Firstly, those muscle groups that remain unaffected generally learn to adapt their function in such a way that they compensate in part for the loss of affected groups. Secondly, the permanently damaged brain area is surrounded by a zone of only temporarily affected tissue, the cells of which regain their function when they have had an opportunity to recover.

Transient ischaemic attacks are similar to very minor strokes. Stroke symptoms appear for a few minutes and then disappear again. A likely cause is temporary SPASM in the blood vessels supplying an area of the brain or temporary pressure upon an artery travelling up the neck to supply the brain, due to getting the neck into an unsuitable position.

ORTHODOX TREATMENT

Surgery is sometimes of great use, when it is possible to seal a ruptured blood vessel or remove a clot of blood. If the source of an embolus can be traced it is sometimes possible to prevent a recurrence. Drugs are sometimes prescribed to prevent further clotting when thrombosis has been the underlying cause. Other approaches include speech therapy, physiotherapy, and occupational therapy.

ALTERNATIVE TREATMENT

Natural medicine

The naturopathic approach would first of all establish the overall vital reserve or vital energy of the stroke patient. A light, nutritious, wholefood diet would be recommended where solid food could be taken, and gentle manipulative therapy carried out with the object of restoring function. Saturated fats in the diet would be substituted by polyunsaturated oil. Gentle exercise as soon as the patient was capable of it would be recommended. Hydrotherapy might be utilized in some patients where the restoration of limb strength and movement might be aided by carefully supervised swimming exercise.

Specific dietary supplements The following daily regimen is suitable both for prevention of strokes in likely candidates and as post-stroke treatment:

- Vitamin E: 400–600iu
- Vitamin C: 500–1,000mg
- evening primrose oil (Efamol): 3g
- lecithin: 5–15g
- fish oils containing EPA and DHA (3g)

A course of pollen would be advisable for its invigorating and healing effects.

Herbal medicine

The herb yarrow is recommended as part of a wider programme, together with other substances which improve the circulation in the extremities and skin, such as elder flowers, rosemary, hyssop, and buckwheat. Nervous restoratives are also recommended, as these help to nourish a debilitated nervous system; examples are damiana, oats, rosemary, lady's slipper, Asiatic ginseng and lavender. Only a trained herbalist has sufficient knowledge and experience to plan the medication in detail.

Aromatherapy

For muscular PARALYSIS, take lavender essence, four drops on a little brown sugar, half an hour before each meal. Also, rub spinal column and paralysed part with the following alcohol preparation: 1 litre 80° alcohol, 40ml essence of lavender, 20ml essence of aspic and 30ml essence of basil.

Homoeopathy

Treatment must be directed by a physician in the early stages.

When the patient is flushed, slow and collapsing, or unconscious; the face is flushed and dark, breathing is heavy, the pulse slow, the pupils dilated; useful to prevent a threatened attack: *Opium*. A basic remedy, to be used when there is either an impending threatened stroke, or weakness of the left side; also bed-sores, a full pulse and noisy laboured breathing: *Arnica*. Useful for the period of paralysis after the acute episode, especially if the paralysis is right-sided and involves the tongue: *Baryta Carbonica*.

Every effort is made to reduce a raised blood pressure, since this is a major precipitating factor of strokes.

Bach flower remedies

Acupuncture

In China this is the standard treatment for strokes: it is applied to both the scalp and the body to aid recovery. Work so far completed suggests that acupuncture increases the blood-supply to the brain. This seems to improve functional ability and acts as a stimulant to recovery after a stroke. A very high success rate is claimed. Practitioners in the West also find acupuncture very useful in helping stroke patients.

Ideally, treatment should be commenced within six months of the stroke occurring; if the damage has been present for more than two years, little improvement can be expected.

Manipulative therapy

Physiotherapy, remedial massage and in some cases reflexology may help.

Relaxation techniques

Biofeedback, autogenics, yoga and meditation might all be beneficial. Autohypnosis, with positive visualization of the healing process at work, may prove helpful.

Exercise therapy

T'ai chi and yoga, as well as being of psychological help, could both be excellent ways of helping a patient regain full use of the muscles. Dance therapy is currently being used to improve the mobility of stroke patients and to boost their self-confidence. In London, classes are held at the Swiss Cottage Community Centre, to which new members are referred by the Royal Free Hospital, St Mary's, New End Hospital or their own GP.[81]

Psychotherapy

This might be applicable to stroke patients with a highly stressful lifestyle which they wish to resume. Learning to relax is vital if a recurrence is to be avoided, so hypnotherapy might prove invaluable here.

Spiritual therapy

Music and colour therapy might be employed to induce a relaxed attitude to life, both during convalescence and afterwards. Aurasoma might prove beneficial. Electrocrystal therapy could be used to boost healing.

X Disorders of the Endocrine Glands and Hormones

The body's main endocrine (ductless) glands are the pituitary, the thyroid, the parathyroids, the adrenals, the pancreas and the sex glands (ovaries and testes). The pituitary, thyroid, parathyroids and adrenals form separate and distinct ductless glands; in other organs only some of the constituent cells are 'endocrine glands' by nature. Examples are the islet cells of the pancreas, the interstitial cells of the testis, and the interstitial cells in the ovarian follicles and the corpora lutea of the ovary.

The *pituitary gland* is situated on the undersurface of the brain. It has two lobes, or discrete parts, the front one being the anterior lobe (or adenohypophysis) and the one behind being the posterior lobe (or neurohypophysis). This pea-size gland is the shape of a greengage and, because it rests in a small depression in the sphenoid bone, above and behind the nasal cavity, certain surgical operations upon it can be performed by approaching it through the nostrils. The anterior lobe of the pituitary gland is the larger of the two lobes and develops in the growing baby from the roof of the mouth. It contains two main varieties of hormone-secreting cells which can be differentiated on microscopy by their different staining properties. The smaller posterior lobe is a downgrowth from the floor of the brain and consists of modified nervous tissue originating as a protrusion of the hypothalamus which acts as a go-between between the endocrine glands and the central nervous system.

The *thyroid gland* lies in the front of the neck, in the midline; the landmark for locating it is the Adam's apple, since the two thyroid-gland lobes lie one on either side of this structure. They are joined at their lower poles by a slim band of tissue that crosses the upper portion of the windpipe. Although each pole of the gland is about 5 cm long, the tissue from which it is composed is very soft and this makes it difficult to feel with the fingertips through the skin. It is, however, richly supplied with blood vessels, and so great care has to be taken to seal off the bleeding points within the gland when it is operated upon.

The *parathyroid glands* consist of two pairs of small pea-like glands situated in the neck behind the thyroid gland and sometimes embedded in its substance.

The anatomical features of the *pancreas* as a digestive gland have been discussed on page 152. Its endocrine structure consists of small clusters of specialized cells scattered throughout the substance of the gland and named the 'islets of Langerhans'. These do not communicate with the pancreatic duct, which collects the pancreatic juice from the rest of the gland, but instead secrete the hormones they manufacture straight into the bloodstream.

There are two *adrenal glands*, situated one on top of each kidney within the abdominal cavity. Each gland consists of two discrete regions—an outer cortex, and an inner medulla.

None of the endocrine glands acts independently of the others. Feedback mechanisms exist between the pituitary and most of the rest, since the pituitary can make and secrete 'trophic' hormones to encourage the function of the others. Their secretions, in turn, inhibit further formation of the stimulating trophic hormone. The blood levels at which this inhibition takes place depend upon the body's requirements. These are gauged—and the appropriate messages passed to the pituitary gland —by the nervous system. Requirements may alter, in some cases from minute to minute, so the state of equilibrium of the body's hormonal levels is a highly dynamic one.

The anterior lobe of the pituitary gland secretes six types of hormone. These are: (a) melanophore-stimulating hormone which acts on the pigment cells in the skin; (b) prolactin, which controls milk-secretion from the breast; (c) growth hormone, which stimulates the growth and development of bone and other tissue in childhood and adolescence, and influences sugar regulation by the pancreas in adults; (d) two gonadotrophic hormones, which stimulate activity in the testes or the ovaries; (e) thyrotrophic hormone (TSH), which stimulates the thyroid gland's secretion; and (f) adrenocorticotrophic hormone (ACTH) which stimulates the adrenal glands to secrete the hormone cortisol.

The pituitary gland's posterior lobe produces two hormones: (a) oxytocin, which stimulates the uterus to develop labour contractions at the end of pregnancy, and stimulates the breast tissue to produce milk; and (b) antidiuretic hormone (ADH), responsible for the kidneys' action in retaining fluid within the body rather than excreting it as urine. This hormone is released and exerts its activity when no fluids have been taken for some time, or excessive amounts have been lost from the body due to heavy perspiration, prolonged vomiting, diarrhoea, or extensive burn injuries. (Its release into the bloodstream is suppressed and the kidneys put out a large volume of urine when the reverse is true, i.e. the blood is slightly more dilute than usual as a result of large volumes of fluid having been consumed.)

The thyroid gland secretes two hormones, thyroxine and calcitonin. Thyroxine contains iodine in combination with an amino acid, and its manufacture and release are stimulated by TSH produced in the pituitary; it increases the body's metabolic rate (i.e. the rate at which the body metabolizes glucose to produce energy). Calcitonin counteracts the effect of the parathormone produced by the parathyroid glands; i.e. it lowers the concentration of calcium in the blood.

The parathyroid glands secrete parathormone, whose action is to raise the concentration of calcium in the blood should the normal level of calcium in the blood be for any reason lowered. Calcium bound to the structure of bone is made more soluble, and is therefore released into the bloodstream.

The islet cells of the pancreas produce two hormones, insulin and glucagon. The function of insulin is to facilitate the passage of glucose from the bloodstream into the cells of the tissues that require it; that of glucagon is to encourage the tissue cells (in particular, those of the liver) to release glucose into the bloodstream.

The cortex of each adrenal gland produces several hormones with similar chemical structures (all are steroids) and three different types of function. Firstly, the hormone group of which cortisol is characteristic regulates the laying-down of fat in the body, suppresses inflammation and allergic reactions, and encourages the synthesis and storage of glucose. Secondly, the hormone aldosterone combats the loss of salt and water from the body in the form of urine, and regulates the balance between sodium and potassium. Thirdly, the sex hormones of both sexes are produced; this function is of less importance than the other two because these hormones are already being made by the ovaries and testes.

The adrenal medulla is considered part of the sympathetic nervous system. Sympathetic nerves function by secreting extremely small amounts of adrenaline and noradrenaline. When these nerves stimulate the adrenal medulla these two hormones are secreted in relatively large quantities, preparing the body for 'fight or flight' (see STRESS REACTIONS).

In the main, the endocrine glands can malfunction in two different ways: they either produce excessive amounts of their hormones (e.g. as a result of tumour formation) or they produce too little (perhaps as a result of lack of stimulation by the pituitary gland, and consequent failure of the appropriate feedback mechanism).

X/1 HYPERTHYROIDISM (THYROTOXICOSIS) AND HYPOTHYROIDISM (THYROID DEFICIENCY)

Enlargement of the thyroid gland is called a goitre. This can be a simple goitre or a toxic goitre; the alternative name for the latter condition is Grave's disease. While there may be very little apparent enlargement, the thyroid's cells are in fact manufacturing and secreting thyroxine at a considerably increased rate, with serious effects upon the patient. One of the most noticeable symptoms is feeling too hot even when the environmental temperature is cool. This is due to the increased metabolic rate that results from excessive thyroxine secretion, while at the same time the body's oxygen requirement is increased, due to the accelerated rate at which fuel (glucose) is consumed (i.e. metabolized) within the body. As a result the heart beats more quickly, and the patient may complain of PALPITATIONS, both because he or she is aware of its increased rate and because its rhythm may be disturbed. Irritability, hyperactivity due to excessive amounts of energy, poor sleep, severe weightloss regardless of the amount of food eaten, and (in women) disturbed menstrual periods are also common features.

Some patients with this condition develop protruding eyes (exophthalmic goitre) due to the presence of an abnormal hormone known as LATS (long-acting thyroid stimulator), which is probably produced in the hypothalmus area of the brain.

The cells of the thyroid gland are, in fact, only rarely the cause of thyrotoxicosis. More frequently, either LATS or an excessive amount of TSH (thyroid-stimulating hormone, produced by the anterior lobe of the pituitary gland) is responsible.

ORTHODOX TREATMENT

Rest is prescribed and the overactive condition of the thyroid dampened down with either iodine or drugs such as carbimazole (Neo-Mercazole) or potassium perchlorate (Peroidin). When the heart is being driven less hard and the consultant feels the time is right, part of the thyroid gland is removed surgically. Beta-blocker drugs, e.g. propranolol (Apsolol, Bedranol), are prescribed for some patients to help relieve the symptoms.

Radioactive iodine can be used to suppress the overactive thyroid cells. These take up the radioactive isotope of iodine as readily as if it were ordinary iodine; when the radioactive iodine is in the gland it kills a proportion of the tissue.

ALTERNATIVE THERAPIES

Natural medicine

A natural wholefood diet would be appropriate, possibly organized by mutual cooperation between a naturopathic doctor and the patient's usual physician. Onions, seafood and vegetables grown organically in iodine-rich soil might be advised. Useful vitamin supplements would include the normal supplementary programme (see page 436) and kelp, which is said to normalize both slightly overactive and underactive thyroid-gland conditions, by reason of its many useful constituents, including iodine.

Herbal medicine

Cabbage, cress and spinach juice are recommended.

Aromatherapy

The following onion preparation is recommended: allow 500g raw onion to macerate for two weeks in 500g of 60° alcohol, and then strain. Take one soupspoonful at the start of every meal. The taste can be improved by adding brown sugar and lemon juice.

Homoeopathy

For thyrotoxicosis accompanied by exophthalmic goitre: *Thyroidinum*. For exophthalmic goitre and thyrotoxicosis, especially when accompanied by palpitations and weightloss: *Natrum Muriaticum*. For simple goitre and for toxic goitres with exophthalmos, where there is a rapid pulse, weightloss and agitation: *Iodum*.

Acupuncture

This has proved useful in some cases of both simple and toxic goitre.

Spiritual therapy

Electrocrystal therapy.

Thyroid deficiency can occur in babies and is due to a failure of the thyroid to develop; it is generally unnoticed at birth. The baby fails to develop mentally and physically as it should, and the untreated condition develops into cretinism. Cretins are intellectually below the level at which formal education can be of any use. Physically, they are short in stature, have thick coarse hair and skin, a fat protruding tongue and a rounded belly. Treatment is by means of thyroxine hormone, and is completely or partially successful depending upon how early the condition is detected and treatment started.

Myxoedema is the name given to thyroid deficiency in an adult; middle-aged women are most often affected. Symptoms include always feeling cold, an increase in weight, dry coarse skin, and poor concentration and intellectual acuity. Characteristically the hair from the outer one-third of the eyebrows falls out and refuses to grow. Some cases of myxoedema are a form of autoimmune disease (see ALLERGY).

ORTHODOX TREATMENT

Thyroxine reverses all the changes of myxoedema in nearly every patient. Examples of thyroxine-supplying compounds are anhydrous thyroxine sodium (Eltroxin) and liothyronine (Tertroxin).

ALTERNATIVE THERAPIES

Natural medicine

A natural wholefood diet to which is added the normal supplementary programme and iodine (if this has been in short supply); this could be taken as an iodine supplement or in its most natural form as kelp. It is also possible that manganese might be deficient. Manganese is essential for the formation of thyroxine by the thyroid gland. Heavy milk-drinkers and meat-eaters tend to be short of manganese. The daily mineral supplement should therefore contain this element. Glandular supplements may also be of use.

Herbal medicine

Kelp would very probably be recommended because of its normalizing effect.

Homoeopathy

The condition can be helped homoeopathically but the choice of preparations would be weighed up carefully by the practitioner, possibly in cooperation with the orthodox doctor.

Spiritual therapy

Electrocrystal therapy.

X/2 DIABETES MELLITUS

'Ordinary' diabetes, is due to a deficiency of the hormone insulin produced by specialized cells in the pancreas. Many diabetics actually produce insulin in reasonably high quantities but are faced with one of two major obstacles with regard to its use: either they have chemical antagonists (possibly antibodies) to insulin in their tissues which destroy the hormone and prevent them from using it, or their cells are incapable of responding normally to the insulin they make (this is especially applicable to liver cells). The effects of insulin deficiency result from the inability of bloodstream sugar to cross the outer membrane of the tissue cells and act as a source of energy. Instead, it collects in the bloodstream where the level gets steadily higher (see HYPERGLYCAEMIA). Above a certain level, the sugar (which is in the form of glucose) 'spills over' into the urine, thereby increasing the volume of urine produced because extra fluid is required to transport the extra glucose. This produces a cardinal feature of diabetes: the passage of large quantities of urine and corresponding thirst.

Since glucose is unavailable to the cells as a source of energy, fat is burnt instead, and so body-fat is lost. But the combustion of fat can proceed only to a certain point due to the absence of certain chemical substances normally produce by the combustion of glucose. The chemicals that *are* formed by the breakdown of fat—ketone bodies —poison the body, causing an acidic state and ultimately COMA; death can ensue rapidly unless insulin is administered.

Another serious effect of diabetic illness is degeneration of the walls of small blood vessels, particularly those of the eyes (see RETINOPATHY) and kidneys. The large blood vessels are especially prone to develop ATHEROMA.

ORTHODOX TREATMENT

There are two main types of diabetes and they are treated differently. Juvenile diabetes starts in childhood or early adult life, and antibodies to insulin may play a major role. This is treated by daily insulin injections and a controlled diet (insulin cannot be given by mouth because it is destroyed in the stomach). Too much insulin can result in hypoglycaemic coma (see HYPOGLYCAEMIA).

Regular testing of the urine is a vital aspect of maintaining a state of health. By and large, an individual's insulin requirement stays much the same from day to day, provided other factors remain steady. A change in diet, more or less exercise than usual, stress and illness all affect the amount of insulin required.

Maturity-onset diabetes (which constitutes over 90 per cent of diabetes mellitus) starts typically in middle-aged overweight people whose problem is one of insufficient effective insulin for their requirements. This sort can often be controlled by diet alone. When it cannot, drugs are available in tablet form which either reinforce the effect of the insulin the patient is able to make or increase the supply the patient manufactures. Examples are chlorpropamide (Diabinese), glibenclamide (Daonil), and metformin (Glucophage). Insulin itself is rarely needed.

ALTERNATIVE THERAPIES

Natural medicine

Evidence is accumulating that much diabetes can be controlled without the use of insulin. Both orthodox and alternative practitioners are becoming aware of this following work initiated by Nathan Pritikin, the nutritional researcher. He gave diabetics a diet containing 80 per cent carbohydrate (nearly all unrefined), 13 per cent protein and 7 per cent fat. (This was in contrast to the old conventional diabetic diet, which was high-fat and low-carbohydrate—mostly refined.) Within a month, half of the maturity-onset diabetics no longer required insulin, and a further 41 per cent had their doses reduced. Of the patients on medication other than insulin, 81 per cent had abandoned their drugs after a month. Regular exercise was included in the regimen.

It is now realized that lowering the fat and increasing the carbohydrate content of a diabetic's diet reduces the need for insulin, while a high-fat diet increases the body's insulin requirement. Fat seems to block the action of insulin, so that a far greater quantity of the hormone is necessary to cope with a given amount of glucose. Constant demands upon the pancreas to produce great quantities of insulin gradually tire it out and make it inefficient. In addition, sucrose (ordinary table sugar) can reduce the efficiency of insulin in controlling blood glucose. Suitable forms of fibre added to the diet, however, diminish this adverse effect of sucrose (although they do not abolish it).

The addition of an exercise regimen, however, freed insulin from these effects of sucrose and enhanced its ability to control blood glucose beyond 'normal' levels, even though sucrose was being taken in the diet.

There are two very important aspects of a diabetic person's overall regimen, therefore: exercise and fibre.

The diet should be low-fat (as in the Pritikin diet) for the reasons given above and because of the increased danger of ATHEROMA developing. Similarly, the carbohydrate content should be high, and certain carbohydrates should be chosen with a view to stabilizing the blood's glucose levels. These include:

- Whole fruit, as opposed to fruit juice (less insulin required, and hunger is more easily satisfied).
- Wholegrains rather than milled grains in bread and cakes; e.g. brown rice requires far less insulin than milled rice flour.
- Foods containing natural gum fibres such as guar gum (some beans) or glucomannon. Fifteen per cent of bread content should consist of one of these types of fibre (add in this proportion before baking). Guar gum can also be taken as a supplement before or with meals; this reduces the insulin requirement. Doctors can now prescribe guar gum in the form of granules marketed under the name of Lejguar.
- Complex carbohydrates (e.g. lentils, wholegrain rice) have a high fibre content and (like the fibres just mentioned) produce a far slower and lower peak in blood sugar level after they have been consumed, thereby demanding less insulin than simpler carbohydrates like potato.
- Also, alcohol—although moderate amounts can safely be taken —should never be drunk on an empty stomach, as HYPOGLYCAEMIA can result.

Specific dietary supplements In his article on diabetes in *Here's Health*[88] Leon Chaitow stresses the pancreatic functions other than insulin production which should be taken into consideration. Allergies, addictions and food sensitivities make extra demands upon the pancreas, so these should be isolated and dealt with as soon as they are suspected. Dietary supplements can also affect the efficiency with which sugar is controlled in the body. Vitamin C enhances insulin's ability to cope with blood glucose by reducing its workload (it also helps to control fat levels in the blood, improves glucose tolerance and protects small blood vessels and arteries from damage; the recommended daily dosage is 500mg).

Chromium and manganese, both trace elements, should be included in the diabetic patient's supplements. Chromium is an important constituent of the 'glucose-tolerance factor' necessary for the proper utilization of insulin; it is present in raw molasses and in brewers' yeast, and is included in a number of mineral supplements available from healthfood shops. Manganese deficiency likewise appears to be involved in the production of diabetes.

Recommended amino-acid supplements include arginine, taurine and glutamic acid, all of which have been found useful for the management of diabetes. Adequate exercise is also a key factor.

Herbal medicine

A number of herbal preparations help to keep the level of sugar in the blood down. These include garlic, goat's rue and fenugreek and foods such as cranberry, coconut, the brassicas, lettuce, spinach and carrot.

Aromatherapy

Rub the area of the spleen with oil and essence of juniper (olive oil with 10 per cent of essence). Also, four drops of essence of juniper on a little brown sugar after each meal.

XI Disorders of the Sensory Organs*

EAR

The ear has three main parts: the outer, middle and inner ear.

The *outer ear* consists of the outer flap (pinna) and the external canal between it and the eardrum. The upper portion is flexible but 'stiff', due to its inner core of elastic cartilage. The lobe of the ear is soft and pliant, containing no inner 'skeleton' to support it. The canal leading down to the eardrum from the pinna is about 3cm long; it is a slightly curved passage which widens out as it meets the drum. The canal itself is lined with sensitive skin bearing fine hairs and secretory cells that produce ear wax.

The *middle ear* lies within the temporal bone of the skull. It is a cavity inside the bone that starts 'inside' the eardrum and ends at a small membrane separating it from the inner ear. Three tiny bones bridge the gap between the eardrum outside and the inner ear within: they are the malleus (hammer), incus (anvil) and stapes (stirrup). At the back of the middle-ear cavity a small hole leads to the mastoid antrum, the 'cave' or space within the mastoid area of the temporal bone. The mastoid is the hard, bony projection to be felt immediately behind the outer ear. At the front of the middle-ear cavity the Eustachian tube opens; it leads down from the middle ear to the back of the nose.

The *inner ear* is buried deep within the temporal bone. There are two main parts to it. The first is the cochlea, a snail-shaped bony structure containing fluid and the organ of Corti and richly supplied with branches of the auditory (hearing) nerve. The interior of the cochlea is divided by a membrane into two spiral compartments. The receiving cells that pick up sound vibrations and pass them on to the brain via the auditory nerve lie on this membrane.

The second part of the inner ear, the vestibular apparatus, is also fluid-filled. It is divided into two parts. The first is the otolith organ, which contains sensitive cells bearing fine hairs to which tiny chalk-like

---

* In this section disorders of the ear and eye are discussed. For information on the nose, skin and tongue see the index.

The Ear and the Eye

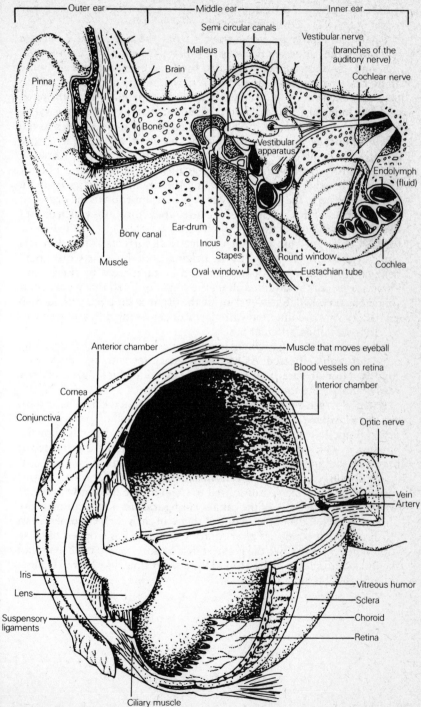

granules are attached. The second is the series of three semicircular canals, lying in three different planes at right angles to one another; they too contain cells bearing fine hairs.

Finally, the *auditory nerve* travels from the hearing and balance sections of the ear across the floor of the skull to enter the brain-stem.

Sound vibrations are concentrated by the pinna and travel air-borne along the length of the canal. When they impinge upon the eardrum they start it vibrating at a certain frequency, depending upon the pitch of the sound heard. The vibrations of the eardrum are in turn passed by successive movements of the hammer, anvil and stirrup bones to the small membrane separating the middle and inner ear. This membrane vibrates as a result of the impulses it receives, transmitting the vibration waves to the cochleal fluid lapping against the membrane's interior surface. The slightest motion affecting the organ of Corti sets up an electrical current, the voltage of which is in proportion to the degree of the movement. High-pitched notes cause rapid vibrations which die out near the beginning of the spiral; the lowest notes get carried to its furthest end. The sum total of the electrical currents is the electrical equivalent of the vibrations of the original sound, so the Corti organ behaves just like a microphone. Sound is interpreted by the brain's identification of the distance along the organ of Corti that a particular sound has travelled. Each level inside the organ is supplied with its own set of nerve fibres connected with the brain, allowing different frequencies to travel along different paths.

The sense of hearing becomes less acute with age, the high notes being most noticeably affected. As hearing degenerates with age, the vowel-sounds of human speech are retained and identified for longer and more easily than are the sounds made by consonants.

Balance is the other main function of the inner ear. The otolith organ's sensitive cells record the direction of the pull of gravity, which depends upon the group of hairs affected; this in turn depends upon the position in which the head is held, and the information is transmitted to the brain, making us aware of our position even when our eyes are shut.

The sensitive, hair-bearing cells inside the semicircular canals record the swirling movement transmitted to them by the fluid in which they are suspended. Because of the canals' configuration, acceleration in any direction has to affect at least one of them (in each ear). Giddiness is an effect of this: it continues after rotary movement has stopped because rotary movement causes the greatest disturbance within the canals and the fluid continues to swirl around for a short time, like stirred tea in a teacup. (See VERTIGO.)

EYE

The eyeball is an almost perfect sphere with a 'stalk' at the back containing the optic nerve. Two factors prevent the eyeball from being perfectly spherical: (a) the nerve stalk, as noted, and (b) the slight bulge in the front in the area of the cornea.

Although the eye is very soft inside, its outer coat is tough and difficult to penetrate. It is called the sclera, and is opaque throughout except over the front part of the eye where it is modified to form a delicate, transparent membrane, the cornea. The sclera is lined with a delicate layer of blood vessels and pigment cells, the choroid, and this in turn is lined by the even more delicate retina, the visual surface of the eye, comprising light-sensitive nerve cells which are all in ultimate contact with the optic nerve.

Immediately behind the cornea is the pigmented ring that gives colour to the eye. This is the iris, and it is the anatomical equivalent of a camera's diaphragm, opening to let in more light when the light in the environment is dim, and contracting to protect the retina from 'overexposure' when the light is bright. The central hole is the pupil.

The lens of the eye is suspended behind the iris by means of small muscles. The space in front of it, the anterior chamber, is filled with fluid called the aqueous humour. Filling the rest of the eyeball behind the lens (posterior chamber) is a watery jelly named the vitrous humour.

The eyeball sits in a protective bony cavity on the front of the skull – the eye socket, or orbit—to which it is attached by six muscles. The eyelids are lined with a fine membrane called the conjunctiva, which covers the front of the eye as well and is continuous with the transparent cornea. This is kept moist at all times by the secretions of the lacrimal gland below the outer part of the upper lid. These tears drain into the nose through a small opening at the inner corner of the eye.

The spherical shape of the front of the eye makes the corneal region, in combination with the aqueous humour behind, an effective convex lens. Light-rays pass through this lens arrangement as permitted by the iris and fall upon the lens proper. This latter is made fat or thin by the relaxation or contraction of the muscles from which it is suspended, and as a consequence, the incoming light-rays are focused onto the retina, at the back of the eye.

There are two types of light-sensitive nerve endings in the retina: cones, which are used in good light and register colour, there being a different type of cone for each of the three primary colours, and rods, which are sensitive to green and blue and function well in poor light. The light-sensitive chemical in the latter is rhodopsin. The ability to see at night depends upon rhodopsin being made as required, and this can take place only when Vitamin A is in adequate supply. The bright light of daytime inactivates rhodopsin and stops its synthesis.

Visual impulses are carried from the retina via the optic-nerve fibres to the visual area at the back of the cerebral cortex, where the impulses are interpreted.

XI/1 OTITIS EXTERNA

The area of the outer ear most liable to problems is the canal leading to the eardrum. Here, wax can collect, boils can develop, and foreign bodies can get stuck (small children often push beads, matchsticks, etc., into their ears and then cannot get them out again). Treatments for the first two conditions are discussed under EAR WAX and ABSCESS; treatment for the third is, obviously, extraction of the offending object.

XI/2 OTITIS MEDIA

Earache due to infection of the middle ear is a common complaint in small children. However, a Scandinavian study has shown that babies fed purely on breast milk are protected against otitis media up to the age of six months, and considerable protection remains for some years after breast-feeding is stopped. By contrast, babies fed from an early age on cows' milk are predisposed to otitis media. It has been suggested that either (a) the Eustachian tubes are damaged by the effects of the cows' milk or (b) human milk contains an antibody not present in other milks, so that bottle-fed babies are deficient in it.[86]

Otitis media is usually due to bacterial infection spreading along the Eustachian tube to the middle ear from the nose, and the pain can be severe. It is caused by pus being formed under pressure within the middle-ear cavity, and pressing upon the inflamed and acutely sensitive eardrum. If the drum perforates, the pressure is relieved and the pain ceases, but the drum may be badly damaged.

An alternative outcome to a ruptured eardrum is infiltration of the pus into the interior of the mastoid bone. This condition can be very dangerous since pus, like any liquid or semisolid, takes the line of least resistance and can in this way reach the interior of the skull. MENINGITIS and brain ABSCESS are rare but possible complications of untreated middle-ear infection.

Pain in the ear can be caused also by dental problems (including teething in infants and the eruption of wisdom teeth in adolescence), throat infections and injuries to the jawbone or neck-bones.

ORTHODOX TREATMENT

Penicillin is commonly given for middle-ear infection (e.g. amoxycillin [Amoxil]), together with ear-drops (e.g. phenazone + benzocaine [Auraltone]).

ALTERNATIVE THERAPIES

Natural medicine

A small child with an acute middle-ear infection would probably have solid foods withheld and be given plenty of cooling fluids, especially freshly squeezed fruit and vegetable juices. A beneficial combination would be 140ml of carrot juice plus the same volume of grape juice. Vitamin supplements would be given as for chickenpox (see **XIII/1**). A gauze plug soaked in an emulsion made from mixing a 40 per cent alcoholic tincture of propolis with olive oil can be helpful.

Biochemic tissue salts   For the fever, pain, throbbing and congestion: *Ferrum Phos.* Alternating with *Ferrum Phos.*, *Kali Mur.* (also good for impaired hearing due to swelling of Eustachian tubes). When there is a thin watery yellow discharge: *Kali Sulph.* Foul matter coming from the ear: *Silicea.*

Herbal medicine

A small piece of cotton wool soaked in garlic (squeezed from a capsule) and inserted into the ear.

Aromatherapy

Drop into the ear (with a small dropper) a little gently warmed olive oil with 10 per cent Borneo camphor and 10 per cent essence of cajeput. Plug the canal with cotton wool soaked in this oil.

Homoeopathy

For a very severe attack with boring pain, fever and sweating, and a badly infected eardrum, symptoms worse at night and better for warmth: *Belladonna*. For very early acute earache, with stinging pain, fever, throbbing due to a chill or temperature change: *Aconite*. For pricking, unbearably violent, severe pain and irritation, red cheeks, patient restless, worse at night and from cold: *Chamomilla*. For severe pain, high fever, often a discharge of pus, with child restless, crying, often sweating and maybe delirious, frequently a specific sensation of icy cold water in the ear (the clearest indication for this remedy): *Mercurius*. For hot, inflamed, painful ear with pains that come and go and are very variable, perhaps a yellow-green discharge, all symptoms worse for heat, patient has no thirst but is very tearful and has a temperature: *Pulsatilla*.

XI/3 MÉNIÈRE'S DISEASE

This disorder of the inner ear affects its two main functions, balance and hearing. Attacks of deafness are accompanied by buzzing in the ears and dizzy spells. The underlying cause is not known but is thought to be associated with a poor blood-supply to the area, accompanied by alterations in the pressure within the ear.

Ménière's disease occurs as occasional attacks rather than as a permanent disorder. A few individuals seem to find their attacks to be precipitated by definite occurrences, such as increased physical and/or emotional stress, and perhaps certain dietary items to which they are sensitive.

ORTHODOX TREATMENT

Drugs for this condition include prochlorperazine (Stemetil), cinnarizine (Stugeron) and buclizine (Equivert).

ALTERNATIVE THERAPIES

There seems not yet to have been any specific alternative remedy directed towards the relief of Ménière's disease. However, the remedies used for the relief of dizzy spells and nausea (see **XII/4**) are likely to help this condition. A salt-free wholefood vegetarian diet has been reported to bring complete relief.[87]

XI/4 LABYRINTHITIS (otitis interna)

INFLAMMATION of the inner ear, or labyrinth. The symptoms are sweating at ordinary room-temperature, NAUSEA, DIZZY SPELLS and a feeling of malaise. The cause is often a viral infection, and the only orthodox treatment is symptomatic. Prochlorperazine (Stemetil) is prescribed for nausea and dizziness; and hyoscine (Buscopan) has proved both free from side-effects and very helpful.

ALTERNATIVE THERAPIES

Natural medicine

A natural wholefood diet would be introduced by degrees, as the patient grew less nauseous. Initially, when the symptoms of nausea, sweating and vertigo were severe, solid food might well be withheld and cold mineral water given as well as freshly squeezed fruit and vegetable juices (140ml carrot plus 30ml watercress juice is beneficial). The normal daily supplement is recommended, when it can be taken.

Biochemic tissue salts   The dizziness may respond to *Kali Phos.*

Herbal medicine

Two pinches of anise infused in a cup of water—one cup after each meal when solid food is taken may help the dizziness.

Aromatherapy

Three drops of essence of chamomile on a little brown sugar when the attack starts, and whenever severe vertigo is experienced (up to three doses daily).

Spiritual therapy

Electrocrystal therapy.

XI/5 GLAUCOMA

This disorder is one of physical damage to the eye, particularly to the optic nerve, due to increased pressure within the eyeball. If left untreated, glaucoma causes progressive visual impairment and ultimately blindness. The chronic type is responsible for one seventh of the total number of blindness cases in the UK.

There are two main varieties of glaucoma. Firstly there is acute glaucoma, in which the symptoms of eye pain, redness and a hard eyeball come on rapidly and distressingly, and require immediate ophthalmic attention in order to save the sight. Secondly there is chronic simple glaucoma, where the pressure within the eye increases slowly, with gradual damage to the fibres around the periphery of the optic-nerve disc at the back of the eye, accompanied by slow impairment of vision around the edges of the visual field. The ultimate result (prior to blindness) is 'tunnel vision', in which the patient can see only things in a straight line in front of the eyes (i.e. in the central portion of the visual field).

Both types of glaucoma result from what is in essence the same underlying cause: failure in the drainage system which removes aqueous humour from the portion of the eye in front of the lens (where it is continuously manufactured).

Early chronic simple glaucoma often goes unnoticed, and is picked up only by chance by an optician or ophthalmologist. The International Glaucoma Association (IGA) designated 1985 'glaucoma year' and made great efforts to bring the facts about glaucoma to the public's attention. Of the total population 1–2 per cent of those over 40 are believed to be affected by early glaucoma, and the IGA are pressing GPs and opticians routinely to test people in this age-group once a year for signs of the disorder.

ORTHODOX TREATMENT

Orthodox doctors treat chronic glaucoma with drugs that reduce the rate of fluid-formation and the acute condition by means of an operation to relieve the drainage problem.

ALTERNATIVE THERAPIES

Natural medicine

Wholefood diet with ample supplies of fresh fruit and vegetables, only a little meat, and supplementary Vitamin C (2–3g daily). Bathe the eyes with cold rue tea, and drink tea made from speedwell. You should keep in touch with your eye specialist and remember to go for checkups. Henry Lindlahr's *Natural Therapeutics*, vol. 2, contains a detailed account of natural treatment for eye disorders.

Homoeopathy

For acute glaucoma: *Aconite*. When the eyeballs seem expanded, large and under pressure, and vision is misty and reduced, pupils fixed: *Opium*. Eyeball feels too large, sharp, shooting pains particularly worse for movement and at night, palpitations often associated: *Spigelia*. Double vision frequent, vision misty and diminished, eyes feel bruised and under pressure: *Gelsemium* (one of the most useful remedies for glaucoma). Intraocular tension raised, intense soreness, watering and PHOTOPHOBIA: *Bryonia*. Useful to diminish the pain and limit degeneration changes: *Phosphorus*. Indicated when the onset is violent and acute with inflammation, dryness and photophobia: *Belladonna*.

Acupuncture

This is claimed to relieve chronic glaucoma at times, but should be carried out only in cooperation with a medical doctor's standard treatment.

Spiritual therapy

Electrocrystal therapy.

XII   Infectious Illnesses

Infection is invasion of the body by harmful (pathogenic) organisms, and the ensuing reaction on behalf of the body. The organisms include bacteria, viruses and virus-like factors, and fungi. They gain admission to the body in a number of ways, including through the air passages and lungs, the mouth and intestine, directly into the bloodstream (e.g. following a cut), and via the urethra and vagina (in the case of vaginal, urethral and bladder infections).

The virulence of the 'infection' as experienced by the patient depends upon the state of his or her immune defence system. Within this context there are two main factors to consider. The first is the capacity of the white cells (granulocytes) to surround, incapacitate and destroy invading bacteria. You can see the result of this effort in the pus that oozes from an infected scratch. Pus is the debris of dead tissue, plus live bacteria and the white cells that are ranged against them. The other factor is the presence or absence of antibodies against the invading germ. For instance, a child who has been infected by mumps once is unlikely to suffer the infection a second time, despite exposure to the virus, as antibodies will have been manufactured against this eventuality (see ALLERGY).

When the immune defence system (IDS) is weak—and alternative practitioners regard this as one of the prime outcomes of chemical, physical and emotional stress factors that we encounter in our environment—it fails to cope with infection as it should, and hence we succumb more readily to colds, 'flu and other illnesses. Orthodox doctors tend to treat infections with antibiotic drugs, and in many instances these are life-savers. However, antibiotics are a two-edged sword: while they deal with the infection they may also weaken the immune defence system's ability to deal with further encounters with germs. They also usually have side-effects, and 'kill off' helpful bacteria we all have in us, with a probable increase in the invasive yeast *Candida albicans*, productive of THRUSH.

The approach taken by alternative practitioners aims at getting to the root of the problem—the weak immune defence system—rather than merely treating infections symptomatically; this is why a naturopathic practitioner will examine lifestyle, exercise, relaxation and diet, as well as stress factors, as causative of a given infection. Medical herbalists, aromatherpists, homoeopathic doctors, do of course provide a certain amount of remedies to alleviate immediate unpleasant symptoms. But the aim of their therapies is to restore the balance of patients' homoeostatic systems—i.e. patients' ability to deal with infections themselves, effectively—and this is directed at the health and well-being of the immune defences. Hence many natural remedies for infection are in fact immune defence strengtheners.

VACCINATION

This is an extremely controversial topic, and feelings run high on the subject, both among orthodox doctors who generally support vaccination (immunization) against infectious diseases, and alternative practitioners who in the main are strongly opposed to it.

The arguments from both viewpoints have been fairly expressed by herbal specialist Simon Mills (February 1984 issue of the *Journal of Alternative Medicine*). He concedes that vaccination is a valid prophylactic against infectious diseases, and that public immunization campaigns have dramatically influenced the incidence of diseases such as smallpox, polio, tetanus, whooping cough and measles. He also pointed out that, due to the scare of brain damage resulting from whooping-cough vaccine, the uptake of the vaccine dropped by 60 per cent and within a year the incidence of the disease had risen by a factor of nine to 50,000 cases, resulting in nine deaths in England.

Taking sides in the argument with those who are against vaccination therefore carries some heavy responsibilities. All the same, the problem remains that blindly stimulating the IDS against infectious illnesses ignores the fact that we all possess potent armoury against the ill effects of pathogens which can succeed in causing illness only under specific conditions. The strength of our natural defences, consisting firstly of the reticulo-endothelial system (RES), which kills invading organisms by white-cell engulfing activity, and secondly of the IDS as a back-up mechanism, should, I think, be enhanced by natural means, rather than by relying upon artificial stimulation of the IDS.

Moreover, each of us is an individual, with idiosyncratic biochemical make-ups and therefore requirements. It is preferable for individual failures of vital resistance to be corrected by natural means (e.g. herbs, homoeopathic remedies) rather than to rely upon 'arbitrary interven-tion'. Mass vaccination also costs a lot of money which could perhaps be better spent upon improving social conditions and nutritional standards. Individual vaccination may still be advisable in certain cases where the person concerned has no interest in pursuing the positive health approach, or where, perhaps, social considerations suggest that the individual's innate resistance is unlikely to cope.

However, there remain other valid strategies from which to choose in appropriate cases. Internationally famous homoeopath George Vithoulkas feels that vaccinations in susceptible people can weaken and distort the vital force, sometimes irreparably. He believes, as do many homoeopaths, that the infectious illnesses against which children are vaccinated will occur only in children who are susceptible to them, and prove dangerous only in those whose vital force has already been weakened by constitutional factors or orthodox methods of treatment. He is of the opinion that vaccinating children is unnecessary if they are treated constitutionally with homoeopathic remedies, since their de-fence mechanisms will then be in a position to deal with the infection; moreover, such children can also be treated when necessary with homoeopathic remedies. Vithoulkas states that, from his own experi-ence, certain disorders such as multiple sclerosis and rheumatoid arthritis have very probably resulted from the practice of vaccination. He thinks that the increased incidence of auto-immune diseases and of

AIDS are also possibly the result of this practice. He claims that vaccinating children damages their IDS and makes them more prone to other disorders such as middle-ear infections, sore throats, colds and chest infections. This state of affairs can, however, be successfully treated homoeopathically. This form of treatment does, however, remove the protection against specific infectious illnesses against which the children have been vaccinated.[89]

XII/1 CHICKENPOX

The virus responsible for this illness is identical with that which causes shingles. It has an incubation period of 14 days, after which the earliest symptoms of a raised temperature and itchy rash appear. The spots appear first on the trunk, and later on the face, legs and arms. They start as small, firm spots which later become inflamed blisters, and these can form permanent scars if the heads are picked off. Chickenpox is highly infectious from 24 hours before the first blisters appear to one week later. It is spread by infected droplets coughed or sneezed from the upper air passages. Dried crusts on the spots are also infectious, and patients should be isolated until all crusts have separated.

Orthodox doctors usually prescribe oily calamine lotion for the spots, and perhaps a paracetamol for raised temperature and discomfort. Antibiotics are unnecessary.

ALTERNATIVE THERAPIES

Natural medicine

Naturopathic practitioners usually regard symptoms of an acute infection as a sign that the body is reacting healthily to threatening disease. This is especially true in the case of children, and most acute childhood illnesses would be treated with fluids only during the acute stage, followed by a light wholefood diet during convalescence. Raw vegetable and fruit juices would be prescribed during the fasting period, and afterwards to speed recovery.

Of particular value would be freshly squeezed orange and lemon juice, sweetened if necessary with a little honey; and 600ml daily of carrot juice, mixed with 140ml of watercress juice.

Specific dietary supplements

- Vitamin A: 10,000iu (consult nutritional expert on dose for a child or baby), 1–3 times daily for five days, then stop for two days
- rose-hip Vitamin C: 500–1,000mg, morning and evening
- Vitamin E: 200–400iu, morning and evening
- multivitamin and mineral supplement, twice daily
- honey, mixed with a little freshly squeezed lemon juice and warmed slightly, helps to relieve accompanying sore throat and cough

Biochemic tissue salts   For fever, heat, restlessness: *Ferrum Phos*. For second stage, when fever has cleared and tongue is coated, spots filled with white substance: *Kali Mur*. When spots are discharging thick yellow pus: *Calcarea Sulph*.

Ionization therapy   This may counter any accompanying stuffiness of the upper air passages, headaches or general feelings of being run-down.

Herbal medicine

Tincture of comfrey is soothing on the spots. Lemon, yarrow, garlic (if the child will take this) and angelica are all recommended for the relief of chickenpox.

Aromatherapy

Three drops of essence of lemon on a little brown sugar, four times daily.

Homoeopathy

The first remedy to be prescribed, in the early stages, for restlessness in mind and body: *Rhus Toxicodendron*. When fever is present, with symptoms of anxiety, fear, thirst, rapid hard pulse: *Aconite*. To help the spots to form, and for cough and cold: *Antimonion Tartaricum*. For excessive itching of the rash: *Apis*.

XII/2 GERMAN MEASLES

This is usually quite a mild illness. The main risk in German measles is the death or defective development which it can cause to an unborn child if it is contracted during pregnancy. The defects include cataracts, heart abnormalities, deaf mutism, mental retardation and micro-cephaly (an abnormally small head). All women should be protected against infection with the rubella virus before becoming pregnant, either by being immune through already having had German measles or by vaccination. However, gamma-globulin (a special protein) can now be given by intramuscular injection to women who do contract the infection while pregnant, and this confers some protection against damage to the baby.

German measles is usually a less distressing illness than ordinary measles (see **XII/5**). It has an incubation period of 2–3 weeks, after which it starts with the patient being off-colour, having a slight temperature and perhaps a headache. The next day, a florid rash begins on the patient's face and his or her eyes can become sore and bloodshot. Enlarged, tender glands can usually be felt with the fingertips behind the ears and sometimes in the neck. The patient is infectious from the day before symptoms start until the day after they have disappeared (they normally last 3–5 days).

ORTHODOX TREATMENT

This includes paracetamol, plenty of fluids, and calamine lotion to soothe the rash if necessary.

ALTERNATIVE THERAPIES

Natural medicine

As for chickenpox (see **XII/1**).

Biochemic tissue salts   For the inflammatory symptoms: *Ferrum Phos.* Swollen glands, cough: *Kali Mur.* alternating with *Ferrum Phos.*

Herbal medicine

An infusion of yarrow, a half-cupful drunk hot three times daily.

Aromatherapy

Three drops of essence of eucalyptus on a little brown sugar, three times daily. Inhalation: to a litre of boiling water add three soupspoonfuls of the following alcohol preparation: a litre of 90° alcohol, 30g eucalyptus essence, 14g thyme, 14g essence of pine needles, 10g lemon essence and 10g lavender essence.

Homoeopathy

When the patient is thirstless, restless and irritable: *Pulsatilla*. For a high fever, full pulse, dry cough, thirst, restlessness: *Aconite*. For streaming nose and eyes, photophobia, sore eyes, moderate fever: *Euphrasia*. When skin is itchy, hot and red, rash slow to clear, with some areas infected and possibly discharging pus; hot body, but intolerance of water on skin: *Sulphur*. As fever is declining: *Arsenicum*.

XII/3 HERPES SIMPLEX

The herpes simplex virus has been mentioned earlier in this book (see V/8). Here we can look at some general therapies.

The dietary approach to genital herpes[68] (herpes simplex II virus) consists of reducing the body's intake of the amino acid arginine (present in carob, chocolate, gelatin, coconuts, oats, wholemeal and white flour, peanuts, soya beans and wheatgerm). At the same time the intake of lysine should be increased; this amino acid is present in considerable amounts in fish, chicken, lamb, milk, cheese, beans, brewers' yeast and beansprouts, as well as in most fruit and vegetables.

Supplements for genital-herpes sufferers include: 0.5–1.5g lysine daily when the virus is inactive and 1.5–3.0g daily when it is active (taken throughout the day), Vitamin C with bioflavonoids (1g daily), vitamins B_6 and B_{12}, folic acid, pantothenic acid, calcium, magnesium, selenium and zinc. Also recommended are vitamins A and E. For individual dosages of all of these it is best to consult a nutritionally educated naturopath.

XII/4 WHOOPING COUGH

The chief symptom of whooping cough is spasmodic, violent coughing, often ending in an attack of vomiting. The characteristic whoop, which may not be present in a mild attack, is produced by the child forcing air into its lungs against the resistance of a closed glottis. The illness is most likely to be serious in small babies, both because of its own virulence and because it can lead to lung damage and to secondary infections such as bronchitis and pneumonia. Orthodox doctors frequently give antibiotics for whooping cough, both against the bacterium responsible for the illness and as a preventative measure against others.

ALTERNATIVE THERAPIES

Natural medicine

As for chickenpox (see **XII/1**).

Ionization therapy   This would be likely to prove very beneficial.

Herbal medicine

An infusion of thyme, made by steeping a small teaspoonful of thyme or a small sprig in boiling water for 10 minutes. Sweeten with plenty of honey and give the child one dessertspoonful three times daily (1 tsp for a baby).

Aromatherapy

An inhalation of eucalyptus as for German measles (see **XIII/2**). Also, garlic ointment or garlic oil squeezed from a capsule and rubbed onto the chest and back.

Homoeopathy

To allay the effects of whooping cough: *Pertussin*. To relieve the paroxysmal cough and vomiting: *Ipecacuanha*.

XII/5   MEASLES

This is generally a mild disease in developed countries and primarily affects 3–5 year olds, but it has a high mortality rate in undeveloped countries where it chiefly affects malnourished children during the first two years of life. The incubation period last for 1–2 weeks, and the first symptoms are a raised temperature, streaming nose and eyes, and a sore throat. Next to appear are the KOPLIK'S SPOTS, and the rash shows up on the third or fourth day of the illness. It consists of red blotches and starts on the face. Provided no secondary bacterial infection is contracted, measles lasts for about one week.

ORTHODOX TREATMENT

This includes paracetamol and advice about giving plenty of fluids. Antibiotics are unlikely to be given unless the child is especially at risk of catching a secondary bacterial infection—such as otitis media (see **XI/2**).

ALTERNATIVE THERAPIES

Natural medicine

As for chickenpox (see **XII/1**).

Biochemic tissue salts   For inflammatory symptoms, fever, red eyes, congestion: *Ferrum Phosphoricum* (continue all the time fever lasts). Main remedy when there is swelling of glands in throat or neck, cough, white coating to tongue: *Kali Muriaticum*, alternating with *Ferrum Phosphoricum* After measles to help recuperation: *Calcarea Phosphoricum*

Herbal medicine

An infusion of marigold flowers, drunk hot, half a cupful three times daily, sweetened with a little honey if desired.

Aromatherapy

As for German measles (see **XII/2**).

Homoeopathy

As for German measles (see **XII/2**). The preparation Morbillimum 200 is useful as a prophylactic and also of value in the ongoing treatment.

XII/6 MUMPS

This infection is typified by swelling of the parotid glands. The incubation period is 14–28 days. The symptoms start with a mild fever and then the painful swelling of the parotid glands on either side of the face. Other salivary glands can become affected, as occasionally can the pancreas and the testicles. A man may become infertile as a result, but this is not inevitable. The symptoms normally disappear after 2–3 days. There is no specific orthodox treatment other than fluids and mild pain-killers, such as paracetamol.

ALTERNATIVE THERAPIES

Natural medicine

As for chickenpox (see XII/1).

Biochemic tissue salts   In the early stages, with fever, pain, vomiting, flushed face: *Ferrum Phos*. Second stage, marked swelling of gland, tender to touch, coated tongue: *Kali Mur*. Excessive saliva, painful swelling of testicles: *Natrum Mur.*, alternating with *Ferrum Phos*.

Herbal medicine

A mouthwash with tincture of thyme. A cupful of marigold tea three times daily, drunk hot with a little honey if desired.

Aromatherapy

Three drops of lemon essence on brown sugar, four times a day.

Homoeopathy

When there is fever, restlessness, pain, thirst in the early acute stages: *Aconite*. When the testicles or breasts are involved *Pulsatilla*. When the right parotid gland is affected, with fever, redness, swelling: *Belladonna*. When the left gland is swollen and red and painful, worse with the cold and damp; also for prevention when contact is suspected: *Rhus Toxicodendron*. If infection complicates the illness (e.g. throat or lung infection, making the mumps attack worse): *Sulphur*. As a prophylactic: *Parotidinum*.

XII/7 POLIO (POLIOMYELITIS)

This is an acute viral infection of the central nervous system, causing permanent or temporary paralysis of voluntary muscle in about two patients in every 100, and no clinical symptoms at all in the majority of cases. A few patients 'in between' suffer from a fever, feeling unwell, a stiff neck, headache and sore back muscles, and sometimes vomiting. These symptoms usually last for 72 hours only. Polio affects people of all ages, and the infection is chiefly passed on by droplets of mucus from the upper air passages.

Vaccination has in many countries, including the UK, more or less eradicated the disease. However, a report appearing in the 25 September 1985 issue of *GP*, said that an outbreak of paralytic polio in Finland the previous winter had been attributed by experts to a possible change in the antigenic structure of the virus. A 'wild' type-3 virus isolated from one paralytic case (known as strain Tampere) could have been responsible. The virus must somehow have slipped through any immunity acquired in the usual way by inactivated virus vaccine. For the time being, the National Institute for Biological Standards and Controls is stressing that travellers to Finland ought to be vaccinated against polio. But, the report stressed, although the incident has potential public health ramifications 'it certainly shouldn't start any hysteria. There is no evidence that the vaccines are not working in general.' There was also 'no evidence to suggest that we will get the Finnish strain in the UK'.

ORTHODOX TREATMENT

Confinement to bed for the mild to moderate cases, which probably will not be recognized as polio (the symptoms are more typical of influenza). Seriously affected cases should be nursed in hospital where special equipment is available should it be needed—e.g. a respirator should paralysis of the respiratory muscles occur.

ALTERNATIVE THERAPIES

Natural medicine

Bed-rest, quiet atmosphere, very light wholefood diet, in early stages probably liquids only by mouth, freshly squeezed fruit and vegetables juices.

Herbal medicine

For the mild to moderate cases, where symptoms are similar to those of influenza, management can be conservative and remedies given to aid fever—1tsp of dried yarrow steeped for 10 minutes in a cupful of boiling water and drunk, sweetened with a little honey if desired. If polio is suspected or confirmed, the patient should be hospitalized and herbal remedies given in conjunction with orthodox medical care. The patient should be kept still and quiet, to avoid the more severe stage developing. Cramp bark is useful—it is a muscle relaxant, possibly acting through the nerves supplying the muscles as well as through a local effect. The herb should be administered by a skilled herbalist. A likely dose is 1–4g of the dried bark three times daily.

XII/8 TUBERCULOSIS

TB is a common infection, causing 1–2 million deaths each year, worldwide. It is contracted either by inhaling *Mycobacterium tuberculosis* bacteria which another sufferer has coughed into the atmosphere or by drinking the milk of an infected animal. In the former case infection starts in the lungs, in the latter in the intestine or throat. From its original location the infection spreads to other organs of the body, in particular the bones, lymph glands and, in women, the reproductive organs.

The commonest form of the disease is *pulmonary tuberculosis* (i.e. TB of the lung). A primary focus starts in the lung, forms a small abscess and either resolves itself, leaving a tiny scar and a positive reaction to the tuberculin skin-test, or, less commonly, spreads, producing a fever. Other symptoms include weightloss, coughing, spitting up blood, night sweats nd malaise.

Other forms include *miliary tuberculosis*, the formation of numerous tiny TB abscesses in other organs of the body as a result of the bacteria being carried there from the primary focus by the bloodstream. Further possibilities are TB meningitis, TB of the bones and joints, TB infection of the skin, and abdominal TB, affecting the intestine and lymph nodes.

ORTHODOX TREATMENT

The standard remedies are the drugs streptomycin, para-aminosalicylic acid and isoniazid; two or all three of them are given together because the bacteria rapidly become resistant to any single drug used on its own.

ALTERNATIVE THERAPIES

Natural medicine

The naturopathic approach to disease has achieved very good results with tuberculosis. Emphasis upon a high-raw wholefood diet, rest and light exercise, relaxation techniques, hydrotherapy and exposure to fresh air and sunlight accord closely with the ideals of orthodox management, and in patients with active tuberculosis an ideal form of management would seem to be a combination of orthodox antituberculous drugs with the naturopathic approach. The latter would very probably reduce the length of time for which the former were necessary.

Ionization therapy

Good results have been reported of the use of ionization therapy in cases of pulmonary tuberculosis.

XII/9   SCARLET FEVER

This disorder is a reaction to infection by haemolytic streptococcal bacteria, often following a little time after a 'strep. throat'. The development of a rash depends upon the balance between toxin formation by the bacteria and the antitoxin defence of the patient.

Scarlet fever starts suddenly with a raised temperature, feelings of being under the weather, inflamed painful throat, white-coated tonsils and lining of pharynx, swollen glands, generalized rash, and a 'strawberry tongue', white at first with red papillae and then peeling to become bright red. The incubation period is 1–3 days, and the illness is commonest in small children, although babies too can be affected. Patients should be isolated for at least a week or until the symptoms have gone. The skin peels off during the second week; this may take several weeks to complete, but the dead skin fragments are not infectious.

ORTHODOX TREATMENT

Careful nursing, bed-rest, fluids, paracetamol and antibiotics to guard against heart and kidney complications.

ALTERNATIVE THERAPY

Natural medicine

As for chickenpox (see **XII/1**). The herbal and aroma therapeutic approaches are as for measles (see **XII/5**).

Biochemic tissue salts   In early stage of fever, sore throat, shivering, quick pulse, perhaps nose-bleed: *Ferrum Phosphoricum*. Chief remedy in scarlet fever, effective when there is a skin rash, white tongue, perhaps protein in the urine: *Kali Muriaticum*. For vomiting of watery secretions, drowsiness and twitching, frothy bubbles on the tongue: *Natrum Muriaticum*. To promote development of rash and re-establish rash if it stops erupting too soon: *Kali Sulphur*. Intercurrently during illness and steadily to promote recovery: *Calcarea Phosphoricum*.

397

Initially during the high fever, and when there is marked excitement: *Aconite*. During the red skin eruption, after *Aconite* has been used (also as a prophylactic—three doses are usually enough to prevent illness): *Belladonna*.

XIII   Cancer

The term 'cancer' describes a large group of disorders, their common factor being uncontrolled tissue growth. All cancers start with a small number of cells losing their ability to divide and multiply according to need; instead, they reduplicate in an uncontrolled and harmful way. Generally the cancerous cells lose many of their specific features of appearance and function and come to resemble the simple, undifferentiated tissue of a developing embryo. Cancerous tissue contributes nothing of benefit to the affected person. If, for example, a kidney becomes cancerous, the cells in the abnormal-growth area compete successfully with neighbouring cells for a supply of oxygen and nutrients, which they demand in large amounts on account of their over-vigorous growth rate. The kidney ceases to function as it should and, sooner or later, symptoms of disease develop.

Cancerous cell growth is beyond the body's normal mechanisms of control (i.e. nervous and hormonal), and the malignant tissue soon outstrips the development of normal nearby structures, spreading well beyond the confines of the original organ. This happens when small groups of cancerous cells become detached and are transported to other areas of the body by the lymph or blood circulation. Here they frequently develop as SECONDARIES (i.e. metastases). Cancer may also spread directly from one part of the body to the other.

Death (in fatal cases) results from a progressive loss of vitality rather than from the effects of the cancerous growth on the tissues of a vital organ. The usual pattern is loss of appetite and weight; increasing weakness and debility; pain, the extent and nature of which depend upon the body areas involved; and often, depression and irritability.

RISK FACTORS

The uncontrolled cell growth that typifies all cancer comes about for a wide variety of reasons. There is no single cause for cancer, and it is likely that several different factors are involved in every case. A family history of malignant disease is certainly a predisposing factor in some people, but other factors, such as stress, personality-type, lifestyle and exposure to recognized causative factors are usually more important than an inherited tendency.

One important physical cause of cancer is ionizing radiation. Sources include ultraviolet light, X-rays and radioactive substances used in medicine and industry: the longer the exposure to a particular source, the greater the chance of developing malignant disease. Another source is nuclear radiation encountered either because of accidental 'leakage' from nuclear-power generation (as happened on a grand scale in spring 1986 at Chernobyl in the USSR) or, of course, because of military testing.

Many substances can cause cancer. They are known as carcinogens, and the most widely recognized is tobacco smoke. Others include coal extracts, soot, some of the lubricating oils, asbestos fibres, arsenic and various chemicals produced during the manufacture of dyes.

Some forms of cancer in animals have been found to be caused by viral infection. It is highly probable that viruses are also responsible for malignant TUMOURS in a number of human cancers, too.

In every case, the factor or combination of factors which causes a cancerous change to take place in human tissues is believed to do so by its effect upon the genetic, or hereditary, make-up of the cells concerned; this effect is known as mutation. As a result of it controlled cellular division ceases and is replaced by wildly uncontrolled division. The mutated cells reduplicate themselves on a massive scale, thereby creating the malignant tumour or 'lump'.

In the case of leukaemia, which is cancer of the white blood cells (see VIII/3), the real equivalent of a tissue tumour is present in the bone marrow and other blood-forming tissues. The white cells fail to mature, and the large numbers of immature white cells released into the circulation retain the ability to reproduce themselves, in contrast to normal, mature white cells, which do not multiply.

Cancer research is looking constantly for other causes for malignant disease. The permitted chemicals with which processed food is sweetened, preserved, coloured, flavoured and textured are under frequent scrutiny; the cyclamate sweeteners, for example, were finally banned because some of their effects were suspected of contributing to cancer. Interest has also been aroused by the possible significance of factors *missing* from our diets. The trace element selenium appears to play a protective role against the development of certain types of cancer, so it is possible to postulate that its absence may well contribute to the evolution of malignant cellular change. Dietary fibre is also widely regarded as protecting those who eat adequate amounts of it from certain bowel disorders, including cancer of the colon. Similarly, diets low in roughage are thought to increase the chances of malignant large bowel disease developing.

TREATMENT

Roughly 50 per cent of all diagnosed cancer cases can now be cured by orthodox means; figures have not yet been obtained for the success percentage of alternative methods of management. The treatment of choice among orthodox doctors is almost invariably to remove the growth surgically whenever possible, together with a good margin of surrounding healthy tissue including nearby lymph glands in case cancer cells have infiltrated beyond the visible limits of the tumour. When the growth is inoperable, or the patient too old or too sick to tolerate major surgery, orthodox doctors adopt such means of growth-control as radiotherapy and the use of drugs aimed at suppressing the multiplication of cancer cells (i.e. cytotoxic drugs). Sex hormones are sometimes able to control the growth of cancer affecting the sexual organs. Sometimes, surgery, radiotherapy and drug therapy are all used together to attempt to cure.

TUMOUR NECROSIS FACTOR

Interest has grown during the past few years in a new agent, tumour necrosis factor (TNF), which, it is predicted, will have specific application to particular types of cancer cell. Several biotechnology companies have succeeded in cloning (reproducing exact doubles of) the human gene which produces this potent anti-tumour agent, and its potential was first recognized in crude preparations given to animals. It has been shown to be effective against a wide variety of malignant cells *in vitro* (isolated from their parent animal), yet to have little or no effect on normal cells. About a third to a quarter of human cancer cells are affected by it, for no apparent reason, according to Dr Nicholas Mathews of the Welsh National School of Medicine, who has been working on TNF in cooperation with the British company Celltech. Included in its successful targets are some forms of melanoma, some leukaemias and some sarcomas.

The TNF molecule needs to be made soluble before it can be given to patients; but it is not expected that this will prove a problem. Even before the commencement of clinical trials, however, some researchers are suggesting that its potential has been exaggerated wildly—as was the case with interferon several years ago. It is not going to prove a 'fantastic wonder drug' that will cure all cancer; and there may be toxicity problems to be overcome. All the same, TNF has to be seen as possibly representing renewed hope for at least some cancer patients.

Before the recent discovery of the TNF gene, the product had been available only as a crude extract prepared by injecting a particular bacterial toxin into animals whose immune systems had been primed with stimulants such as *Mycobacterium bovis*. The large white macrophage cells that attack bacteria invading the human bloodstream are believed to be the source of TNF, but its mode of action is not as yet known.

Both the TNF produced as just described and TNF made by cloning the appropriate gene have produced 'significant necrotic responses' in mice with deliberately induced sarcomas, whether the agent was injected into the tumour itself or into the mouse's bloodstream. In addition, 50 per cent of mice with transplanted adenocarcinoma (a common kind of carcinoma in humans) were cured by TNF compared with 0 in a control group; the TNF here was produced in a gene present in the bacterial species *Escherichia coli*.

TNF is known as a 'monokine', one of the many substances—including lymphokines such as the interferons—which are produced naturally by the immune system in response to viral attack. About six of these natural products are being investigated by biotech companies.

ANTICOAGULANT THERAPY

There is evidence that some abnormalities in blood coagulation found in breast cancer and other tumours may favour tumour spread. At present, knowledge of clotting defects in cancer patients is sketchy; but animal studies have shown that anticoagulants can reduce the incidence of secondaries from the original cancer tumour and reduce tumour growth. A major forthcoming study of the blood-clotting system of cancer patients could lead to a new form of cancer treatment, anticoagulant therapy. The study, projected to start at Glasgow University, is aimed at scrutinizing the many clotting defects in cancer patients to discover whether there is any pattern which will point to a persistent fault. If such a fault were correctable by anticoagulant drugs it could lead to a reduced rate of spread of tumours and therefore a better outlook for cancer patients.

A US trial on men with small-cell lung cancer showed a small but statistically significant increase in survival if they had anticoagulation therapy in addition to cytotoxic drugs. But the Glasgow study will be the first study for research on breast-cancer patients.

ALTERNATIVE ANTICANCER APPROACH

Alternative therapists often agree with the surgical removal of a malignant tumour, but generally warn patients against radiotherapy and highly toxic tumour-killing drugs on the grounds that these are very dangerous and generally unnecessary. Usually an eclectic approach is considered most beneficial, and cancer-control centres such as the Bristol Cancer Clinic include diet control, psychotherapy and meditation and visualization techniques in their choice of management.

Diet, in fact, plays an enormously important role in the alternative treatment of cancer and, although it is unwise from every point of view to claim 'cures', a number of cancers have been found to stop growing —and some to disappear—when patients adhere very strictly to a suitable regimen.

Basically the naturopathic approach is adopted; i.e. wholefood eating with, generally, the omission of red meat, animal fats and dairy products. Great emphasis is placed upon organically grown, raw or lightly steamed vegetables and raw fruit, and their juices. The 'vitality factor' present in freshly picked organic garden produce, though indefinable in scientific terms, is valued very highly, and seeds and sprouts, as well as sprouting grains, are included in the daily quota of raw food.

Two diets of special relevance in this context are the Bristol diet and the macrobiotic diet; these are discussed in more detail on pages 435 and 433.

Other naturopathic aspects of most alternative cancer treatments include taking an overview of the patient's lifestyle, personal habits (smoking? drinking?), stress factors and personality-type. Advice is given with respect to the solving of personal problems and the reduction of stress-factor bombardment. Gentle exercise is encouraged wherever this is possible, and psychotherapy prescribed wherever this might help reduce internal conflict. The applicability of visualization and meditation techniques to overcoming cancer are also discussed on pages 489–98, respectively.

Spiritual therapy

Both electrocrystal therapy and spiritual healing can prove helpful.

PREVENTION

There are three chief aspects to cancer prevention:

- Avoiding contact wherever possible with proven carcinogens such as tobacco smoke, asbestos, substances containing arsenic, etc.
- Adopting a lifestyle aimed at maintaining you in a state of positive, optimal health (see NATUROPATHY, Part III).
- Being aware of early warning signs, which should be investigated as soon as they appear. Seven cardinal signs put forward by New York's Metropolitan Life Insurance Company are: (1) the failure of any sore to heal; (2) a lump or thickening in the breast or anywhere else; (3) unusual bleeding or discharge; (4) any change in a wart or mole; e.g. increased hairiness, bleeding, surface irritation, increase in size; (5) difficulty in swallowing, or persistent indigestion; (6) persistent hoarseness or cough; (7) any change in usual bowel habits.

XIV   Disorders of the Mind

Many theories have been propounded about the human mind and how it works. Inevitably, many of the ideas put forward conflict with one another. It is widely accepted, though, that Freud's idea of different psychic levels was essentially accurate. Initially, in the 1890s, he described the *conscious* and *unconscious* regions of the mind, the latter having the greater capacity (an iceberg is sometimes used as an analogy of their relative proportions, the conscious being symbolized by the small part of the iceberg projecting above the water and the unconscious by the other 90 per cent, hidden from view below the surface). Next came Freud's topographical theory with the notions of conscious, preconscious and unconscious regions, which he described in *The Interpretation of Dreams* (1900). The *conscious* is concerned with moment-by-moment awareness of self and surroundings, with recall, planning, calculating, feeling and deciding. The *preconscious* contains all the memories and sense impressions which are not present in our conscious all the time, but which can be reintroduced into the realm of conscious awareness without undue effort. The *unconscious* is the deep reservoir of repressed memories and sensations in which are stored hidden memory patterns of every single event that we have ever experienced. Also within the unconscious are our more primitive impulses and fantasies.

Twenty-three years later Freud introduced his structural theory in *The Ego and the Id* (1923). The ego corresponded with the conscious and the id with the unconscious; also involved was the superego, the equivalent of the principle of 'conscience'.

The structural theory is considerably more complex than the topographical one. It is a 'hybrid that attempts to combine biological, experiential and interpersonal dimensions. For example, by Id is meant the basic biological aspect of the psyche, the inherited instinctual and constitutional aspects which we share to a large extent with other higher primates.'[90] Also fundamental to Freud's theory was the identification of the *id* with the pleasure principle and sexual gratification with its strongest motivating force.

The *ego* is concerned with rational thinking, external perception and with movement. It is basically the 'mediator between the needs and demands of the inside world and the realities and opportunities of the outside world. In performing this refereeing task it has to heed the Super-ego.'[90]

The *superego* is formed from the impressions made upon us by the moral code and standards of behaviour adopted by our parents or whoever looks after us, and later through our relationship with teachers and other authority figures.

In order to understand how these elements of the mind function in practice imagine a young baby requiring to be fed. He (or she) will be motivated entirely by the id (or primitive instinct level) and scream loudly until he receives what he wants. At a slightly later age, he will have developed some of the ego principle, which will enable him to 'weigh up', against his internal needs, the expediency of screaming for what he wants. His mother might, for instance, become very irritable when he yells and either (a) push his bottle towards him or (b), conversely, ignore him. Experience will have taught him that the 'best' thing to do when he is hungry is to grizzle quietly rather than scream, or to toddle off to find his mother and pull at her skirt. If this almost invariably produces a hug and a nice drink his ego will pick this up and guide him in the behaviour best fitting the situation.

Several years later, as a small child, at an instinctual (id) level he may desire to take her handbag when she is not looking and pull all its contents out on the floor. His ego, however, will quickly make him aware that Mummy will be very cross—hence it is 'wiser', with respect to his own welfare, to leave the bag alone. His superego may also be prompting him to leave well alone *because* Mummy has said that it is naughty to disturb other peoples' things and because he wishes to obey her and please her. An interesting example of the malfunction of the superego, is its repression of feelings and impulses—a repression which can then produce symptoms of mental illness. For instance, Freud cites the case of a woman who wanted to hit her therapist and, instead, developed a 'paralysed' left arm.

While psychoanalytic theory refers to the different levels of the psyche in terms of id, ego and superego, *transactional analysis theory* (described in Eric Berne's book *Games People Play*, 1966) expresses them in terms of 'child', 'adult' and 'parent', respectively. There is a basic correspondence between the primitive child in us and the id; a clear one between the ego and the adult, rational part of us; and a clearer one still between our superego conscience and the 'parent' within us. This makes the idea of internal conflicts easier for most people to understand: '... conflicts between Super-ego and Id ... would make little sense to most patients; to talk of conflicts between the parent and child parts within us makes sense to most people.'[91]

The concept of different layers of the psyche is shared by all psychodynamic schools. Conflicts may arise between the conscious and unconscious, the ego and the id, secondary-process thinking (rational and logical, and characteristic of the conscious) and primary-process thinking (illogical and irrational, and characteristic of the unconscious), and the principles of pleasure (id) and reality (ego). Other dualities between which conflict may arise are present and past, instinct and culture, and the outer world (external reality) and the inner world (psychic reality). Jung described the contrast between the outer 'persona' mask which we present to the world and the 'shadow' or darker side of our natures which we seek to conceal. Winnicot (1960) and Laing (1960) have described the 'false self' which hides the inner 'true self', and Berne, as we have seen, has referred to the adult concealing the child.

Although the description of personality dynamics so far refers to the isolated individual with his interacting ego, id and superego, and his perception of external reality, this of course is a hypothetical 'model' since the truly isolated individual does not in reality exist. This model is in fact a system within a larger system, the family, which in turn is within an even larger one, society.

When talking about an individual person's impulses, the idea of psychic energy is useful. If you think of the id, for example, as exerting a force and the superego as exerting an opposing force, it helps to understand their mutual relationship to one another and to the mediating ego which strives to bring about the most satisfactory resolution between the two.

When considering the influence of early relationships on the interactions between two people, the *object relations theory* is more pertinent. This was developed in the 1950s and 1960s, and to the proponents of this concept (Fairbairn, 1952; Guntrip, 1961; Winnicott, 1965; Balint, 1968) the primary motivational drive in the human being was the seeking of relationships with others. They considered Freud's emphasis on sexuality as the pleasure-seeking drive to be too much centred upon the individual and his or her gratifications. Instead of the infant and developing child seeking sexual pleasure through sucking the breast (oral phase), the retention and passing of motions (anal phase), and fingering his genitals (genital phase), they saw the developing person seeking relationships with others (initially the mother) through means appropriate to the different stages of development. Hence sucking the breast (and suckling the baby) represents a relationship of mutual satisfaction to the two participants.

Just as there are numerous theories seeking to explain the structure and function of the mind, many exist to account for the development of mental and emotional disorders. Here the orthodox and holistic views find a meeting point, for it is generally agreed by most workers in this field that mental illnesses result from a combination of physical and psychological causes aggravated by environmental factors, in particular stress.

For the sake of convenience and familiarity, in discussing mental disorders we will generally refer to Freud's view of mental illness as resulting from unresolved conflict during the oral, anal and genital phases of the developing psyche.

XIV/1 SCHIZOPHRENIA

The psychoses (or psychotic illnesses) are of two types: they can be organic, and result from injury to the brain, as in delirium and dementia, or they can be functional, existing in people with apparently perfectly normal brains. The characteristic feature of psychotic illness is that patients lose touch with reality. Their thoughts and perceptions are disordered in a fashion that cannot be explained simply in terms of an idiosyncratic though normal response to experience. Moreover, the disturbances are sufficiently severe to affect patients' appreciation of the world and the relationship of events within it.

Schizophrenia affects about 1 per cent of the adult population throughout the world. It starts in adolescence and, while many patients show certain personality characteristics prior to suffering from schizophrenia, such as excessive shyness, or a pronounced tendency to avoid social activities and dwell upon religion or philosophy (the so-called SCHIZOID PERSONALITY), at least half are apparently perfectly normal beforehand. Typical mental changes at the onset of the illness (besides emotional unrest and confusion, common to many mental conditions) are abnormal mental experiences and disturbed modes of expression.

Hallucinations, illusions and delusions are common among the former: examples are a deluded belief that the patient is, say, Charles I, and delusions about bodily control, the well-known 'passivity experience'. Sufferers from this latter symptom feel that they are being controlled by some outside power which forces them to walk, speak or move about in a particular way. They often hear 'voices' which direct their behaviour or call out derogatory remarks or threats. Delusions of being persecuted (PARANOIA) are also common.

Disturbances in modes of expression include abnormal language, in which answers to questions are frequently rambling, verbose and 'off-key'. Thoughts are expressed in vague terms and frequently lack obvious direct connection with one another (the 'flight of ideas' symptom). Words may be ill chosen, and the patient makes no attempt to clarify points when questioned further. Emotional expression is disturbed, incongruity being a common feature. Schizophrenics might say, for example, that they are being poisoned—yet roar with laughter while talking about it. Catatonia can occur, in which the patient occupies one position for hours on end, motionless and silent.

The cause of schizophrenia is unknown. There is a strong genetic predisposition to the illness. Freud saw it as a result of unresolved conflict at the oral stage of psychic development; R. D. Laing regards it as a self-protective mechanism, which guards the individual from the continuing effects of severe family stress. The Schizophrenic Association of Great Britain (SAGB), on the other hand, attribute the illness to malnutrition and to food allergies (many schizophrenics have digestive problems, including GLUTEN INTOLERANCE and recurrent HYPOGLYCAEMIA).

Doctor Vicky Rippere, clinical psychologist at the Maudesley Hospital, London, tries to help her patients both by psychotherapy and by identifying allergies and improving their nutritional status (i.e. condition). She confirms that word about the link between diet and mental illness is spreading, and would like to see nutrition included as a routine part of the psychiatrist's initial patient assessment.[92] She comments: 'If nutrition training came within the general medical curriculum, then I think I would have no patients left.'

ORTHODOX TREATMENT

Drugs belonging to the phenothiazine group—Largactil (chlorpromazine), Stelazine (trifluoperazine)—keep the symptoms under control and shorten the length of attacks. Other frequently used drugs are Depixol (flupenthixol), and Modecate (fluphenazine), which is given in injection form at regular intervals as maintenance treatment. Psychotherapy is used in suitable cases.

ALTERNATIVE THERAPIES

Natural medicine

Wholefood diet, worked out by nutritional experts after glucose tolerance, gluten tolerance, and cerebral food and environmental-chemical allergy tests have been carried out. Other relevant investigations are tests for altered perceptual functioning (such as the Hoffer-Osmond diagnostic test, which is said to appraise the illness far more effectively than a psychodynamic interview), and lab tests for thyroid function, liver and biochemical profiles, and hair mineral analysis.

A high-protein low-carbohydrate diet which forbids alcohol and caffeine and which is supplemented by mega-doses of vitamins B_3, B_6, C and E has proved successful in some cases under the care of the North Nassau Mental Health Center. This megavitamin treatment is known also as 'orthomolecular psychiatry', and is used in this way for schizophrenics because its proponents regard the disorder as a genetically inherited biochemical disturbance. This is a pragmatic and empirical approach—but it is claimed to work. Other vitamins whose lack may 'cause' schizophrenia include thiamine, biotin, Vitamin B_{12} and folic acid. Schizophrenics with low histamine levels are usually given 2g of folic acid; zinc can be prescribed if the hair mineral analysis indicates a high level of copper; PABA (para aminobenzoic acid) is used for some patients. Supplementation with the amino acid methionine is also used to treat schizophrenia.

Orthomolecular psychiatrists agree that disturbed family relations and personal conflicts may contribute to the illness, but maintain that the primary defect is a biochemical one.

This type of treatment is part of a broad-ranging programme which includes the use of orthodox drugs, ECT and psychotherapy if and when necessary. However, the earlier natural therapy is instigated the more likely is a complete recovery to take place—with, thereafter, a lifetime maintenance diet and vitamin supplementation.

Homoeopathy

This can prove very helpful. Examples of remedies include *Belladonna, Stramonium, Hyoscyamus, Tarantula Hisp.*

Psychotherapy

This must be of a supportive rather than an exploratory type, initially, with some cautious exploratory therapy in suitable cases after the acute episode has resolved itself.

Spiritual therapy

Colour therapy; music therapy. Soul-directed therapy claims to aid schizophrenia, *but may prove highly traumatic*. Other possible techniques include Aurasoma and electrocrystal therapy.

XIV/2 MANIC-DEPRESSIVE PSYCHOSIS

A psychotic illness in which the patient's mood swings from mania, characterized by elation and supreme self-confidence, and severe depression (see **XIV/3**), characterized by sadness and self-loathing. The illness tends to be episodic, with attacks of mania and depression interspersed with periods of apparent mental health varying in length from weeks to years. The attacks may be of one kind only—i.e. single or repetitive periods of depression (the commoner manifestation)—but attacks alternately manic and then depressive, or repetitively manic, are not uncommon.

During an attack of mania patients appear almost to be on a drug 'high'. They talk very rapidly, flitting from one subject to the next, get extremely excited, and have very poor concentration. They get themselves into difficulties by making unrealistic promises and/or absurd business deals, acting in a sexually promiscuous way, spending vast sums they do not possess, and perhaps do foolish things like insult their employers or colleagues at work. They are easy to anger and can become physically violent if thwarted.

The mania varies from a state of mildly elevated mood to one in which speech is incoherent and incessant activity and failure to sleep can cause exhaustion. This condition is called delirious mania and is a medical emergency.

The feelings of persecution that can arise in the manic phase, when patients in a state of ebullience suddenly grow angry because they think they are being unfairly picked upon, stem from the DELUSION that they are so important that they must be under scrutiny by forces such as foreign powers.

During the depressive episodes patients look and feel miserable. They complain of having no confidence in themselves and, when questioned, may reveal a lack of self-esteem ranging from feelings of inadequacy to a conviction of absolute wickedness. The self-blame aspect of the depressive episodes is often expressed in delusions that some appalling (but deserved) punishment is about to be meted out to them.

This last trait distinguishes the manic-depressive patient who is in depressive phase from a paranoid schizophrenic, who believes that he or she is being unjustly persecuted (see XIV/1). The delusional ideas can exist on a grander scale still in some patients, who are completely convinced that they are cursed by God or are responsible for earthquakes and other disasters. Other delusions may be that a part of their body is rotting away, or that everyone around them loathes and despises them.

Physical symptoms commonly accompanying the depressive phase of manic-depressive disorder include disturbed sleep patterns, weight-loss, poor appetite and constipation. Suicide is a recognized possibility with severely depressed patients and, when this risk has been assessed, such a patient may require a spell of hospitalization for his or her own protection or that of others (homicide is also a possibility in cases where patients are convinced that their whole family is damned).

A predisposition to manic-depressive psychosis can be inherited. There is a seasonal tendency for the attacks to occur during the spring and autumn and, while many attacks occur for no apparent reason, many seem to be precipitated by an environmental disturbance such as severe emotional stress (see STRESS REACTIONS).

ORTHODOX TREATMENT

Hospitalization, as noted, is prescribed where necessary.

Manic episodes are often well controlled with lithium salts, which can prevent or reduce the severity of the attacks. Blood measurements of lithium levels should be a regular feature of treatment because of lithium's toxic side-effects (mental confusion, TREMOR, even COMA) and its limited therapeutic range. Depressive episodes are generally treated by drug therapy (tricyclic antidepressants, or monoamine oxidase inhibitors—MAOIs). ECT can be used in conjunction with or instead of these drugs.

ALTERNATIVE THERAPIES

Natural medicine

A wholefood diet worked out by a nutritional expert for the patient as an individual, after similar tests to those described for schizophrenia (see XIV/1) had been performed. A review of lifestyle, with special reference to the elimination of stress factors. A high proportion of raw foods in the diet have been reported to induce a feeling of mental and emotional balance and stability.

Specific dietary supplements Dietary supplements likely to help the depressive (and perhaps the manic) phases include the following vitamins and minerals: folic acid; Vitamins B_1, B_3 and B_6; Vitamin C; Vitamin E; calcium pantothenate; zinc; calcium; and magnesium. Essential-amino-acid supplementation with DLPA (D-L-phenylalanine), which is very useful in pain relief, has been found also to have an antidepressant effect. However, L-phenylalanine alone in a dose of 100–500mg daily seems to be preferable for the treatment of straightforward depression (caution must be used with the higher doses in the presence of raised blood pressure); the course is continued for 1–2 weeks.

Hydrotherapy This has a definite application in the treatment of depression. Daily cold baths to stimulate the circulation are sometimes prescribed, following reports of the benefit achieved from the immersion in cold water of the limbs of depressed patients. In addition, regular outdoor exercise can be very beneficial in depression.

Biochemic tissue salts For depressive phase: *Kali Phos.* alternating with *Natrum Mur.*, in a dosage of four tablets every 2–3 hours.

Herbal medicine

For depression: a cup of hot rosemary tea, 2–3 times daily, made by infusing two pinches of the leaves of the herb in a teacup of boiling water. One pinch of valerian may be added.

Aromatherapy

To treat depressive phase: essence of chamomile, 3–4 drops on a little brown sugar, three times a day between meals. Also, rub the spinal column with the enriched oil, made as follows: sunflower seed oil, enriched per litre with 50g of borneol, 100g essence of chamomile, 20g essence of rosemary and 50g essence of sage.

Homoeopathy

For suicidal depression alternating with mania, and delusions of power or grandeur; poor circulation and nervous muscular twitching: *Agar-*

icus. For mania with swearing, loss of control, irritability, or a dream-like deluded state: *Anacardium orientale*. For depressive phase, with restlessness and delusions, fearfulness, and sometimes great impatience; absolute certainty of beliefs: *Medorrhinum*. For acute manic-depressive state, sharply alternating between the two phases; burning heat and redness, especially of the face; all stimuli worsen the condition: *Belladonna*.

Relaxation techniques

Biofeedback can be used to enable patient to achieve and maintain a good state of physical relaxation.

Exercise therapy

Yoga asanas, to flex and stretch the body and calm the mind, should be used under expert guidance only. Dance therapy might be prescribed to suitable patients.

Spiritual therapy

Music therapy; colour therapy. Electrocrystal therapy can help manic-depressive psychosis, as can Aurasoma.

Another class of mental disorders consists of the personality disorders and the neuroses. Here we shall discuss depression, anxiety (**XIV/4**), hysteria (**XIV/6**), phobia (**XIV/7**), obsessive-compulsive disorders (**XIV/5**), and anorexia nervosa (**XIV/8**). Firstly, however, we should look at what we mean by the terms 'personality disorder' and 'neurosis'.

PERSONALITY DISORDERS

Sometimes people are said to suffer from 'personality disorders' on the grounds that they get on less well with other people and within their natural environment generally, than do most of us. The personality traits involved are numerous and sometimes vague, and certainly not always definable in terms of mental illness.

The SCHIZOID PERSONALITY is a definable entity, and may lead to the development of schizophrenia (see **XIV/1**), just as the highly emotionally volatile sort of person may one day suffer from manic-depressive psychosis (see **XIV/2**); but again these traits are markers of a predisposition and do not in themselves constitute illnesses. The *psychopathic personality*, however, is definitely abnormal, and the affected individual is identifiable by being a chronic social misfit who would not be diagnosed as 'insane' but would be identified by his abnormal, irresponsible and socially unacceptable behaviour. Aggression, extreme insensitivity to the feelings and needs of others, and a childhood in which isolation figured prominently are characteristic features of this type of personality disorder.

NEUROSES

The neuroses, or neurotic illnesses, include depression (**XIV/3**), anxiety (**XIV/4**) and hysteria (**XIV/6**). Some authorities say that they are easier to link with a history of early conflict than are the psychotic illnesses. They differ from the psychoses in that patients have insight into their own illnesses (i.e. accept that they are ill in some way, and can see their symptoms *as* symptoms of an underlying disorder requiring treatment). Unlike psychotic patients, neurotic patients do not lose contact with reality.

XIV/3 DEPRESSION

A multiplicity of factors are seen by many workers to contribute to the development of depressive illness: they include genetic predisposition; a biochemical abnormality involving the neurotransmitter chemicals in the brain (which pass nervous stimuli from one nerve cell or neurone to another); the effects of early conflict, arising during the oral stage of infant development; and the effects of stress (see STRESS REACTIONS) in terms both of major life-events (such as bereavement, giving birth) and of daily stresses encountered in life today.

Two main types of depression are recognized: endogenous, which arises for no reason apparent to the sufferer; and exogenous (or reactive), arising from an obvious factor such as bereavement or (especially) divorce, but representing an exaggerated response to the event in normal terms.

The features of depression include intense misery and self-doubt; self-blame, and notions of unworthiness—without, however, the DELUSIONS associated with the psychotic state of manic-depressive disorder (see **XIV/2**). Patients suffering from severe depression are typically lethargic, apparently dull-witted and often unable to respond to psychotherapy in the initial stages. A total lack of psychic and physical energy is a characteristic symptom, and patients are often unable to cope with work, study, running the home, etc.

There are also physical symptoms associated with a general 'depression': constipation; sleep disorder (a tendency to sleep excessively, or to wake up early or fail to fall asleep at night); poor appetite; weight-loss; headaches; a bad taste in the mouth; and tearfulness.

ORTHODOX TREATMENT

This includes (a) psychotherapy; (b) the use of drugs—tricyclic or tetracyclic antidepressants (including imipramine [Tofranil] and clomipramine [Anafranil]) and the monoamine oxidase inhibitors, or MAOIs (tranylcypromine [Parstelin] and phenelzine [Nardil]); (c) electroconvulsive therapy (ECT).

ALTERNATIVE THERAPIES

Natural medicine

A wholefood diet would be a prerequisite of naturopathic treatment, as junk food is one of the environmental stresses that can help to precipitate depressive illness, combined with a stressful lifestyle and poor nutritional status. Applied kinesiology might be employed to detect food allergies, and possibly to correct them. Exercise, hydrotherapy and dietary supplements might also be prescribed (see under X/2).

Zinc often works very well in simple neurotic depression, and should be included as part of a total supplement programme. A likely dose is 30mg of the chelated mineral daily.

The amino acid tryptophan has been used with success to treat certain forms of depression (it achieves better results in neurotic than in manic depression). *It must not be taken by any person also taking MAOI anti-depressant drugs or within three weeks of their finishing a course of them.* The dose is 3g daily with a small carbohydrate meal (i.e. not with protein), plus 1g daily of nicotinamide (Vitamin B_3). When the effects of tryptophan on depressed patients were compared with those of the tricyclic antidepressant drug imipramine (Toranil) results were apparent sooner in the drug-treated patients but tryptophan produced highly statistically significant improvements.

Also useful is propolis tincture, 4–5 drops on a sugar lump, 3–4 times daily.

For guidelines on biochemic tissue salts, herbal medicine and aromatherapy see the relevant discussions under XIV/2.

Homoeopathy

Useful for neurotic depression. For emotional tearful depression in an irritable personality, pragmatic rather than intellectual, worse for sympathy: *Natrum muriaticum*. In an intellectual person, not very emotional, worried about future: *Lycopodium*.

Acupuncture

This can be useful in cases of neurotic depression.

Psychotherapy

Analytic and supportive psychotherapy, the former when the patient is sufficiently capable of responding.

Exercise therapy

Yoga; dance therapy.

Relaxation techniques

Biofeedback; possibly autogenic training; autohypnosis for appropriate patients.

Spiritual therapy

Colour and music therapy; art therapy; electrocrystal therapy; Aurasoma.

XIV/4 ANXIETY

Anxiety neurosis is a very common illness in our society—5 per cent of the adult population suffer from an anxiety state, and 30 per cent of physical illnesses reported are accompanied by anxiety of clinical proportions. Like depression (**XIV/3**), anxiety is considered to result from a combination of contributive causes: a possible genetic predisposition; environmental and life stresses play a large part in its generation; and, according to Freudian theory, a major psychological cause is unresolved conflict during the genital stage of psychic development.

The symptoms are of four different types: (a) bodily tension, with shakiness, trembling, eyelid-twitch, restlessness, inability to relax, muscular aches and pains and fatigue; (b) overactivity of the autonomic nervous system, resulting in sweating, pounding heart, cold clammy hands, dizziness and tingling in the hands and feet; frequent passing of water is another sign, as are DIARRHOEA, racing pulse, lump in throat, upset stomach and flushing; (c) 'apprehensive expectation' whereby patients feel constantly apprehensive without knowing the cause and worry and brood, anticipating that something dreadful is going to occur; (d) the symptoms collectively known as 'vigilance and scanning', which may cause patients to feel on edge so that they have difficulty in concentrating, sleep badly, and feel exhausted when they wake up.

Depression (**XIV/3**) very frequently coexists with anxiety, and sometimes requires treatment aimed specifically at alleviating it in addition to the treatment designed to relieve the anxiety. When the diagnosis is in doubt, orthodox doctors normally treat as for depression in preference to anxiety. Other conditions which may confuse the clear diagnosis of an anxiety state include PANIC ATTACKS, which can occur as isolated incidents or exist as part of a generalized anxiety disorder; phobia (see **XIV/7**); and obsessive-compulsive disorders (see **XIV/8**). These last two conditions are specific clinical manifestations of anxiety neurosis, as also is hysteria. The basic orthodox and alternative treatment of anxiety is given under OBSESSIVE-COMPULSIVE DISORDERS.

XIV/5 OBSESSIVE-COMPULSIVE DISORDERS

Repetitive, irrational actions or thoughts which torment the sufferer and from which he or she is unable to free himself or herself. Obsessive behaviour and/or thought-patterns can constitute a single neurosis or exist as an aspect of a more complex neurosis. They can also appear as a symptom of more serious psychiatric disorders. An example of obsessive-compulsive behaviour is the uncontrollable need to check that water is not flooding all over the bathroom floor: while 'knowing' that this is not so, a person obsessed with the fear that it might be would be compelled, perhaps a dozen times before being able to leave the house each day, by an inner demand to investigate the state of the bathroom and to make certain that the taps are turned off.

ORTHODOX TREATMENT

Careful case-history taking and, if necessary, biochemical tests, would enable the doctor to distinguish between (a) true anxiety disorder, (b) variations on the theme of anxiety such as these conditions, and (c) physical conditions which might occasionally mimic anxiety; these latter include thyrotoxicosis, paroxysmal atrial TACHYCARDIA, HYPOGLYCAEMIA, and habitual coffee-drinking (providing an excess of caffeine).

Treatment includes the important elements of listening, discussion, explanation and reassurance. Psychotherapy, possibly behavioural therapy, may be prescribed. Drugs are prescribed for patients with either (a) severe anxiety or (b) mild to moderate anxiety whose symptoms do not respond to reassurance. Examples are well known tranquillizers such as diazepam (Valium); chlordiazepoxide (Librium); lorazepam (Ativan); and propranolol (Inderal), which acts by relieving the physical symptoms of anxiety.

ALTERNATIVE THERAPIES

Natural medicine

Complete revision of the patient's diet, response to stress, exercise routine and relaxation routines would take place. A wholefood diet would be instigated, together with a full dietary supplementation programme of vitamins and minerals. The diet would be likely to contain a high proportion of raw ingredients. Applied kinesiology might be employed to detect food allergies and possibly to treat them.

Specific dietary supplements　A high potency stress-B complex should be taken daily; of special importance are thiamine (B_1), B_6 and pantothenic acid. In addition, Vitamin C helps guard against stress, Vitamin E aids brain cells to obtain sufficient oxygen, and zinc, calcium and magnesium are helpful. (The mineral supplements should be chelated in all cases.) The essential amino acid tryptophan helps in the treatment of anxiety as well as depression (see **XIV/3**).

Raw juice therapy　140ml lettuce juice with 140ml carrot juice, twice daily and before retiring.

Biochemic tissue salts　*Kali Phos.*, four tablets every 2–3 hours, alternating with *Ferrum Phos.* in same dosage.

Herbal medicine

A pinch of hawthorn flowers, infused together with a fig and a prune in a cup of boiling water for 10 minutes.

Aromatherapy

Four drops of sweet-marjoram essence on a little brown sugar after every meal.

Homoeopathy

For sudden panic attacks: *Aconite*. For more prolonged anxiety with periodic panic attacks: *Arsenicum Albium*. For agoraphobia: examples of remedies include *Aconitum, Arnica, Arsenicum*. For claustrophobia: examples of remedies include *Argentum nitricum* and *Carbo vegetabilis*. For fear of eating out in public (a common phobia): *Lycopodium, Gelsemium*. For fear of the opposite sex: *Pulsatilla, Ignatia, Calcarea*.

Acupuncture

This can be helpful in restoring a sense of balance and tranquillity.

Reflexology

This can help to relieve severe anxiety.

Psychotherapy

Supportive and later exploratory psychotherapy; behavioural therapy. Hypnotherapy, following straightforward analysis or hypnoanalysis, can cure phobias.

Exercise therapy

Yoga, dance therapy.

Relaxation techniques

Yoga, biofeedback, autogenic training, autohypnosis.

Spiritual therapy

Colour, music and art therapy might all help, as might Aurasoma and electrocrystal therapy.

XIV/6 HYSTERIA

This is a neurotic behaviour disturbance in which symptoms and signs of physical or mental ill-health are imitated more or less unconsciously for subconscious reasons. The aim is always one of personal advantage to the patient. The assumed disorder may be a full 'conversion hysteria', and consist of paralysis of an arm or leg, loss of voice, loss of sight or hearing, or some other dramatic condition. Less florid manifestations include hysterical fits, amnesia and sleepwalking.

Hysteria is thought by some psychologists to result, like anxiety (**XIV/4**), from unresolved conflict at the genital stage of development. However apparently serious the physical or mental symptoms of an hysteric, these are totally remediable provided the right course is taken in psychotherapeutic treatment.

ORTHODOX TREATMENT

The sooner the diagnosis is made, the better the chances of recovery because the more doctors hesitate, and the more frequently the patient undergoes X-rays, blood-tests and other investigations, the more firmly rooted the hysterical symptoms become. Treatment methods include psychotherapy and a brief course of tranquillizers; for psychiatric pain, intravenous injections of small doses of sodium amylobarbitone (a barbiturate) are sometimes very effective.

ALTERNATIVE THERAPIES

Natural medicine

Wholefood high-raw diet, with supplements to help deal specifically with anxiety. Exercise programme where appropriate to help deal with unreleased tension; and appraisal of lifestyle, in order to pinpoint stress areas in general and the major precipitating stress factor(s) in particular.

Use of raw juices, biochemic tissue salts, dietary supplements and herbal medicine is as for Anxiety (**XIV/4**).

Aromatherapy

Essence of valerian, three drops on a little brown sugar between meals.

Psychotherapy

Hypnotherapy in particular can prove helpful.

Relaxation techniques

If the hysteric can be persuaded to undertake these and is able to do so, gradually learning the art of relaxation could prove very helpful.

Spiritual therapy

Art, music and/or colour therapy may be employed to aid recovery; also Aurasoma and electrocrystal therapy.

XIV/7 PHOBIA

An incapacitating fear of an object or situation which does not really warrant such a reaction. The patient's personality type unconsciously determines the mechanism adopted to deal with the anxiety (which is termed 'free-floating', meaning that the patient cannot attach it to a cause). The development of a phobia is one of the three possibilities, the other two being (a) PSYCHOSOMATIC illness and (b) 'externalization and identification', in which the anxious person becomes deeply engrossed in the worries and problems of others, due to the unconsciously projection of his or her anxiety onto something tangible. A phobia equally substitutes the 'known for the unknown', giving the free-floating anxiety something to latch onto; but this does not deal any more adequately with the underlying problem than do the other two methods, and can be extremely distressing and incapacitating.

Two common phobias are *agoraphobia*, a terror of wide open spaces, and *claustrophobia*, a dread of being shut in a small space. Others are great fear of spiders, heights, illness, cats and thunderstorms. All are due to the same underlying problem, and are different symbolic expressions of it, chosen by the unconscious mind of the individual.

For treatment see under XIV/5.

XIV/8 ANOREXIA NERVOSA

This is a potentially hazardous condition, the chief feature of which is profound loss of weight; it is a type of neurosis. Besides refusal to eat, restless energy is often prominent. There is usually an accompanying loss of menstrual periods, as well as personality changes, particularly noticeable in individuals (usually women but occasionally men) who are normally happy, outgoing and cheerful. There is a tendency to become moody, depressed, antisocial and withdrawn, and to spend many hours alone in preference to mixing with friends. Anorexic patients, it is thought, basically resent their inevitable maturation into adults, and reject food as a symbolic rejection of adult sexuality.

The anorexic is unlikely to admit to being ill, and equally unlikely to agree either to see a doctor or to eat more. Attempts by family members to force the issue will probably make matters worse, because a prime cause of anorexia nervosa is stored resentment and anger due to earlier family clashes, and repeating them once the illness has started only reinforces the underlying trigger. Family pressure may indeed result in the patient resorting to methods other than simple food-avoidance in order to lose weight. Possibilities include deliberately induced vomiting after meals (known as *bulimia*) and taking massive doses of laxatives to induce severe diarrhoea and reduce the absorption of food.

As well as unexpressed anger, anorexia is believed also to be due to a distorted body-image (the anorexic sees herself as fat, however much weight she loses), and possibly to malfunction of the pituitary gland in the brain. It has been suggested that an inability to utilise Vitamin A and a deficiency of the mineral zinc might also be contributive to the illness. In this connection, it is interesting that a recent American study has shown zinc to be necessary for the maintenance of normal concentrations of Vitamin A in the blood plasma.[93]

Anorexia nervosa is becoming more common than it once was. It is thought that in the UK as many as one in 250 schoolgirls may suffer from it.

ORTHODOX TREATMENT

Treatment is vital, as patients who remain untreated or who fail to respond may very well die, either from malnutrition or from associated conditions such as potassium deficiency, hypothermia and dehydration. The usual approach is to win the patient's confidence, persuade her to go into hospital away from friends and family members, and start a refeeding programme supervised by experienced nurses. Daily records of the patient's weight are kept, and the patient is warmly complimented on tiny gains. Early meals are supervised by one of the nursing staff. As soon as the patient is well enough, she is discharged from hospital and psychotherapy is started, to discover and to help her to overcome the underlying problem.

ALTERNATIVE THERAPIES

Natural medicine

Many alternative practitioners would agree that a patient is best off in hospital in the early stages. A naturopath would recommend a wholefood diet with a high raw element where the patient was capable of taking this, probably supplemented by freshly squeezed fruit and vegetable juices, especially in the early stages. A full supplementation programme of vitamins and minerals would be added as soon as the practitioner considered this desirable.

Homoeopathy

Remedies include *Thuja*, *Natrum muriaticum* and *Cannabis ind*.

Exercise therapy

Dance therapy is useful for adolescents with neurotic illnesses and a tendency to be antisocial.

Psychotherapy

Supportive psychotherapy and counselling at first; possibly analytic psychotherapy later. Biofeedback, autohypnosis or autogenics could prove helpful once the patient had started to respond to psychotherapy.

Spiritual therapy

Colour therapy; art therapy; Aurasoma; electrocrystal therapy.

XIV/9 AUTISM

This form of mental illness in children was recognized first in 1943 and is as yet not understood. About one child in 3,000 seems to be affected. Autistic children give the appearance of being cut off from the rest of the world, preferring contact with toys or anything mechanical to any form of contact with people. They neither give nor respond to affection, will not establish eye-contact, and have a tendency to pick up and carry out stereotyped mannerisms repetitively. They are neither mentally retarded, blind nor deaf, but their perception seems to be at fault, because, although they can hear sounds perfectly well, they are unwilling to attempt the mimicry that normal children perform in learning how to speak. Hence, speech is generally retarded and a difficult problem to solve. When they do learn to speak they often speak of themselves in the third person. The Director of the Institute for Behaviour Research in California, Bernard Rimland, believes that the mechanism underlying autism involves the inability to give meaning to incoming stimuli due to an incapacity to relate such stimuli to relevant stored information.[94]

Frequently the only sign of emotion in autistic children is the occasional TEMPER TANTRUM. There is no known 'cure' but, as the condition is becoming easier to diagnose, the quality of special care and management of autistic children is improving.

When hair mineral analysis was carried out using the scalp hair of 28 autistic children and 18 controls, the only major difference between the two groups when concentrations of 16 nutrient minerals and 7 toxic minerals were measured was that the autistic group had significantly lower magnesium in their hair.[95]

A number of theories exist about the relationship between magnesium levels and autism. One is that there might be a functional deficiency of vitamin B_6, since magnesium is required for the activity of this vitamin in the body. Others include the effect of magnesium on neurotransmitter metabolism, and the fact that some of the children had been on anti-psychotic drugs which decrease both calcium and magnesium levels in the blood. Hair mineral analysis might be usefully included as a routine test in childhood autism.

Leon Chaitow comments at the end of this report[95] that hair mineral analysis is a useful tool but is inadequate when used alone for the forming of a definitive diagnosis. It provides a useful piece of information, to be interpreted in conjunction with other evidence of the individual's nutritional status. He points out that 'autism, as with so many psychiatric conditions, would seem to be increasingly amenable to some degree of nutritional intervention'.

Excess copper or iron has also been suggested as a possible cause of autism. This might come about during the first six months of life through inadequate production by the liver of the normal copper-binding protein ceruloplasmin or of the iron-binding protein ferritin. The function of these proteins is to join up with their respective metals and keep them in solution in the blood, thus preventing excessive absorption. It has been postulated that, if either were produced in inadequate amounts, excessive absorption of the relevant metals could occur, thus affecting the brain and possibly causing autism. Heavy metals such as mercury or lead could interfere with ceruloplasmin or ferritin synthesis.[96] It is known that high levels of copper in the tissues or blood may be an important factor in the generation of a number of clinical syndromes, including paranoid schizophrenia, depressive illness, senile dementia, hyperactivity in children and autism.

ORTHODOX TREATMENT

Drugs such as Melleril (thioridazine hydrochloride), plus psychotherapy.

ALTERNATIVE THERAPIES

Natural medicine

A wholefood diet that strictly eliminates all forms of processed foods and synthetic additives is suggested. The total content of carbohydrate (especially of the refined type) should be low. Applied kinesiology might be employed for the detection of hidden food allergies.

Vitamin and mineral supplementation has been used successfully in treating the underlying causes of autism in many children.[97] These nutrients work by correcting imbalances rather than by disguising them, and so take effect slowly: 3–6 months is the minimum time for maximum changes to be manifest. Parents should not give up because progress is gradual and at times apparently static. Supplements that have been used in autism include, in particular, vitamins B_1, B_2, B_3, B_6, pantothenic acid, deanol (a natural compound introduced by Pfeiffer in 1957, which acts as a biochemical stimulant, though without side-effects or the risk of dependency developing), glutamic acid, manganese, zinc, magnesium and sulphur (as in egg-yolks).

Psychotherapy

Dr Rachel Pinney, author of *Bobby—Breakthrough of an Autistic Child*, has invented a technique called 'creative listening' to help disturbed children, including autistic ones. In this method, the child is watched playing and allowed to do as he or she wishes, within certain limits of safety and propriety. He or she is given undivided attention and listened to with complete concentration. The 'taker' of the session makes running comments on what the child is doing, but never seeks to interpret his or her activities, nor to ask questions about them. Playing, acting out tensions freely, and even being shown how to laugh at his own problems were part of the technique which transformed Bobby, the subject of Pinney's book. Pinney has a clinic in the East End of London. The pamphlets *Creative Listening* and *Children's Hours* are available from the Children's Hours Trust, 28 Wallace House, 410 Caledonian Road, London N7 8TL.

Exercise therapy

Success has been reported with dance therapy.

Spiritual therapy

Music therapy is used for autism, as is electrocrystal therapy.

PART THREE

Introduction

The demand for alternative therapies has increased substantially over the last few years. Many theories have been advanced to explain this; but few constructive attempts have been made to assess the facts. However, a recent in-depth study carried out at the Centre for Alternative Therapies in Southampton has proved both valuable and highly informative. The centre, run by Dr George Lewith and Dr Julian Kenyon, not only offers a range of alternative therapies but also has good teaching and research links with Southampton University. The survey was carried out by two medical students seconded to the centre for six months; their objective was to evaluate commonly preconceived ideas about why patients seek alternative therapies.[98]

This is a summary of their findings, many of which substantially dispel a number of commonly held notions on the topic:

- Awareness of alternative therapies and of what they have to offer was a far more important factor than bank balance in determining a patient's choice between orthodox and alternative therapies (of the patients seen at the centre, 20 per cent pay only a £5 consultation fee on account of low income).
- Pain is the single most important complaint for which patients require treatment, accounting for 45 per cent of the presenting symptoms. Most patients had had their problems for a long time (on average nine years).
- Nearly all patients had seen their own GPs and often a specialist as well; most found their GPs helpful and understanding, implying that they were in no way dissatisfied with the NHS. Only 3 out of 65 patients had bypassed orthodox medicine, and about 30 per cent had in fact been referred to the centre by their GPs.
- Only one patient in four felt that their GP had rushed them while one in five felt rushed when seeing the doctors at the centre. (This is directly contrary to the prevailing wisdom!) Interestingly, the same patients who felt rushed by their GPs also felt rushed when seeing the

centre doctors. Treatment outcome was not affected by this variable.

- Two-thirds of the patients interviewed expected a great deal from the alternative treatment, and believed alternative therapies to be very effective. Their expectations correlated with treatment outcome, in that, if they believed they were going to recover, their chances of doing so were greatly increased.
- Approximately half of the patients involved were being treated with manipulative therapy and acupuncture, and the rest with either herbal or homoeopathic medicine or a food-exclusion diet. At follow-up, 59 per cent felt their condition had improved significantly. It can generally be expected that physical (manipulative) treatment will achieve results more rapidly than medical treatment directed at internal illness. Only 19 of the 33 patients at follow-up had actually completed their treatment; the report believed that, had the follow-up taken place a few months later, many more of the patients would have noted a significant improvement in their conditions.
- The patients (like the vast majority of patients seeking alternative treatment) were *chronically* (rather than acutely) sick. The report suggested that this implies that orthodox medicine is most likely to fail with chronic illness, 'almost certainly because it's looking for symptom-suppression rather than attempting to define the cause of the illness and treat it' and that 'the philosophies behind alternative medicine may indeed be more powerful at dealing with chronic illness than conventional medicine'.

A year before this report was published a major survey[99] was commissioned by Swan House Special Events (backed by Newman Turner Publications) into the relative popularity of a number of alternative therapies; patients were also asked to rate the effects of the therapies they had tried (in herbal medicine and vitamin therapy there was obviously a large element of self-treatment). Questions were directed to the 'man in the street', and 2,000 people took part. A summary of the findings is shown in the table.

The alternative therapies discussed in succeeding pages are subdivided into (a) those directed primarily at the body, (b) those directed primarily towards the mind, and (c) those recognizably directed most of all at Man's spiritual faculty. It must be borne in mind, however, that according to the principle of holism all three parts of Man are inextricably interrelated, and, whatever the primary direction of any given

Types of therapy	personally tried (%)	satisfied (%)	dissatisfied (%)
Herbal medicine	12	73	18
Vitamin therapy	7	65	12
Osteopathy	6	73	14
Massage	6	82	9
Homoeopathy	4	66	16
Meditation/relaxation	4	83	12
Acupuncture	3	50	47
Chiropractic	2	68	19
Healing	2	68	16
Hypnotherapy	2	43	50
Psychotherapy	2	75	12

holistic therapy, the whole of Man's tripartite nature is inevitably feeling the effect.

The therapies selected for inclusion are all likely—judging by research findings, anecdotal accounts of patients who have experienced them, or my own personal experience—to be of genuine therapeutic value to those who seek them; also, all are available in the UK.

Therapies of the Body

NATURAL MEDICINE

The basic types of natural medicine discussed in this book are naturopathy (including hydrotherapy), ionization therapy, Bates's eyesight training, and biochemic-tissue-salt therapy.

NATUROPATHY

Natural therapists in general believe that illness results from our losing touch with the innate instincts that prompt us to exercise, eat, drink and combat stress as we should. This being so, they recommend as natural a lifestyle as possible in order to re-establish the communications link between our conscious awareness and our long-silenced instinctual knowledge. The term 'naturopathy' is generally accepted as referring to treatment based on simple, natural lifestyle principles.

Naturopathy is a distinct system of healing, based upon clearly defined principles of theory and practice the essence of which can be traced back at least to c400BC, when Hippocrates demonstrated the treatment of disease by natural methods. One of the pioneers of modern naturopathy was Dr Henry Lindlahr, author of *The Philosophy of Natural Therapeutics*, who believed that a full understanding of the meaning of health must form the basis of our understanding of disease.

Naturopathic medicine is founded upon three basic principles. Firstly, the body has the power to cure itself due to its inner life-force (or vitality) and to natural instinctual wisdom. The concept of the life-force or vital force is fundamental to naturopathic theory and practice; and the aim of therapeutic procedures is to stimulate the body's natural healing power and encourage it to work as it should.

Secondly, the appearance of the symptoms of a disorder are tangible proof of the life-force at work. Health is a state of dynamic equilibrium between Man's biochemistry, mechanical structure and mental attributes, the energy of the system being drawn from the inner life-force; disease is a state of imbalance arising when one of these three factors becomes unstable:

- *Biochemical upset* is apparent in the body's fluids (blood, tissue fluid, urine, digestive secretions, bile) and is due to an inadequate or harmful diet, inadequate excretion of waste products by skin, lungs, liver, kidneys or bowel, or poor circulation.
- Man's *mechanical structure* (skeleton, ligaments, tendons, muscles) can cause imbalance when the posture is poor, joints are underexercised or misused, the spine is out of alignment or the muscles are held in a tense and strained position due to stress and anxiety.
- *Psychological factors* can cause imbalance when stress is not counterblaanced by relaxation but allowed to cause chronic depression, anxiety or other problems.

The third fundamental principle of naturopathy is that it adopts a *holistic* approach to health. This has much in common with the second principle, for all three of Man's essential 'components'—body, mind and spirit—are considered when a disorder arises: the patient is considered as a whole person, not simply in terms of that part of the body displaying symptoms. Moreover, the aim of naturopathy is to eliminate the root problem, not just the symptoms, and therefore many aspects of the patient are taken into consideration when diagnosis and treatment are being considered—e.g. inherited weaknesses, previous medical history and present general state of health.

Consultation

At first this may seem very similar to a consultation with an orthodox doctor, but more time is usually spent in taking a case history and some of the questions asked may not at first appear relevant to the patient. This is because the naturopath is trying to assess not so much a specific disease-entity as the overall functional capacity of the patient, his or her nutritional status, and the degree of vigour or depletion of the life-force within. Examples of such questions might be how the patient's symptoms are affected by environmental heat or cold, the time of day, geographical location, the weather, and certain types of food and drink.

Besides carrying out a physical examination and routine diagnostic tests involving, for example, the blood and urine, or X-rays, the naturopath may also use supplementary diagnostic procedures not generally adopted by orthodox practitioners. These might include constitutional assessment, iridology, hair analysis, radionic analysis, medical astrology, palmistry, Kirlian photography and electrocrystal diagnosis.

Treatment

In a 1964 Naturopathic Commission draft sponsored by the British Naturopathic and Osteopathic Association, the following therapies were defined as of primary importance in the naturopathic treatment of disease: fasting, dietetics, hydrotherapy, natural hygiene, structural adjustment, and explanation.

Fasting The majority of curative fasts are prescribed for 3–7 days. Permitted liquids include mineral or boiled water and fruit or vegetable juices. Fasting is considered to differ from starvation by the absence of severe hunger. Its value is considered to lie in the rest given to the digestive organs, in the elimination of toxins, and in stimulation to subsequent recovery.

Fasting should be carried out under professional guidance only. Its effects can be unpleasant: they have been described in terms of a 'fasting acidosis'. When this occurs, the rate at which the body gets rid of uric acid is reduced, and hypoglycaemia is a prominent feature. The symptoms may include depression, poor concentration, loss of appetite, a bad taste in the mouth and bad breath (partly due to the presence of acetone), a furred tongue and irritability. This stage passes with an 'acidotic crisis' (akin to a 'healing crisis'), and the symptoms then resolve themselves.

Fasting is particularly likely to be recommended for acute conditions; e.g. febrile illnesses such as childhood infections, tonsillitis, bronchitis and influenza (there is a traditional saying: 'Feed a cold, and starve a fever').[100]

The Guelpa fast is often recommended. Known also as the 'saline fast', this is a modified fast which depends upon an initial loading dose of saline to intensify its action.[100] It is recommended for patients for whom a total fast is inadvisable, and has a powerful cleansing action. It lasts for three days. The source of saline is Epsom salts taken in the morning of the first two days.

Dietetics The most usual diet for naturopathic doctors to prescribe is a balanced, natural, wholesome diet (i.e. a wholefood diet), although other controlled diets are given for specific disorders.

The wholefood diet is simply what it says: it has nothing added and nothing taken away. It avoids processed foods, food items containing anything artificial (e.g. synthetic colouring matter, preservatives, flavourings, thickeners, emulsifiers) and foods from which useful, wholesome ingredients have been extracted by a 'refining' process (e.g. white flour and pasta and bread made from it, white rice and white sugar).

The naturopathically favoured wholefood diet presents a balanced selection of natural foods. It is typically low in sugar, even the natural brown variety, and products containing sugar of any kind. It is also generally low in salt, but permits the use of salt substitutes based on potassium rather than sodium. The consumption of alcohol should not exceed two glasses of wine daily (or equivalent); and coffee, tea and cola drinks should either be drunk in very limited quantities, if at all. Herb teas, freshly squeezed fruit and vegetable juices and spring or boiled tap water are approved. The diet is low in animal fats, and encourages the use of substitutes such as polyunsaturated-fatty-acid plant oils and their products: these include safflower and sunflower oils for cooking, margarine high in polyunsaturates instead of butter; even these should be used only in moderation. The diet favours the use of skimmed milk, low-fat cheese and yoghourt in place of their high-fat counterparts; and recommends offal, oily fish (their oil content protects against heart disease) and poultry as sources of animal protein; meat and poultry, should be from organically reared animals, and all fat and skin should be removed. Only three (free-range) eggs should be eaten per week.

Baking, grilling (with a minimum of oil) and steaming are much preferred to frying and roasting, and vegetarian savouries should form the main meal at least once or twice a week. Pulses (beans, lentils), brown rice, other grains (millet, barley, oats), organically produced vegetables, wholemeal bread and baked potatoes (including their skins) are advocated: these are excellent sources of complex carbohydrates which satisfy hunger, keep the blood-sugar level from soaring (as happens with simple-sugar-containing foods), and supply a sufficiency of natural fibre.

Many naturopaths have for a long time favoured the inclusion in the diet of a high proportion of raw fruit and vegetables, nuts, seeds and sprouts—i.e. the high-raw diet. The importance of this dietary alteration was brought to the public's notice by the book *Raw Energy* (1984), by Leslie and Susannah Kenton.

Examples of modified diets favoured by naturopathic practitioners are described in the next few pages.

The Schroth cure stimulates the metabolism: fluid-intake is reduced, and cold-packs are placed on the skin to promote skin elimination. The diet's three-day cycle is repeated for 2–3 weeks. The Schroth cure is specially recommended for catarrh, chronic skin conditions and conditions in which fluid retention and effusions are present (e.g. rheumatoid arthritis). Features of the diet include a high proportion of complex carbohydrates (porridge, dry wholemeal toast or rolls), and no fluids on the third day.

The Hay diet is based on avoiding certain food combinations and selecting others, according to the principle that various foods require different conditons for digestion to occur satisfactorily; e.g. protein and starch are never eaten together since protein digestion needs an acid environment and starches require alkaline secretions. Also incompatible are starch and acid fruit. The full details of and the thinking behind the Hay diet can be found in a number of recent books.[101] It was originally intended as a way of eating for everyone, but it is prescribed therapeutically by naturopaths for people suffering from digestive problems.

In *mono-diets* the diet is for a number of days restricted to a single type of food in order to saturate the patient's system with the nutrients it contains. The *grape cure* is the best known fruit mono-diet: 2.75kg of grapes are permitted per day, with water and apple- or grape-juice to drink. It is recommended for hypertension, heart disorders and fluid retention. The *rice diet* consists of 250–300g of rice daily, boiled or steamed. A little liquid and a little fruit are permitted, and sometimes other grains such as millet. It is used for heart complaints and obesity.

The *macrobiotic diet* is based rather upon ethical/philosophical beliefs than upon naturopathic principles, but a naturopath may well prescribe a macrobiotic regimen for a particular patient because of its curative properties.

The basis of macrobiotic eating is the recognition that foods fit into two categories, Yin and Yang, according to their properties. These two qualities both oppose and complement/counterbalance each other. At opposite ends of a vast spectrum, both universal and cosmic harmony and personal human health (physical, mental and spiritual) are dependent upon Yin and Yang remaining in a state of balanced equilibrium. Yin foods are acidic in quality, grow in a Yang environment (hot, dry), tend to contain a high proportion of water, and have an aromatic smell; the plants in this class generally grow above ground-level. Examples of Yin foods include tomatoes, durum wheat, beef, pork, whelks, oysters, yoghourt, cream, butter, bananas, citrus fruit, pineapples, honey, molasses, margarine, dyed quick-brewing tea, coffee, and sugared drinks. Yang foods grow in a cold, wet (Yin) environment, are alkaline in nature, and tend to be sour or salty; Yang plants tend to be drier, shorter and harder in quality, and are often found growing below the soil. Examples are: fertilized eggs, pheasant, turkey, herring, shrimps, sole, buckwheat, millet, wholewheat, watercress, carrots, parsley, onion, Halloumy goat cheese, goat milk, Fetta sheeps'-milk cheese, Edam cheese, apples, strawberries, cherries, blackcurrants, sesame oil, maize oil, sunflower oil, ginseng tea, mu tea, herb teas and spring water.[102]

Disease is believed to occur when the principles of Yin and Yang are out of balance. Balance can be restored in a particular person along macrobiotic lines by discovering whether he or she needs more or less Yin or Yang food and making the appropriate dietary adjustments. By and large, Yang foods, being alkaline, are favoured as more conducive to health; but—as in all applications of the holistic principle—the individual person, with his or her own specific physical, spiritual and psychological identity, is what above all else needs to be considered.

It is only fair to point out that the macrobiotic diet has been severely criticized in the UK press as 'rigid, unpalatable, and useless for treating the diseases for which it is recommended' (*Observer*). On the other hand, many patients, including cancer patients, have much to say in its favour. Those who described it as a failure to the *Observer* had returned to orthodox treatment after a 'very short time'. As the Public Relations Officer of the Community Health Centre pointed out, anyone wishing to get results must follow the diet for some months.

Vegetarian diets—many of which permit the inclusion of eggs, dairy products and fish—are often followed for the ethical reason that it is wrong and unnecessary to kill animals for food. Other people simply dislike all forms of meat, are made ill by meat, or feel healthier when they refrain from eating it. Yet others become vegetarian for a mixture of the two convictions. A naturopath would be likely to suggest omitting meat from a patient's diet if he or she considered that this would be of benefit. Many sufferers from arthritis, both rheumatoid and osteoarthritis, are said to gain relief from excluding both meat and dairy products from their diets.

A naturopath might suggest that a patient follow a *vegan diet* if a total absence of animal products seemed to be what the patient required. In fact, true vegans use nothing of animal origin—no fur clothing, leather goods or ornaments made from feather, bone, ivory, teeth or parchment. Their ethical principle is 'dynamic harmlessness'. Like vegetarianism, the vegan diet has been criticized as nutritionally deficient, but this seems to represent a hasty judgement by the omnivorous critics since it is possible to obtain the right kinds of protein in the correct amounts by using certain combinations of wholegrains, pulses, nuts and seeds. One of the main criticisms of veganism has been the likelihood of Vitamin-B_{12} deficiency. However, although for a long time animal products were the only known source of B_{12}, it is in fact supplied also by *Spirulina*, a blue-green alga (type of seaweed) used as a staple food by the Aztecs and now being developed as a high-protein food supplement rich in minerals and vitamins.

The Bristol Diet has come to be known as the 'Bristol Cancer Diet', but this is an unattractive and misrepresentative name, since the diet was originally designed by its innovator, Dr Alec Forbes, to prevent the development of illnesses and to encourage a positive attitude towards good health. The original version was modified for use by cancer patients when Forbes left the NHS and helped to set up the Cancer Help Centre in Bristol.

However, although the diet has been carefully based upon the raw-vegetable diet many people have used in recent times to cure themselves of cancer, it is useful for many other conditions. To do the diet justice and to understand fully the information Forbes supplies it is advisable to read this book, *The Bristol Diet* (1984).

Vitamin/mineral supplements

Many naturopathic therapists would recommend vitamin and mineral supplements to their patients, and many people buy these anyway because they feel that their diet lacks them. Generally speaking this is true, because it is virtually impossible for most of us to ensure that everything we eat is balanced, organically grown, sufficient in minerals and vitamins and totally free from additives. A second reason why supplements are an excellent idea is that they help to combat two of our major health enemies—(a) stress, and (b) pollution derived from the atmosphere, our diet, and other sources. The following starter programme is suggested by Earl Mindell as the foundation for general good health in his *Vitamin Bible*.

Take the following twice daily:

- a high-potency capsule or tablet of multiple vitamins with chelated minerals (time-release to be preferred)
- Vitamin C, 1,000 mg, with bioflavonoids, rutin, hersperidin and rose hips
- high-potency chelated multiple mineral tablet/capsule

He makes suggests the following daily regimen for a woman, aged 19–50:

- high-potency multiple vitamin and mineral capsule or tablet (time-release type if possible)
- Vitamin C, 1,000mg, with bioflavonoids
- Vitamin E, 400iu in dry form

   one of each of these with breakfast, and also with evening meal if necessary

- 3 RNA–DNA 100mg tablets
- 1 multipe digestive enzyme, when needed
- stress-B-complex, morning and evening, if stress conditions exist

For men in this age group Mindell suggests: the first four items as for a woman and

- 2 multiple minerals
- lecithin granules, 2tbsp or 9 capsules
- stress-B complex as for a woman.

Mindell emphasizes that his suggested regimens are not intended as medical advice and are not prescriptive. He is in favour of checking with a nutritionally orientated doctor or therapist before commencing a supplement programme unless the person concerned is in good health; and mentions special precautions with respect to supplement-programme modifications in the case of people suffering from thyroid disorders, diabetes, Parkinson's disease, blood clotting disorders, hypercalcaemia, heart disorders, high blood pressure, pernicious anaemia, hormone-related cancer, convulsions, glaucoma, peptic ulcers, impaired liver function, kidney disease and Wilson's disease, and for patients taking steroid drugs.

Hydrotherapy   This is a very complex subject, and so I will give only a few examples of the application of external hydrotherapy (internal applications include enemas, colonic irrigation and inhalation).

Cold applications initially constrict blood vessels and are useful for pain and inflammation. The secondary effect of cold-water application is dilation of the blood vessels (provided the application was brief); this increases the circulation to the area, bringing oxygen and nutrients and removing waste.

Prolonged cold applications have reflex effects due to stimulation of the sympathetic nerve ganglia in the vessel walls. An example is a prolonged cold footbath which causes contraction of the vessels of the womb and may help to counteract haemorrhage from this organ.

The primary effect of hot applications is excitation of the brain and nervous system; the secondary effect is depressant through reflex action. Prolonged application increases heat-production and may led to exhaustion either locally or generally. Benefits to be obtained include increase in the white-cell count and decrease in the red. Prolonged application over abdominal areas increases gastric and liver secretions. Raising the body-temperature includes the following benefits: anti-bacterial effect, antiviral effect, and stimulation of immune response.

Alternate hot and cold applications ('contrast bathing')—in particular a brief hot application followed by a shorter or equal cold one —have an excitatory effect. The overall effect is one of excitation with increased circulation to the area.

Finally the Moor bath and the Sitz bath must be mentioned. The first contains a peat extract and is said to be of value in chronic inflammatory pelvic and genital conditions, as well as in infertility caused by ovarian insufficiency. The overall success rate in treating the latter in a number of clinics is claimed to be as high as 47.5 per cent. Moor baths are also useful in rheumatic conditions.

The Sitz bath is one in which the patient sits immersed to the waist in hot or cold water while the feet are put in water of a contrasting temperature. Sitz baths are recommended as beneficial in cases of prolapse, gynaecological problems, piles and diverticulosis or diverticulitis. The warm water should be about 38°C and the cold about 16–22°C.

Cold-water wading was recommended during the 19th century by the famous Sebastian Kneipp for the treatment of depressive illness.

Fresh air and sunlight too are used for their therapeutic properties. Air baths are prescribed for disorders of the air passages and lungs, and ionized air (see page 447) is held to be beneficial to health. Sunlight and artificial radiant heat are used to cause sweating in the treatment of anaemia, rheumatic complaints, neuralgia and neurasthenia. Colour therapy is employed by some naturopaths, primarily for its calming effect (e.g. blue) or its stimulatory effect (i.e. red). Adequate exposure to natural, full-spectrum light is also encouraged, especially in patients who are obliged to spend part of their lives under artificial lighting.

Natural hygiene   This includes (a) general body-care; (b) the practice of moderate but regular physical exercise; (c) the cultivation of a positive approach to life, and (d) health, relaxation techniques, etc.

Before taking up aerobic exercise it is always advisable to start with a nondemanding type of movement that gradually reintroduces the body to the *feel* of deliberate exercise, stretches and improved posture; suitable types are yoga, dance therapy and T'ai chi, all of which are discussed later. Suitable relaxation techniques, also discussed later, are yoga and meditation, autogenic training, biofeedback and auto-hypnosis. When the patient is depressed and/or finds it very difficult to cultivate the essential positive attitude to life and health, referral to a psychotherapist might be made.

Structural adjustments   The naturopath seeks to balance and integrate the spine, muscles, ligaments, tendons and joints of the patient, and may choose referral to an osteopathic practitioner, a chiropractor, a teacher of the Alexander technique, a reflexologist, a practitioner of applied kinesiology/touch for health, or a masseur (for therapeutic massage). These specialities are discussed on pages 447–81.

Comment

Orthodox medical views are compatible with some of the naturopathic philosophy. The existence of the life-force is obvious; and the body clearly has self-healing powers (e.g. growth of new blood vessels to reroute blood circulation when a major vessel becomes blocked; mending of a fracture). Conventional doctors may not explain health as an abundance of the life-force principle in balanced harmony between biochemical functions, physical body structure, and psychology, but the sense of the holistic approach—the consideration of physical, mental and emotional/spiritual factors when diagnosing and treating disorders—is becoming more and more widely accepted.

Fasting is likely to be considered detrimental by many orthodox doctors. However, the benefits of the 'solid-juice fast' phase of Alec Forbes' Bristol diet are slowly becoming known. In addition, the Hay diet, the grape fast, vegetarianism, veganism and even macrobiotics have aroused their share of interest among conventional medical practitioners and have their supporters among them.

Little can be said against the principles of wholefood eating as recommended by naturopaths everywhere. Orthodox medicine is now aware of the vital part that food and drink play, for better or worse, in our health. The avoidance of large quantities of fat in the diet—especially of saturated fat—has been a basic dietary principle urged by naturopaths for many years.

Alternative diagnostic techniques

Space allows only a brief discussion of a selection of the alternative diagnostic techniques which a naturopathic doctor might use.

Constitutional assessment (biotypology)

The constitution, or biotype, provides a useful general guideline in the diagnosis of patients. The fundamental principle of recognizing the person's individuality is never overlooked; nevertheless, certain varieties of physical constitution can be related to proneness to certain types of disorder.

Patients' constitutions are classified as endomorphic, mesomorphic or ectomorphic according to body-build. Endomorphs tend to be plump, with softly rounded contours and big digestive organs. Mesomorphs tend to be heavy, with a rectangular outline due to bulky muscles, large bones and ample connective tissue. Ectomorphs are long and thin; they are often envied by mesomorphs and particularly by endomorphs as naturally slim individuals who can eat what they want and never gain weight. Their brain and central nervous system are also larger in relation to body-mass than is the case with the other types.

This approach, refined by Herbert M. Sheldon into a sophisticated system involving numerical scores and the classification of temperament,[103] tends to be used by naturopaths nowadays in its simplest form. They assess the physique category into which a patient fits, and use this as one of many reference factors in deciding the individual's most likely health hazards and nutritional requirements.

Iris diagnosis (iridology)

Iridology is concerned with the general appearance of the eyes and the detailed appearance of the coloured iris. Investigation may be carried out using just a torch and a magnifying glass or with the greater sophistication of custom-made photographic equipment, from which slides are made, the diagnosis being carried out by examining details on a well lit screen.

The theory that the iris inspection is useful for diagnostic purposes is about 100 years old; it arose independently from two workers, one Hungarian (Ignatz von Peczely) and the other Swedish (Nils Liljequist). Dr Bernard Jensen pioneered the art of iridology in the USA, and developed a comprehensive iris chart showing the representative areas within the iris of the various bodily organs.[104]

The irises are said to reveal not only the patient's present state of health (or vital reserve or energy state, as naturopaths express it) but also to provide information about past disorders and tendencies to develop future ones. The iris's colour and texture are believed to provide information about genetic tendencies and innate constitutional well-being. Other signs indicate degrees of 'toxic encumbrance' (i.e. the degree of toxic-material accumulation) or of inflammation, within the various organs and systems of the body. Generally, however, abnormalities in the iris's appearance indicate the type of pathological change that has occurred rather than its extent; and inherent weaknesses in certain organs rather than specific diagnoses as orthodox doctors recognize them. The basic concept of iridiagnosis is hard for orthodox doctors to credit; nevertheless, Lindemann has shown it to compare favourably with conventional methods in detecting intestinal problems, heart disorders and tuberculous lung infections, among other conditions.

Comment

Orthodox doctors include an inspection of the eyes in a full physical examination, and mentally note whether the patient's eyes are clear and bright or whether the whites are bloodshot, productive of discharge, or tinged with yellow, as in jaundice. The pupils too are examined for reflex activity in different intensities of light; and the patient's ability to focus and decipher large and small objects is noted.

Two important changes associated with the iris are recognized by conventional medicine. One is the 'arcus senilis', the outer white rim that appears around the periphery of the iris in elderly people. The other is the golden-brown or green Kayser Fleischer ring of deposited copper that appears around the perimeter of the iris in patients suffering from a rare metabolic disorder called Wilson's disease. It is unlikely that the concept of different areas of the iris corresponding to various areas and organs throughout the body would be acceptable to many orthodox doctors.

However, for some years the British School of Iridology has maintained a successful working relationship with a private medical practice in South Kensington, London, whose orthodox doctors may refer patients for iris diagnosis followed by treatment by natural methods. A fuller account of this successful cooperation can be read in the November 1985 issue of the *Journal of Alternative Medicine*.

Hair analysis   This procedure consists of obtaining 1g (2tbsp) of hair from the patient, preferably from the nape of the neck close to the skin; in the case of bald patients, body hair from other areas can be used. By means of a computer-controlled technique known as atomic-emission spectroscopy it is possible to assess the levels of 22 minerals present in the hair.

The development of this technique stems from the recognition that it is difficult to base assessments of mineral deficiency or excess upon symptoms, since imbalance produces such variable effects. Minute amounts of most minerals are required for optimum health, but modern food-processing techniques can cause a gradual deficiency of essential elements. Possible deficiencies include those of iron, magnesium, potassium, zinc, vanadium and selenium. Moreover, because our environment in the West is becoming increasing polluted with toxic substances, many of us may slowly accumulate undesirable minerals in our bodies without being aware of the fact: likely candidates are lead and, in some instances, copper.

Caution has to be exercised, though, against making inviting but invalid diagnostic conclusions. An unusually high level of calcium in the hair may mean not an excessive amount of calcium in the body but increased calcium excretion due to hormone imbalance. For this reason, interpretation of the results is carried out in the light of knowledge of present and recent dietary intake.

Ratios of one mineral to another are also taken into account. Zinc, for instance, may be within the range of normality but, if there is an accompanying raised level of copper (as often occurs premenstrually), a zinc supplement may be indicated.

Comment

The value of hair-mineral analysis as a diagnostic tool has its staunch supporters and severe critics among both alternative practitioners and orthodox doctors; certainly the interpretation of the results is still in its infancy. However, the examples of hair analysis' usefulness are impressive and will surely increase in number as more is learned about metabolism and the hair.

It is worth mentioning here that a high proportion of hyperactive children have been found to be zinc-deficient, and responsive to zinc treatment;[105] that in the USA, clinical trials have indicated that a raised level of copper in the body can be highly suggestive of increased tendency to coronary thrombosis;[106] and that certain types of dementia seem to be related to an excessive amount of aluminium within the body.[107]

Radionics

Radionics is a diagnostic and healing technique based upon the determination of a patient's energy patterns, utilizing a sample provided by the patient. The sample is usually hair, but saliva or a drop of blood from the fingertip are also acceptable. Here any comparison with either hair analysis or orthodox tests ends, however, because the testing performed upon the sample (or 'witness') by the radionic practitioner is in no sense biochemical. It is performed by a specially trained and very sensitive radionic therapist who tunes in to the vibrational state or rhythm of the patient by means of the 'witness' and a specially designed 'black box'. A complete picture of the patient's whole system, inherent strengths and weaknesses and vital reserve (present energy state) can be built up. The state of health ('vibrations') of individual systems, such as the kidneys, ureters and bladder or the digestive system, can be elicited, once the 'witness' has been obtained, simply by dialling the relevant number on the box's dial.

Radionics was the brainchild of Albert Abrams, an orthodox doctor and specialist in neurology born in San Francisco in 1863. The diagnostic techniques he described were investigated and accepted by the Royal Society of Medicine in 1924,[108] and the work was continued with further discoveries and advances in long-distance treatment and improved accuracy. It should be stressed, however, that some modern observers regard radionics as pseudoscientific; indeed its practice is banned in the USA.

Radionic diagnosis is particularly compatible with naturopathy because they share the same basic philosophy that equates health with harmonious and balanced life-force. Radionics is unlikely, though, to become widely accepted among orthodox medical doctors.

Medical astrology

An astrologer asked by a naturopath to shed further light upon the condition of a patient would first draw up the person's horoscope by drawing a birth chart, using details of the time, place and date of the person's birth. Each Sun Sign tends to be associated with a proneness to certain disorders (Scorpios, for example, tend to have problems with disorders of the reproductive organs), but a professional astrologer specializing in medical astrology would go a great deal further, making a detailed examination of the natal planetary positions in order to pinpoint which disorders ought particularly to be considered.

Astrology is regarded by many people the world over as a serious and complex science. Degree courses are available in astrology in the USA, and soon may become so in the UK also. At the same time it is still regarded by many people either as nonsense or as a wicked and superstitious practice. Astrology indicates trends, shows general patterns, and suggests the likelihood—even sometimes the extreme likelihood—of certain events, but it never purports to be predictive of actual occurrences, and any fairground astrologer making claims to the contrary should be dismissed as a liar.

Medical astrologers provide useful information by drawing the therapist's attention to an inner need, usually for the recognition and expression of some latent quality which needs integrating into conscious awareness. This is because they see disease as resulting mainly from inner conflict between our astrologically patterns tendencies, which prompt us towards a certain lifestyle and career, and the way of life, marital partner and job we often end up with.

Comment

Hippocrates believed that cosmic forces played a prominent role in the generation of physical and mental disorders. The connection between physical diseases and the movement and configuration of the planets at the time of a patient's birth ceased to be considered seriously after the Renaissance; all the same, people continued to believe in a definite connection between planetary aspects and mental illness.

Our word 'lunatic' comes from the belief that people's mental disorders grew worse at full moon; and there are still many people

443

(some of them doctors) who continue to believe in this association today: outbreaks in violent and criminal behaviour have been reported by some as coinciding almost invariably with the full moon.

The use of horoscopes as a diagnostic aid and treatment guide was pioneered by the Swiss psychologist and psychiatrist Carl Jung. The research of Michel Gauquelin (author of *The Cosmic Clocks* [1969]), a psychologist and statistician at Strasbourg's Psychophysiological Laboratory, has done much to establish faith in astrology as a valid art and science; attempts to disprove his findings are generally accepted to have emphasized their validity, and the famous and influencial psychologist Professor Hans Eysenck evaluated Gauquelin's work and found it to be valid.[109]

Palmistry

Research into palmistry as a serious dignostic tool had little effect until the general recognition that the palms of 75 per cent of Down's syndrome victims bear a 'simian crease'. Other palmar-line configurations connected with various disorders have since been discovered, and it is a mixture of this type of information and the intuitive power of the palmist that can prove of value as a diagnostic aid.

Palmistry is, however, unlikely to become a recognized orthodox diagnostic tool. Nevertheless, it is possible and even probable that further discoveries will be made in connection with the configuration of palmar creases and certain physical and mental disorders.

Kirlian photography

This is a photographic technique involving the generation of a high-frequency electromagnetic field which interacts with the energy field surrounding living things to produce light; in this way images can be created on photographic film. These appear as a coloured 'aura' surrounding the living object photographed, often a small area of a person, such as a hand or a fingertip, or the leaf of a plant.

There are three very interesting things about the images captured. Firstly, the 'aura' bears great similarity to the coloured light halo (or aura), which psychic individuals claim to see. Secondly, the Kirlian 'aura' bears witness to the naturopathic belief in life-force—a reduction in whose quality and quantity naturopaths look for in the presence of physical and non-physical disorders. Thirdly, the wave of life-force captured in Kirlian photographs dims as the subject loses strength and vitality, and regains a healthy brightness once health is restored.

Kirlian photography is usually said to have been discovered by accident in the 1950s by Russian electronic technician Semyon Kirlian; it is now thought that the phenomenon was first observed and demonstrated by a Russian engineer, Yakov Narkevich-Todko, in 1898. Enthusiasts of this technique claim that it can be used to detect both psychological and physical disorders before the onset of tangible symptoms. There are many sceptics of its applicability to diagnosis, among the criticisms being the variable results obtained and the establishment of parameters by which they may be interpreted.

The procedure consists of obtaining a photographic handprint, and it has been shown possible to get a repeatable result with the same subject, given the same conditions. Critical factors include the pressure on the photographic plate, temperature, air humidity, voltage waveform and consistency, duration and frequency of discharge, and consistency of the film.

Disturbances in the energy field are evident on film both when the subject is sick in some way and when he/she/it is developing a disorder without as yet showing symptoms. In the well known 'phantom-leaf' experiment an energy image of a whole leaf can be reproduced even though part of it has been cut away seconds before (although one worker has reported that she can achieve the phantom-leaf effect only once in every 100,000 experiments).[110] In fact, it is possible, by placing merely the central stem in the Kirlian device, to obtain the energy image of a whole cluster of leaves.

These dramatic effects are repeatable if much patience is exercised —and if *the plant has been organically grown*. Organically grown and raw foods show far higher energy levels than processed or cooked items.

Comment

A scientifically controlled study at the Charing Cross Hospital Medical School confirmed the existence of the human aura which can be viewed by Kirlian photography. Normally blue and even, with no marked breaks of spikiness[110] in healthy, calm people, it has been found to change colour and sometimes shape when the subject is depressed, excited or stressed, ill or developing a disorder, feeling emotionally stimulated, or taking alcohol or drugs. Besides these factors, the Charing Cross team found that the state of ionization of the air was also critical: if the atmosphere was positively charged, subjects' auras were greatly influenced. The main problem the team encountered was the impossibility of distinguishing the specific case of an abnormal aura by looking at the effects on film.

The trial director, Robin Williams, also pointed out that many people who buy Kirlian apparatus may not be aware of its dangers unless it is properly earthed, since enormous voltages (perhaps 35,000V) are involved.

Williams did not accept statements by some researchers that cancer tissue has a distinct energy form demonstrable at a very early stage. He believes the state of the aura is directly related to perspiration, which in turn is closely related to health, disease and emotion. There may also be a relationship between the aura and acupuncture points (see pages 463–4) because Kirlian photography does illustrate an energy field and the pictures repeatedly showed little dots in the position of acupuncture points.

Electrocrystal diagnosis   This is a very recently developed technique linked with electrocrystal therapy (see page 497). It was invented by a biologist, Harry Oldfield, who produced the equivalent of Kirlian energy-field photographs in a different form. He analysed the energy field (around living subjects) with which he was already familiar through Kirlian photography. He found that it contained electromagnetic components at both radio and audio frequencies as well as at those of light, thus permitting sound-sensitive devices to be substituted for photographic film in investigation of the human energy field. His apparatus, which works on a 9V battery, is used to generate an electromagnetic field in the human body. Like the stimulating device used in Kirlian photography, this field reacts with the natural human energy-field to produce a detectable—in this case audible—response.

Oldfield found that the whole energy field of each person responds to the stimulus of one basic frequency and its harmonics. The fundamental frequency differs from person to person, and is barely audible even to the subject whose surrounding energy field is radiating in every direction. It is an 'electromagnetic resonance—a fluctuation in the energy field rather than a physical movement'.[111]

While the patient holds an insulated transducer in one hand, the therapist scans the stimulated energy-field at various points on the patient's body with a sensitive probe, after first tuning the generator to a healthy control area such as the inner aspect of the elbow. This is done in order to obtain the peak response of that person's own particular resonance. The result is then translated into visible form as two green lines on the screen of an oscilloscope. One of these represents the energy being channelled into the body, and is more or less stationary; the other represents the energy which the body re-emits in a particular area, and therefore alters its shape according to the energy level of the area or

446

organ being scanned. Any area which is out of harmony with the whole organism and lacks vital force responds relatively less vigorously to the induced frequency.

Experienced and intuitive (users of this scanning technique are generally able to detect past and present weaknesses from the scan, and to foretell likely future health problems. Many GPs have been surprised and impressed by the accuracy of the diagnoses made in this way.

Certain energy patterns have now been associated with certain disorders. Orthodox doctors, as well as naturopaths and other practitioners interested in 'non-invasive' diagnostic techniques (i.e. ones not involving invading the interior of the body in any way), are using the technique themselves. Its diagnostic scope has led naturally to its therapeutic application, electrocrystal therapy (see page 497).

IONIZATION THERAPY

A naturopath may suggest this as an adjunct in the treatment of a large number of disorders. Ionization therapy is usually carried out in the patient's own home, and consists of the use of an electrical machine which gives the molecules of air in the atmosphere a negative electrical charge (i.e. 'ionizes' them).

Air is a mixture of gases, most of whose molecules are electrically neutral. Neutral air molecules and negatively charged ions are beneficial to those who breathe them. Conversely, a preponderance of positively charged ions or a shortage of negative ions has been proved harmful. Negative ions are destroyed by fumes, dust, cigarette and other types of smoke, and other forms of atmospheric pollution. Positive ones are actively created as an effect of central heating.

Deliberately increasing the supply of negative ions in the air has been found very helpful to patients suffering from respiratory disorders such as asthma, bronchitis, catarrh, sinusitis and hay fever. It also enhances the sense of energy and vitality of people accustomed to experiencing those conditions that upset the balance of useful air ions.

Comment

The results of controlled trials into the effects of ionization have contained two items of major importance from the point of view of orthodox medicine (and of holistic therapies): firstly, ionization therapy has no ill effects; secondly, the performance of subjects in standard tests was maintained at a high level when the volunteers were subjected to negative ionization (when exposed to a normal atmosphere

447

or to a positively charged one, their performance rose in the morning and the afternoon, and fell in the evening).[112]

There is every reason to hope that air ionization may become a standard adjunct to other types of orthodox therapy for appropriate patients in the future. Advertisements for ionizers for use in the home are frequently to be found in health magazines such as *Here's Health* and *New Health*.

BATES'S EYESIGHT TRAINING

Poor eyesight in people with basically healthy eyes is most commonly due to longsightedness (hypermetropia) or to shortsightedness (myopia).

Poor eyesight in the elderly should be particularly carefully checked in case either diabetic eye disease or glaucoma is the underlying cause. However, 'normal' ageing eyesight (presbyopia) is not associated with any underlying disease process. Glasses and contact lenses are usually prescribed by orthodox practitioners to overcome the problems of 'natural' visual defects, but naturopaths feel that these aids can in many cases be avoided. They prescribe a balanced diet and eye exercises based on those devised by Dr W. H. Bates, a US ophthalmology specialist working in the early part of this century. In 1919 he published his own alternative ideas and findings in a well known best seller, *Better Eyesight Without Glasses*, described for UK readers in 1929 in a book of the same name by Harry Benjamin.[113]

The Bates regimen attaches much importance to regular relaxation of the eye muscles, to proper lubrication through blinking, to hydro-therapeutic measures (e.g. splashing the eyes with water regularly), to specific focusing exercises, to the use of the visual imagination and memory, and to the repetition of a visual movement known as 'shifting'. Treatment sessions are usually frequent at first, as the aim is to establish a degree of improvement right from the start. Bates's eyesight training is offered by qualified practitioners who advertise in the press and Yellow Pages and in magazines such as *Here's Health* and *New Health*.

Comment

Even orthodox consultant ophthalmologists are ready to admit that the entire mystery of sight has yet to be totally unravelled. There is no definite proof that Bates's training techniques *cannot* produce great eyesight improvement in some people. Unfortunately, however, its possibilities tend to be ignored by orthodox practitioners.

BIOCHEMIC TISSUE SALTS

The possible link between diseases and an imbalance or deficiency of essential minerals was first propounded in the 1870s by Dr W. H. Schuessler, a German homoeopathic physician. The fundamental principles of his approach can be summed up as follows:

- the human body contains 12 essential mineral salts, which have to be in a correct state of balance for the healthy functioning of bodily cells, and therefore for the overall health of the body
- disturbance of this balance in any way causes illnesses to occur
- the normal balance of these tissue salts can be re-established by taking the appropriate mineral salts, known as the Schuessler Remedies

Schuessler termed his therapy 'biochemistry'. For obvious reasons, however, the adjective 'biochemical' is never used when referring to Schuessler's remedies, which are instead described as 'biochemic' tissue salts.

Naturopaths and other bolistic therapists often prescribe salts. They can be bought from pharmacists and healthfood stores, and are prepared in homoeopathic potencies. It is quite safe to buy and use them as a home remedy although, if you are receiving treatment from any type of practitioner—orthodox or holistic—it is best to seek his/her approval first.

Examples of the biochemic tissue salts and the disorders for which they are indicated include:

- *Calc. Fluor.* (fluoride of lime) gives elasticity to connective tissue —indicated where too much tissue 'stretch' has occurred (e.g. piles, ruptures, strained tendons). Suggestive symptoms include cold sores at the corners of the mouth; cracked tongue and lips; and a tendency to form fissures and skin cracks.
- *Calc. Phos.* (phosphate of lime) helps build new blood cells and to strengthen bones and teeth—indicated for poor circulation, wasting disorders, skin eruptions and in convalescence. Specific disorders for which it may be prescribed include iron-deficiency anaemia; fractured bones; decaying teeth; and slowness of teeth to appear in the growing child.
- *Kali. Mur.* (chloride of potash) aids metabolic processes—indicated for congested conditions such as those producing catarrh (e.g. asthma, bronchitis), a white or grey furred tongue (e.g. throat infections, tonsillitis, croup), or for certain types of jaundice.

449

Comment

There is no doubt that most of us lack certain natural and vital inorganic mineral salts; nor that many of the activities of our cells are dependent upon the correct balance of a variety of salts both inside them, in solution in the blood plasma, and in the tissue fluid bathing them. However, Schuessler probably went overboard in claiming that *all*—or even most—diseases are due specifically to tissue-salt imbalance, and in believing that all disorders are capable of correction by appropriate supplementation of these salts. Most orthodox doctors have consequently gone just as far in the other direction, attaching little or no credence to Schuessler's claims.

Regardless of these extremes of opinion, though, biochemic tissue salts either work or they do not. So far as I am aware, no actual research has been carried out into their efficacy, but many people claim to derive much benefit from them. Moreover, since homoeopathic remedies indubitably 'work', we need not be put off biochemic tissue salts solely because of the extremely low concentrations in which they are used. In short, salts in common biochemical use by our tissue cells may very well benefit them when administered as a form of treatment. The author of a definitive work on biochemic tissue salts[114] states that the administration of the Schuessler remedies should not necessarily be regarded as a full treatment for a disease or its symptoms, but rather as a part of the treatment in connection with 'such other measures as may be deemed necessary by the physician'.

HERBAL MEDICINE

The term 'herbal medicine' correctly refers to any form of medicine or medical treatment relying mainly upon the use of herbs; strictly, therefore, it includes both aromatherapy and Bach flower remedies. I have used the term in Part Two to denote the type of herbal medication you would expect to receive from a medical herbalist, or to obtain for yourself, either by gathering or buying the herbs and preparing them or by purchasing the commercially prepared product. In the discussion below aromatherapy and Bach flower remedies are treated separately (see pages 453 and 455).

A massive amount of traditional belief and folklore surrounds the origin of herbal medicine. Probably the best known herbalist of all time is Nicholas Culpeper, an apothecary with a special interest in the use of herbs who practised in London's East End 400 years ago. Culpeper was (and still is, to a certain extent) criticized for his conviction that there was a close relationship between astrology and the efficacy of herbal preparations. This is evident from the text of his most famous work, today known as *Culpeper's Herbal*, which is regarded as *the* English herbal.

Plants in their natural state are used by medical herbalists wherever possible, since it is thought that the plant as a whole organism is in perfect balance, and use of it offers both buffering action (counteracting possible unwanted effects) and synergistic action (enhancing the desired effects). Although herbal preparations are used both in the form of patent remedies and as herbal prescriptions for the removal of symptoms, professional herbalists do not regard this as their main function. Certainly, though, it is better for many patients to use a mild herbal tranquillizer for 'nerves' than a pharmacological synthetic compound such as diazepam (Valium), or to treat an upset stomach with, say, slippery elm rather than a standard antacid. That aside, true herbal medicine is, like naturopathy, regarded today as essentially holistic.

Because of its development from worldwide origins lost in prehistory, there is no fundamental philosophy from which herbal medicine can be said to have grown. Nevertheless, its theory can now claim as a foundation the recognition of vital force or life-force, with its self-healing ability. It is this ability to correct inner imbalance that herbal medicine sets out to encourage and bolster whenever the need arises.

Recent investigations of lunar cycles on plant growth, as discussed by Culpeper, together with interest in medical astrology and biorhythms, suggest that there is much hidden knowledge about the power of plants to be uncovered. Barbara Griggs, a well known medical herbalist, has pointed out how intricately Man and plants interrelate; and in many people's experience plants are sensitive to atmosphere in a home and to notice and affection. The energy fields of plants and humans are believed to interact to the mutual benefit of both organisms.

Consultation

When medical herbalists take a case history they ask about allergies, stress factors, diet, emotional life and associated harmony or tension, inner feelings of disturbance or tranquillity, exercise habits and past health record. They also examine the patient, taking urine samples, blood pressure, pulse and temperature, where appropriate. Their examination and the diagnostic aids used are similar to those utilized by a GP, but they may include also alternative diagnostic aids such as iridology or radionics. Diagnosis by a medical herbalist is less likely to

451

be expressed in the conventional manner—e.g. 'chronic bronchitis', 'spastic colon'—being more probably couched in terms of the pathological mechanism(s) involved—e.g. 'chronic inflammation', 'muscular spasm'.

Treatment

Herbal treatment is selected according to what aspect of health is considered to be most in need of support. The underlying cause ('primary lesion') is identified, wherever possible, and advice given on all those aspects of the patient's lifestyle the herbalist feels would profit from an overhaul. Wholefood diets are very likely to be recommended. The overall aim is sufficient correction of body functions for normal homoeostatic regulation to take over. Herbs are selected for their ability to encourage the return of such fully functioning homoeostasis. Stephen Fulder[115] mentions the following classification of the essential features of herbal remedies:

- Challenging qualities, which provoke protective responses from the body. For example, *Aloe vera* gel soothes inflamed skin and mucous membranes, diminishes pain and irritation and promotes healing. Others cause the kidneys to make more urine than usual (diuretic properties), or irritate the bowel lining to cause the bowels to move.
- Body-process directing qualities. For instance, hawthorn (*Crataegus oxyacantha*) increases the blood-flow in the coronary arteries and slows the heart rate, and is therefore very useful in cases of heart failure. Another example is ginseng root, which helps combat stress by improving the ability of the adrenal cortex to respond optimally.
- Eliminatory properties, which encourage the excretory activity of skin, liver, lungs, kidneys and large bowel, and the function of the circulatory system.

Comment

Although most pharmaceutical research has been aimed at exploiting plants as sources of (a) new compounds or (b) precursors for the synthesis of orthodox drugs, many practitioners—orthodox and herbalist alike—feel that a 'much broader picture of the total chemistry of the herbal plant' needs to be established. So wrote Dr William Court in a major feature on herbal medicine in the GPs' weekly newspaper *Pulse* (20 October, 1984). He suggested that clinical trials should be carried out, under controlled conditions and 'bearing in mind the holistic philosophy of herbal medicine', to establish both the safety and efficacy of herbal treatments. He stated that adequate standards of the quality of herbal products need to be established along the lines already laid down by some specialist companies. Users of herbal medicines need more and better advice, such as better labelling and improved education of retailers. Efficacy, safety, standardization and regulation of supply should all be considered as priorities for any future rational use.

The majority of medical herbalists would very likely agree with part—or all—of this opinion, but it has to be pointed out that carrying out the controlled trials envisaged by Court might prove very difficult. If the explanation for the curative effect of herbal medicine is the beneficial interaction of the life-force energy fields emanating from plant and Man (rather than the 'total chemistry of the herbal plant'), what exactly *can* clinical trials achieve which do not recognize the nature of the efficacy they set out to test?

Notes on preparation

Herbs can be prepared for self-administration in a number of ways —from a simple infusion or decoction to poultices and powerful enemas. The reader is directed to Maurice Messegué's *Health Secrets of Plants and Herbs* (1981), which provides a mine of extremely useful information on the gathering of individual herbs, instructions on all the methods of preparation, and many remedial recipes. Pure, organically grown herbs and plants are emphatically recommended. In the absence of specific instruction it is safe to modify quantities and to make more or less as you require, keeping the quantities in proportion.

AROMATHERAPY

'Aromatherapy' was once the term applied to stimulation of our sense of smell to produce a healing effect. The name was first used 60 years ago to describe the medicinal use of essential plant oils as stimulants. Although a few references show that something of this type of therapy was known to the ancient Greeks, it was not until some 400 years ago that essential oils were seriously employed to treat illnesses. We have to thank for this two Germans, Conrad Gesner and Hieronymus Braubschweig, who independently wrote books on 'distillation' which referred to the healing properties of essential oils. Since then, essential oils have been used to treat a very wide range of disorders, in much the same way as have other herbal preparations.[116] Two Frenchmen, René Maurice Gattefosse, author of *Aromatherapy* (1928), and Dr Jean Valnet, who wrote a book of the same title in 1964, are very largely responsible for the revival of the art that has occurred during the last few decades. About 1,500 French doctors have taken a 2–3 year post-graduate training course in phytotherapy (another name for the medicinal use of plants) in which aromatherapy figures as a significant subject.[116] Of particular interest to French aromatherapists is the utilization of the striking bactericidal properties of essential oils which may one day seriously challenge the use of antibiotics since, besides their efficacy, the plant oils are free from side-effects.

Diseases which have been treated successfully with essential oils are mentioned in Valnet's book *The Practice of Aromatherapy* they include various types of cancer, tuberculosis, diabetes, urinary- and gall-stones, anaemia, osteitis (inflammation of the bone) and gangrenous appendicitis.

About 200 essential oils are extracted on a commercial basis.[116] Of these about 60 have well known curative properties; they are the ones commonly used by aromatherapists. Of the remaining 140, 40 are unlikely to be of interest, 50 are being researched, and 50 are merely variations on other oils (e.g. spike lavender and true lavender).

Consultation

A full case history is taken, including details of stress factors, personal habits such as smoking and alcohol consumption, and past medical history. Present problems are asked about. The therapist thus gains a notion of the underlying cause and ideas for appropriate treatment.

Some aromatherapists may ask for a 'tally'; this may be a lock of hair or even a piece of paper bearing the patient's handwriting. The therapist would place this 'tally' in the centre of a dowsing disc and dowse with a pendulum to find (a) the most appropriate oil for the patient concerned, and then (b) the best form of applicaton.

Treatment

The oils may be bathed in, injected, inhaled, and/or given as compresses, douches and enemas. The commonest routes of administration, though, are by mouth and through the skin. Taken orally, the oil is usually excreted in the urine. Dosage has remained more or less constant since the time of Gesner and usually consists of 1–10 drops. Modern aromatherapy textbooks recommend 2–4 drops for all essential oils, three times a day after food. The oils do not usually taste very nice, so it is best to add the drops to 30ml warm water with 1tsp honey, or to drop them straight onto a little brown sugar.

When correctly used for a massage the oils are always diluted. The best strength of the solution is 2.5 per cent, which equals one drop of essential oil for every 2ml vegetable oil (thus a 50ml bottle of vegetable oil should have 25 drops of essential oil added to it). The therapist massages a large area of skin in the appropriate body region.

Comment

Robert Tisserand[116] has added that the basic difference between herbs and plant essences is the 'ethereal nature of oils', their very volatile constituents which give them 'a profound effect on the mental/emotional level, an effect comparable to the Bach flower remedies'. As this effect can be even more profound than the action upon the body, 'aromatherapy lends itself to a holistic mind/body approach which goes beyond normal practice'. Clary sage, for instance, helps lighten the mood in depressive illness; and aromatherapy is especially suited to the treatment of psychosomatic and stress-related disorders.

It must be mentioned that taking the oils orally is discouraged by some practitioners: they claim the membranous linings of the digestive tract are too sensitive, and stress that some oils should not be taken with certain drugs. However, Valnet prescribes them by mouth, and Tisserand defended the practice in a letter to the *Journal of Alternative Medicine* (June 1984); he said that, using the standard LD_{50} test by which oral preparations are judged, *all* essential oils come into the two groups 'safe' (90 per cent), and 'marginal' (10 per cent). (The other possible groups are 'toxic' and 'very toxic'.)

Tisserand is preparing an *Essential Oil Safety Data Manual* with the support of doctors and pharmacists and the interest of the DHSS. It will list all the known hazards of oils used in aromatherapy. Among them are those involving the skin—e.g. dermal toxicity, skin sensitization and phototoxicity. Such hazards involve only a very small group of oils, but should be known about as these oils are dangerous, even diluted, if used for skin massage.

BACH FLOWER REMEDIES

This system of treatment uses 38 remedies, 37 of which are derived from wild flowers and one of which—Rock Water—is pure water collected from a rocky stream. It was invented by Dr Edward Bach. His view of disease was that it resulted from disturbance of the mind and emotions, and that therapy should properly be directed towards the inner causative conflict, not towards the outward physical signs of disease. For several years he practised as an orthodox physician, holding posts at University College, London, and at the School of Immunology. However, he became distressed at the many defects he saw in orthodox diagnosis and treatment, and in March 1919 accepted the post of pathologist and bacteriologist at the London Homoeopathic Hospital.

The homoeopathic principle defined by Hahnemann (see page 457), of treating the patient and not the disease and of using natural substances to effect a cure, impressed Edward Bach profoundly. He directed his attention to studying patients' personalities rather than their list of symptoms, and combined this knowledge with his extreme sensitivity to the natural properties of plants, of which he had an intuitive knowledge.

The techniques he invented rely on capturing the essential energy concentrated within the flowers, just as drops of rain or dew absorb the properties of the flower petals to which they cling when irradiated by the rays of the sun. Bach made up his remedies in the same way, preparing them naturally by reliance upon the four 'elements' Air, Earth, Fire and Water. Freshly picked flowers were placed on the surface of a glass bowl of (natural) water and left in the sun for three hours, the energy released into the water from the petals by the action of the sun being the 'stock' from which the diluted product was made up. An equal volume of brandy was added to preserve the stock and to keep it clear; then it was bottled. [117]

The healing properties of these remedies is explained in terms of Bach's conviction that emotional and personality problems are the basic cause of disease, and the relationship of the latter with the powers of nature. Orthodox drugs often relieve symptoms but they do not remedy the underlying mental and emotional disturbance that Bach felt should, rather than the symptoms, indicate the type of remedy required. He believed that this emotional disharmony and instability was best cured by the subtle energy given off by plants.

Consultation

Far more attention will be paid to your inner feelings, conflicts and emotional problems than to your physical disorder. You will be encouraged to talk about your hopes, fears, anxiety or depression as freely as you can, and to recognize and face up to feelings you may have kept hidden from your conscious awareness.

Treatment

You will be prescribed the appropriate re dies and advised how to take them. Much application of Bach flow remedies is in the form of self-help, though, and you can either make the remedies yourself or obtain them from the Dr Edward Bach Centre (see Appendix for address). Treatment can be obtained at the centre, as can detailed books on the therapy. The remedies are available singly or as a complete set of 38, or made up as a greaseless ointment with a homoeopathic base.

If you do make them up personally, prepare the 'stock' as described above, and then dilute this by adding five drops of the liquid to every 30ml of pure water you use. Finally bottle this. The remedies are usually drunk, the dose being five drops in 1tbsp of water, 2–3 times daily, or more often if the need is felt (they are absolutely harmless). They can also be used as a lotion, compress or fomentation, or added to a bath.

Children, young babies, animals and even plants can benefit from treatment. To dose plants, place two drops of each remedy you choose in a bottle.[118] Use about 5ml (1tsp) of the mixture to 5 litres of water, and make a spray to go round the root of the plant.

Comment

It seems that the problem Edward Bach left for his followers to overcome after his death (1936) was the aura of mysticism with which he had enshrouded the explanation of his treatment. He spoke of the plants having the power to 'elevate our vibration' and draw down spiritual power, cleansing mind and body and healing. This may well be the case; but vague and mystical explanations do little to further the general acceptance of a relatively new therapy. All the same, there is no reason to suppose that the therapy might not be highly effective in a number of people. Many people already accept that herbs exert their healing power by an interaction between their energy fields and ours. Bach's approach may be seen as an extrapolation of this.

HOMOEOPATHY

Homoeopathy is a system of medicine based upon the principle of treating 'like with like'. This means that the medication chosen for a particular patient would, if given in large quantities, produce the very symptoms of which he or she is complaining.

Homoeopathy was founded by Dr Samuel Hahnemann, an 18th-century German physician and chemist. In common with naturopathic belief, Hahnemann recognized the error of orthodox medicine which, in so many instances, treats symptoms only. Current European medical practice was, in fact, favouring some particularly harsh, not to say distressing, forms of treatment—e.g. bleeding, purging and the use of potent sedatives and stimulants. Surgical operations were still being performed without the benefit of anaesthetic or, for that matter, hygiene.

Hahnemann was convinced of the body's ability to heal itself, and—again like naturopaths—regarded the symptoms of disease as evidence of the body's self-curing activities. In the later editions of his world-famous book, *Organon of Rational Healing* (1810) he spoke of the body's 'vital force', which he saw as responsible for the body's natural healing processes. A further parallel with naturopathic philosophy may be seen in his conviction that disease resulted from the vital force becoming imbalanced, and that the function of treatment was the restoration of balanced harmony.

He adopted a holistic approach which placed the whole individual patient under the powerful lens of diagnostic scrutiny. He sought a system of treatment designed to enhance the body's innate self-restorative efforts, instead of merely dampening them. He experimented with a wide range of natural remedies derived from animal, vegetable, mineral and sometimes biological substances, and in so doing he rediscovered the 'like cures like' effect known to the ancient world. The analogy has been made (for its explanatory value only!) between homoeopathy and vaccination. Vaccination of a small dose of, say, tetanus toxoid will cause the body's immune system to form specific antibodies against further chance encounters with the real thing. Similarly, homoeopathic medication stimulates the body, mobilizing more of its innate healing capacity, and thus effecting improvement and frequently a cure. And Hahnemann soon discovered that, the smaller the dose, the more potent the effect.

In preparing the medicines, 'mother tinctures'—crude alcoholic extracts of the plant or other material used—are made and repeatedly diluted a hundredfold. The first hundredth dilution of the mother tincture is termed 1C; the second (2C) is a hundredth dilution of the 1C preparation. This dilution process is called 'trituration'. The preparation is then shaken vigorously by hand or machine many times over. This was essential to the 'potentizing' of the remedy, in Hahnemann's view, and is still a vital part of the preparation of homoeopathic remedies.

Understanding how diluting a remedy can possibly increase its potency has proved a major problem for orthodox doctors and others investigating homoeopathy. In fact, precisely how the remedies work is not known; but theories place much emphasis upon the molecular energy of the active compounds, which is built up during the grinding and shaking stages of preparation. What is finally given to the patient is a very low concentration of the substance in a state of high energy.[119] This then stimulates the body as mentioned above.

Consultation

The first consultation is likely to be lengthy (an hour or longer). To the homoeopath it is vital to see the whole person within the context of his or her personal environment, and to be aware of stress factors, habits, feelings and personality type. Details of possible interest to the homoeopath might include patients' like or dislike of milk, their reaction to heat or cold, their liking or fear of the dark, and whether they are placid and calm in the face of danger, or inclined to panic.

Treatment

When enough is known about the patient and the symptoms have been considered, the homoeopathic doctor can then use his skill in matching the patient to a specific medicine. This is chosen on the grounds that it makes people *of that particular type* feel as the patient is presently feeling. Thus, influenza occurring in three different patients (one a self-opinionated young man of literary bent and histrionic disposition, with small, red eyes; the next a 50kg hazel-eyed fair-haired woman of timid temperament and creative disposition who quickly becomes discouraged; and the third a year-old toddler with red hair and a dreamy disposition) would be treated with three quite different remedies. Similarly, the same remedy might be used for very different indications (e.g.: shingles; restlessness at night, accompanied by great apprehension; and excessive thirst, with a dry mouth and throat—all *Rhus toxicodendron*), provided certain factors within the patients corresponded to this remedy choice.

Some homoeopathic practitioners are also orthodox doctors (in 1983 there were about 550 such doctors in the UK). Besides holding medical degrees they are also members of the Faculty of Homoeopathy, which keeps a register of qualified practitioners. They can be consulted under the NHS, and can issue NHS prescriptions for homoeopathic remedies. There are also five homoeopathic hospitals in the UK, where patients receive both homoeopathic and orthodox treatment.

There are also lay practitioners, most of whom study part-time with the Society of Homoeopaths. Lists of qualified lay homoeopaths can be obtained from this society, from the Hahnemann Society, or from the British Homoeopathic Association.

Self-help is also possible, but it is essential to follow package instructions carefully and to consult a homoeopathic practitioner if symptoms prove worrying or persistent.

Comment

The Blackie Foundation is an independent medical charity set up 14 years ago by Margery Blackie, the Queen's late physician, in response to the growing call for scientific evidence of homoeopathy's benefits. It is currently involved in an extensive research programme, one of its main aims being the establishment of a structured laboratory system to ensure that any findings can be reproduced.

Recent work has included the investigation of lead homoeopathic preparations to help clear the body of accumulations of this toxic metal; extremely dilute homoeopathic preparations have been used. Other metals to be similarly investigated have included copper, zinc and aluminium.[120]

Other biological, chemical and physical experiments suggest that, despite the lack of detectable substances in homoeopathic remedies, specific physical changes may occur in the solvent which might have important therapeutic effects. Early work by Paterson and Boyd found that the Schick test for diphtheria was changed from positive to negative by the oral administration of alum-precipitated toxoid in a dilution of 10^{-x}, or with *Diphtherium* (a homoeopathic preparation of throat swabs from diphtheria patients) in a dilution of 10^{-x}.

Recent research has shown that potencies of arsenic (7C, 9C and 15C) caused elimination from rats that had been artificially poisoned with this element. Injections of alloxan (9C) have been shown to reverse the tendency of large doses of the same substance to produce diabetes in rats. And—also in rats—phosphorus (7C and 15C) appeared to reverse the toxic liver damage caused by carbon tetrachloride (a dry-cleaning agent) when compared with control animals.

Boiron and Luu-Dang-Vinh at the Faculty of Pharmacy, Montpellier University, demonstrated by means of a Raman laser that substances with homoeopathic potency (even when no material substance was apparently present) had specific molecular cluster arrangements within the solvent, and specific stereophysical deformations in the alcohol itself. These physical changes can be destroyed experimentally by ultrasound, by irradiation and/or by high temperatures (120°C).[120]

A useful booklet published by the Homoeopathic Development Foundation, *Homoeopathy for the Family*, often on sale in healthfood shops, gives comprehensive instructions with respect to self-treatment. For more serious conditions it is strongly recommended that a qualified homoeopathic physician be consulted.

ACUPUNCTURE

Acupuncture is a technique of stimulating points on the surface of the body by inserting needles, applying heat (moxibustion), applying fingertip pressure (acupressure), or a combination of these. Modern innovations include the use of electromagnetic fields, polarized light and low-power lasers.

It is one of the oldest forms of treatment, and dates back to at least 2697BC when the Father of Acupuncture—Huan Ti—became Emperor of China. Together with his physician Ch'i Po, Huan Ti worked out the principles of anatomy and health on which the theory and practice of acupuncture are based. The result was a book on the subject, *Nei Ching* (*The Yellow Emperor's Classic of Internal Medicine*). Acupuncture was unknown in Europe until the 17th century, when stories of it were brought back by missionaries returning from China. Little notice was then taken, however, and it was not until the late 1950s that the general public became aware of the art (although it had been practised in the UK for years by a few Chinese experts for Chinese patients). Then a number of alternative therapists learned as much about the subject as they could and began to practise it. By the 1960s, acupuncture had started to flourish.[121]

According to its underlying philosophy, acupuncture works by harmonizing the vital force or energy. This energy the Chinese call *Ch'i*, imbalance of which they regard as the cause of both physical and mental disease. *Ch'i* is regarded as running along invisible lines (meridians) within the body. Its course along these meridians is satisfactory and unimpeded when a person is in a state of balance (i.e. healthy). When, however, the two great opposing yet complementary principles—Yin and Yang—become unbalanced within a person the inner harmonious rhythms of biological, mental and spiritual function are upset. *Ch'i* ceases to flow freely along the meridians, and the effects of imbalance become apparent (i.e. symptoms of illness become noticeable).

Yin and Yang are essential elements in all traditional Eastern philosophy (see page 434). They are polar opposites, present in all things, and evidence of them is everywhere apparent to the practised eye. Obvious examples of their manifestation include heaven and earth, male and female, night and day, heat and cold, activity and passivity, and dryness and wetness. Within the healthy body, degrees of Yin-ness and Yang-ness are forever varying slightly: they are in a fluctuating yet balanced state, like a trapeze artist walking along a tightrope. A false step, though, will cause the tightrope walker to topple to one side in such a way that his previous balance cannot be regained and he falls to the ground. Equilibrium has been lost and balance upset; this is analogous to the acupuncturist's view of disease. The art (and the objective) of the acupuncturist is to diagnose the cause of the imbalance and to restore harmony and health. This he or she does by unblocking clogged-up meridian channels, and releasing *Ch'i* to flow freely once more.

Acupuncture also links man with the rhythms of nature and the universe. This, and the Yin and Yang aspects of the main body organs, together with the elements with which they are associated, comprise a complex aspect of oriental acupuncture philosophy. An acupuncturist considers all such interactions when assessing a patient and deciding upon treatment. 59 meridians are recognized, and about 1,000 acupuncture points.[122] These points are specific points along the meridian channels at which stimuli of the types mentioned above will have maximum effect.

Acupuncture is unlikely to be effective in conditions where irreversible tissue damage has taken place but, where tissues and organs (and the emotions) can be improved, it is likely to be helpful. Many diseases have been mentioned in this connection; the following list is taken from Dr George Lewith's book *Acupuncture* (1982): sprains, fractures (after the bones have been set), osteoarthritis, rheumatoid arthritis (in its chronic stage), headaches, migraine attacks, recovery period following a stroke, trigeminal neuralgia, and the neuralgia which can follow shingles. Other responsive conditions mentioned by Dr Lewith include: certain psychological disorders including depression and anxiety, and *possibly* schizophrenia; certain varieties of nerve paralysis; hiatus-hernia symptoms and stress-related indigestion; peptic ulcers; possibly gall-stones and piles; bowel infections; possibly Crohn's disease and ulcerative colitis; bronchitis and asthma; angina and some cases of irregular heart rhythm; hypertension; obesity (especially when due to a strong desire to eat much of the time) and drug-addiction (including smoking and addiction to hard drugs). Acupuncture can also be used as a reliable form of anaesthesia.*

* Where acupuncture is mentioned in Parts One and Two as a possible source of relief or cure for disorders which are not included in the above list, it has been mentioned in such contexts in other literature.

Consultation

The first consultation may last for an hour or more. The therapist is likely to be interested in the history of the present disorder, past disorders, medical history of both parents, stress factors and lifestyle. He or she will note also the condition of the nails; the skin colour; the nature of the voice; the state of the tongue, eyes, breathing, posture and emotions; and the patient's body odour.

Diagnosis is based on five colours and five smells. Examination of the pulses is also a very important and highly developed art in acupuncture practice: there are six of these to be felt in each wrist, one for each of the 12 main meridians, and each associated with a vital organ. Each of these 12 pulses is purported to have one of 24 different qualities. By feeling the pulses in turn, the acupuncturist will be able to establish which meridians are blocked (thus preventing the free flow of *Ch'i*) and whether Yin or Yang is in excess.

Treatment

The acupuncture points are located by touch or with an instrument that measures the Chinese 'inch', which is in fact different for each patient. The sterile needles (usually 2–6) are then inserted and left in place for about 20–30 minutes. They may be left undisturbed, rotated or pumped up and down to stimulate the point. (Alternatively, a low-frequency electric current may be used for the stimulation.)

When more reinforcement is needed, 'moxibustion' is performed. Usually needles are inserted and a small cone of moxa (dried mugwort) is placed around the head of each needle; the patient's skin is protected from falling ash by small card discs. The moxa is ignited and this generates enough heat down the needle for a pleasant warmth to be felt. This technique helps to clear the meridian channels, and to reinforce the flow of *Ch'i*.

The number of acupuncture treatments depends upon both the nature of the disorder and the patient's responsiveness. A common number is six, but one is sometimes sufficient and 24 or more may be needed for slowly responding conditions. The immediate effect of an acupuncture treatment is often described as one of great exhilaration. Other people say they feel very sleepy.

Acupuncture is available under the NHS. Many GPs have trained, and there are also hospital departments which offer it. The British Medical Acupuncture Society has a list of doctors who have trained in acupuncture, but lay practitioners may well be easier and quicker to find. Registers of qualified acupuncturists can be obtained for a small fee from one of the colleges that train them, such as the British Acupuncture Association or the British College of Acupuncture.

Comment

Acupuncture points have been identified by electrical properties rather than as discrete anatomical features. They have a high voltage relative to surrounding skin. Over 4,000 loci with the electrical properties of acupuncture points have been found on the body surface. The traditional 1,000 points have been found to correspond to a subset of these loci, which can be located with appropriate electrical apparatus. Meridians have also been located by their identifiable electrical properties.[123]

Orthodox doctors have found further verification of the existence of meridians, in that unrelated problems may respond to a single treatment, or a treatment may cause quite remote side-effects, the relationship becoming evident only when the meridian pathways are considered. For example, the removal of a knee cartilage can cause stomach problems because the operation-scar cuts across the stomach meridian.

Many profound physiological and biochemical changes are now known to be induced by acupuncture, the most widely known being that of the release of hormone-like chemicals called endorphins. These have a multiplicity of functions, two important ones being the relief of pain and—in certain circumstances—the elevation of mood from depression to optimism.

Auricular acupuncture

The external ear offers a complete set of acupuncture points corresponding to various parts of the body. The most enduring results from acupuncture treatment are said to be achieved by using body and ear points in combination.[123] The ear (auricular) points can be detected as areas of low resistance, but only when a disorder is present; they are not found in healthy subjects. Auricular acupuncture is the first choice of acupuncture treatment for acute conditions. Many orthodox doctors who accept acupuncture reject auricular acupuncture.

Acupressure and Shiatsu

The art of stimulating your acupressure points to give yourself relief from certain disorders may be learned either from an acupuncturist or from a book. *Shiatsu* was once the Japanese form of Chinese acupressure, but today it incorporates a number of aspects of other therapies, especially massage and applied kinesiology/touch for health (see pages 472 and 475). In the West *Shiatsu* has become practically indistinguishable from Acupressure. A good book on acupressure is *Acupressure Techniques* (1978) by Dr Hans Ewald.

MANIPULATIVE AND POSTURAL THERAPIES

Physiotherapy is prescribed every day by orthodox doctors for a wide variety of disorders affecting the muscles, bones, tendons and nerves, and is regarded as an essential aspect of conventional medicine. Other forms of manipulation are gradually gaining acceptance, however, especially osteopathy, chiropractic and massage. Reflexology is becoming accepted very much more slowly.

Alternative therapies based upon manipulation and postural correction are regarded by practitioners as affecting the patient in three possible ways: the physical consequences of the treatment; the psychological impact; and the mobilization of the life-force or vital energy.

REFLEXOLOGY

Reflexology (known also as 'zone therapy' and 'compression massage') is a system of diagnosis and treatment carried out by exploring the feet (sometimes fingers and occasionally tongue) of the patient and then massaging relevant areas of them. It is probable that the ancient civilizations of China and Egypt used a form of curative foot massage; and similar approaches to disorders are noted in primitive cultures today.

Reflexology has its modern origin in the USA in the present century, when Dr W. Fitzgerald and his colleagues discovered in the 1920s that the human body is subdividable into energy zones corresponding with sensitive areas on the feet. This knowledge was developed into a type of therapy in the USA by Eunice D. Ingham, who was responsible also for mapping out exactly where the various parts of the body are represented on the feet. Finally an English nurse, Doreen E. Bayley, studied under Eunice Ingham while visiting the USA and set up the Bayley School of Reflexology when she returned to the UK, where it became established during the 1960s.

The theory upon which reflexology rests states that 10 invisible energy channels run from all over the body to the feet, and that disorders are due to blockages of one or more of these channels. The various energy terminals in each foot are examined, and the blocked channels identified. Appropriate foot massage of these 'reflex areas' can then be carried out to unblock the obstruction and allow the energy to run freely. This constitutes a return to health.

How reflexology works is not yet understood. However, reflexologists claim that the massage manipulates the body's intricate stimulus-response system, and that its effects are mediated by electrical impulses triggered by pressure on the foot. It is said to be able to improve almost any disorder. It is not, though, a magical panacea for all ills, and does not aim only at the relief of symptoms. Reflexology is holistic in its approach, because it tones and harmonizes the energy flow throughout the entire body, resulting in greater vitality and well-being.

Particularly susceptible to the curative effects of reflexology are said to be back pain, hay fever, migraine, sinusitis, some kidney and heart disorders, high blood pressure, hiccups, hot flushes, asthma and arthritis.

Consultation

A case history is normally taken, although some therapists prefer to diagnose 'feet first' and do not require details of health disorders before making their exploration. In addition to generalized tenderness in either or both feet, which often occurs when the patient's overall health is bad, the reflexologist feels for small, grainy, crystalline deposits below the skin in the various reflex areas. Their presence is diagnostic of blocked energy channels and poor circulation of the vital energy; they also indicate the reflex areas in which stimulation is required.

Treatment

Tender areas are compressed and grainy deposits gently but firmly broken down by the massaging action of the therapist. To start with, the therapist may well induce the patient to relax by gently rotating the feet round and round, clockwise and then counter-clockwise, and then repeating the circular motion with the big toes. The feet are then worked upon, starting always with the left foot, partly because the main vessel of the lymphatic system (the thoracic duct) is stimulated by this action to release toxic residues. Once the deposits have been broken down they are believed to be absorbed by the body and disposed of in sweat or urine.

The massage may be very gentle, or deep and very strong, causing some discomfort, even momentarily severe pain. This type of pain is often described as 'unpleasant but nice'.

Major factors in the production of blocked energy channels are inner tension and anxiety, anger and other negative emotions.

Comment

The concept of every part of the body having a representative area on the foot is on the surface incompatible with established anatomical and physiological fact. Few orthodox doctors appear to take reflexology seriously—yet acupuncture was ridiculed for years before conventional medicine found means of satisfying itself that acupuncture points and meridians exist.

OSTEOPATHY

Osteopathy is a form of joint manipulation which corrects and maintains the functioning of the body's framework. It began as the discovery and invention of Andrew Taylor Still, an American, at the end of the last century. Still became increasingly disillusioned with the shortcomings of current medical practice and found that he could cure certain disorders by manipulation. One of his first patients was a child affected by dysentery, a disease which at the time claimed many lives.

Still felt that understanding the structure of the body in relationship to its use was the only viable foundation for the understanding of disorders. He grew to believe that good health depends upon the unhampered, normal functioning of the spinal column, and that disorders largely originate when part of it is misaligned. He explained this by pointing out that the spinal column encloses the spinal cord, which is affected when part of the bony cage around it is displaced in some way. The spinal cord, in turn, works in close association with the autonomic nervous system, responsible for much of the regulation of our bodily functions. Hence Still formulated the idea—and began the practice—of firstly identifying the trouble spot within the spinal vertebrae, and then correcting the vertebral malposition by manipulation. This, he maintained, freed the body's built-in self-regulating mechanism to put whatever disorder was present to rights. In addition, he defined the three basic precepts of osteopathic theory:

- the body is capable of healing itself
- good health is the result of structural integrity
- disease essentially stems from misaligned structure[124]

467

Still also described the 'osteopathic lesion'. The existence of such lesions has been called into question mainly because no actual vertebral displacement is necessarily implied by the term. In fact the lesions represent unbalanced tension and strain in and around the spine and its muscles, resulting in confused nervous impulses reaching the spinal cord. Alternatively, an osteopathic lesion may be due to oversensitivity of the spinal nerves which in turn affect joints, ligaments and muscles, and the blood vessels associated with the organs and tissues supplied by these irritable nerves.[125]

Osteopathy is, like naturopathy and most other alternative therapies, holistic: it sees patients very much as individuals with different weaknesses, strengths, needs and capabilities. It treats the patient, not the disorder, setting out to restore harmony to the whole organism, physically, mentally and spiritually through both physical manipulation and lifestyle counselling.

Consultation

The osteopath takes a full case history, including details of the present symptoms, and past illnesses and injuries. He is likely to enquire about stress factors (emotional and physical), lifestyle, habits and the amount and type of exercise taken. The physical examination which follows includes tests of muscle, joint and nerve function. Posture and breathing are noted. Signs of abnormal function and of degenerative disease are looked for, and blood and urine tests may also be required.

Osteopaths are trained to develop a high degree of sensitivity in their fingers, and they can sometimes detect changes in the texture of body tissues that fail to show up on X-ray. This method of examination is called palpation, and it includes exploration of muscles, ligaments, tendons, fascia (type of connective tissue) and joints.

Treatment

Osteopath's decide upon treatment once they have decided what constitutes for that particular patient the optimum in harmony and balance, to what degree he or she is off-centre, and what factor or factors are preventing his or her homoeostatic mechanism from re-establishing order. The type of manipulative treatment employed may be very gentle or firmly thrusting, depending upon the wide variety of factors that go to make up both a patient's constitution and his or her requirements. The 'high velocity thrust' many people associate with osteopathic treatment is normally painless, if dramatic, although the breaking down of 'adhesions' can be uncomfortable.

The patient will be advised about the type of exercise to take, postural corrections to make, and other lifestyle changes that promise to be beneficial.

Comment

It has been reported that in the UK some 77,000 new patients consult a registered osteopath (RO) every year, 52 per cent of whom are complaining of lower-back pain; this is not surprising when one considers that every working day 88,000 people are off work with backache!

A report in the *Journal of Alternative Medicine* in May 1985 described six months of weekly osteopathy helping to transform a brain-damaged child of five. The orthodox diagnosis was one of 'slight brain damage or mild cerebral palsy', and the effects were speech difficulty and inability to run or to step up a pavement kerb. Her family took Sian to the British School of Osteopathy's Children's Clinic, which has a record of helping similarly affected children, and she was treated by gentle manipulation to relieve the tensions caused by early stress. At the time the report was made, the child could 'run, jump, sing and chatter!'.

Other disorders, besides back problems, which respond well to osteopathy include rheumatism, arthritis, migraine, tension, headaches, bronchitis and menstrual problems. Also helped in some cases are allergies, constipation, cystitis, varicose veins, infertility, impotence, non-anginal chest pains ('false angina'), and the symptoms of hiatus hernia.

Cranial osteopathy

Cranial osteopathy is an additional osteopathic technique used by many osteopaths as a supplement to their more usual methods. It was developed by an osteopath, William Sutherland, before the turn of the century, and its aim is to diagnose and treat disorders through exploring the rhythmical pulsation of the cerebrospinal fluid. This fluid is contained within the hollow cavities of the brain and within the connective tissue protecting the spinal cord, which it bathes.

Cranial osteopathy is a very gentle technique, and depends upon both sensitivity in the fingers and a degree of intuition. The rhythmic flow can be picked up by a skilled practitioner on the skull and in the region of the pelvis. Slight pressure changes can be made by means of the hands, resulting in benefit in a variety of disorders, including epilepsy, Ménière's disease, deafness, migraine, fractious small babies who have had a difficult birth, and some cases of autism. Visual disturbances and tinnitus consequent upon a head injury can also be helped in some instances.[126]

CHIROPRACTIC

This therapy is defined by the British Chiropractors' Association as 'an independent branch of medicine specializing in the diagnosis and treatment of mechanical disorders of the joints, particularly those of the spine, and their effects on the nervous system'. Like osteopathy, chiropractic developed in the West around the turn of the century, being founded in 1895 by an American, David D. Palmer. The clinical case which caused him to consider the possible benefits of manipulation was one of deafness. A janitor in the building where Palmer worked had been deaf for years after bending over awkwardly and feeling something 'give' in his back. Palmer located the spot, and replaced the misaligned vertebra, thus restoring the man's hearing. Palmer spent the rest of his life researching and working for the recognition of the therapy that grew from this result.

The chief differences between chiropractic and osteopathy are now said to be mainly academic. Chiropractors are more apt to use X-rays then are osteopaths, and the latter use more soft-tissue techniques (manipulation of the soft skeletal structures) and more joint mobilization. A further point[127] is that time-honoured osteopathic manipulation uses more leverage, therapeutic force being applied some distance from the target joint. Chiropractic manipulation relies less on the mechanics of leverage and is likely, for example, to be applied to two adjacent vertebrae, and use a quick pushing movement to alter their relevant position.

Chiropractic theory sees vital energy or the life-force in terms of a Universal Intelligence which directs the self-correcting mechanisms present to some degree in all living things. Within Man this occurs *via* the central nervous system and the spinal and cranial nerves. Even minute displacement of the vertebrae which enclose and protect the spinal cord is capable of compromising the function of a nerve, with the result that the organ or body area it supplies will be adversely affected.

Like osteopaths, chiropractors regard the body as potentially self-healing. They see their task as that of freeing trapped nervous tissue, thereby enabling the Universal Intelligence to carry out its self-corrective functions.

Chiropractic theory places emphasis upon the nerves and the organs they supply, while osteopathic theory concentrates ultimately upon the blood vessels and circulation. Some osteopaths and chiropractors claim that these theories are of historical interest only while others maintain their traditional beliefs.

Consultation and treatment

The chiropractor takes a full case history, including details of present disorder, past disorders and injuries, stresses and lifestyle, including amounts and type of exercise taken, occupation and recreation. This is followed by a physical examination, with particular attention being paid to posture, to discover any indications among the vertebrae of dislocated or subluxed (i.e. minimally dislocated) joints or of misalignments. Having examined the patient's posture the therapist tests reflexes, passively moves and rotates joints, and assesses tissue tone. Two diagnostic instruments may then be introduced—the neurocalometer and neurocalograph—which identify small variations in temperature on corresponding sides of the spinal column indicative of spinal-nerve inflammation. Finally, X-rays will be taken.

In addition to the kind of manipulative movements already described, the chiropractor will advise the patient about weight-reduction, suitable exercise, perhaps about diet and almost certainly about posture, gait, lifestyle modification and relaxation methods.

Comment

About half the patients visiting a chiropractor want treatment for a back disorder. Other conditions which this therapy is able to treat include neck pain, headaches, sciatica and other leg pains, hip and knee problems, shoulder and arm pain, pins and needles and 'odd sensations' in the limbs, and pains and stiffness in the ankles, feet and elbows. Migraine, catarrh, the pain of sinusitis, digestive problems, menstrual disorders and constipation may also be helped.

With respect to research, more is now being done in this field. Stephen Fulder[128] writes that one medical study of specific chiropractic manipulation versus other orthodox medical treatment was carried out and reported in the *Lancet*. Comparable groups of patients with back problems were treated by doctors and by chiropractors. Results showed that chiropractors were somewhat better at restoring function than were orthodox physicians; also, they saw their patients more frequently and over a shorter period than did the doctors.

The *Journal of Alternative Medicine* reported in February 1984 that chiropractic and osteopathy were breaking through into mainstream medicine in a research project being undertaken with the cooperation of the orthodox medical services. The British Chiropractors' Association had completed a two-year feasibility study funded by the Medical Research Council, and this was likely to lead to bigger things.

To find a qualified chiropractor, write to the British Chiropractors' Association, who will send a register of association members on receipt of a 9 × 6 SAE. The letters DC after a practitioner's name mean Doctor of Chiropractic.

REMEDIAL MASSAGE

Remedial massage is less of an independent therapy than a useful adjunct to other varieties of healing, both conventional and alternative. Massage as such—except where it is included in physiotherapy—is not available under the NHS, yet most orthodox doctors would readily agree about its therapeutic value.

In contrast to osteopathy and chiropractic, which are primarily concerned with spinal and other joints, the beneficial effects of remedial massage are directed towards the soft tissues of the body, such as the muscles, ligaments and tendons. It is useful in rehabilitation following war wounds, sports and exercise injuries, and strokes; and can be used with equal success either to stimulate or to relax the subject.

Consultation

The therapist discusses the purpose of the massage with the patient, and will often enquire about recent or present illnesses, exercise, recreative and sporting activities, when these are relevant.

Treatment

Masseurs often own a special massage table, although some prefer to work on the floor (rarely on an ordinary bed or sofa, because these do not provide sufficient support). Four main movements are used.

- Effleurage is frequently used to start with as it consists of a stroking motion which, when performed gently, relaxes the superficial muscles. Oil is often used, and the technique may be combined with aromatherapy by the inclusion of an essential oil. In this way the patient both inhales the essence of the plant and absorbs its therapeutic properties through the skin. If effleurage is performed energetically it has an invigorating effect.

- Pettrisage, in which the soft tissues are kneaded like dough with the object of relaxing knotted tense muscles, helps also to stretch contracted tissues.
- Friction, small, circular movements against the bone, using a reasonable amount of pressure, is aimed at the deeper tissues to relax muscular tension spots.
- Tapotement involves stimulatory movements which improve muscular tone and strength.[129]

Massage is not generally considered suitable for patients with: acute inflammation (e.g. the acute stage of rheumatoid arthritis) or fever, although it can be very useful during the recovery or ensuing chronic stages; serious heart disease (e.g. congestive cardiac failure, or just after a coronary thrombosis); thrombosis, including thrombophlebitis and phlebothrombosis, where an embolus might be set free into the circulation; or severe skin rashes, both infective and non-infective. In most other cases, especially those involving a considerable element of stress, remedial massage is very beneficial. The City and Guilds Institute keeps a list of approved colleges offering courses in both beauty therapy and massage, if you wish to check on qualifications and training.

Comment

Massage is an holistic form of treatment in that patients usually benefit physically, mentally and spiritually. The first type of benefit is obvious. Many patients speak of an improved sense of well-being, which includes better mental alertness and greater energy. Spiritual benefits are likely to result from the use of aromatherapeutic oils, just as they do from colour, art and music therapies (see page 493). They may also result from the psychophysical rapport that often develops between the patient and a skilled and sympathetic therapist.

THE ALEXANDER PRINCIPLE

The Alexander principle is a form of educational therapy aimed at improving a patient's overall mental and physical well-being by the improvement of his or her posture. The therapy originated when an Australian dramatic actor, F. M. Alexander (b.1869), investigated the reasons for his loss of voice during stage performances. He discovered that he had the habit of tossing his head back in an unconscious effort to throw his voice to the back of his audience. This compressed his vocal cords, and reduced the timbre of his voice. Simply trying to counteract

473

the effect by pushing his head forwards had a similar effect, and the problem was only overcome by his standing and walking about in as natural a manner as possible.

He eventually overcame his natural tendency to revert to the old, bad habit by consciously correcting his overall posture, without strain and tension, and permitting his head and neck to assume their natural position. He passed on what he had learned firstly to other actors, about both voice improvement and the general health improvement which he attributed to the new, correct use he was making of his body as a whole and integrated organism.

At the turn of the century, he left Australia and taught the principles he had formulated in both the USA and the UK. Firstly, although he agreed with the importance which osteopathy and chiropractic attach to a correctly aligned spine, Alexander attributed faulty vertebral positioning to habitual misuse of our bodies rather than to any fault inherent in structure. This misuse consists of adopting physical positions while sitting, running, standing or lying down which our bodies were never constructed to adopt. As inevitably happens when misuse becomes chronic, overall functioning is adversely affected.

Secondly, Alexander believed that long-term misuse affects a person's overall well-being, including, besides the obvious physical aspects, both mental and spiritual factors.[130]

Consultation

A teacher of the Alexander principle will take a case history from the patient, and note past and present complaints, illnesses and past injuries. Much attention will be paid during the consultation to posture, signs of stress and attention, timbre of voice, unconscious mannerisms, signs of a stiff and awkward gait, and overall appearance of health or lack of it.

Treatment

Treatment consists of a series of lessons in the Alexander principle, the number relating to the seriousness of the underlying disorders and to the response of the patient. The object is to train the patient to relinquish old habits which—*because* they are habits—'feel right', and, gradually, to adopt better postural habits. Common bad habits include slouching, slumping in chairs, sitting at a factory bench, office desk or work table in a chair of the wrong shape and height, and tensing muscle groups unnecessarily.

Patients may be asked to visualize how they would be standing were they in perfect health and very physically fit; and to adopt the habit of constant correction, bearing this ideal model in mind. This, with sufficient persistence, eventually breaks old habits and replaces them with new ones, thus renewing the efficiency of the whole body.

The approach is unarguably a holistic one, as the benefits aimed at—and usually achieved—are physical, psychological and spiritual.

Typical patients requiring Alexander technique lessons include those with health problems (often, of course, musculoskeletal) which orthodox practitioners have treated unsuccessfully. Some are people feeling below par without knowing exactly the reason. Other conditions known to have responded to Alexander-principle training include hypertension, spastic colon, asthma, trigeminal neuralgia, osteoarthritis, frequent headaches and persistent lassitude.

Comment

Dr Wilfred Barlow, who studied the Alexander technique, collaborated with Professor J. M. Tanner of the Institute of Child Health to investigate the effects of the training on a group of 50 music students. They compared these students' postures over a nine-month period with that of a group of matched drama students given routine gymnastic training and admonishments to correct particular faults. Dr Barlow found that 'the figures showed a marked postural improvement in the Alexander group and a deterioration in the other group'.[130]

APPLIED KINESIOLOGY—TOUCH FOR HEALTH

Applied Kinesiology (AK) is a form of diagnosis and healing based on human touch, used not for massaging or correcting joing misalignments but for stimulating the body's flagging energy or life-force. AK practitioners believe that various forms of muscular weakness occur prior to the symptoms of a disorder actually appearing; and that what may appear to be muscular tension in, for instance, one group of muscles, may in fact be weakness in the counterbalancing muscle group.

AK originated in 1965 from the findings of a Detroit chiropractor, Dr George Goodheart, who discovered that standard tests for muscle strength and tone which he performed routinely on his patients reflected also the energy state of inner organs such as the heart, bowel, kidneys and bladder. He saw a functional connection between specific muscle groups and the energy pathways represented by acupuncture meridians, and developed a system of diagnostic and curative techniques based on both chiropractic and acupressure.

One of his pupils, Brian Butler, subsequently brought Touch for Health to the UK. In this technique, lay members of the public are taught the basic principles of AK so that they can utilize it for themselves as a preventive measure against future disorders.[131]

Goodheart developed diagnostic techniques for identifying joint malfunction, lesions of the spine, disorders of the organs within, psychological effects on the function of the body as a whole, nutritional needs and allergies. Treatment is carried out by activating appropriate muscles in such a way that muscle balance is restored and the flow of energy throughout the entire body revitalized.

Consultation

A therapist would take a case history including details of the present disorder, and observe posture and muscle tone in great detail. Any areas of asymmetry would be noted, as would be instances of muscular weakness and tension. Disorders are viewed as malfunctioning energy pathways, and the appropriate muscle groups would be tested with this in mind. Questions would very probably concern diet and any known food allergies.

Treatment

All the noted abnormalities of tone, strength and symmetry are corrected wherever possible, for the aim is not simply to relieve a particular set of symptoms but to restore balance to the entire person. The muscular testing is usually carried out with the patient lying or sitting down, the therapist examining first one side of the body and then the other. A group of muscles is initially tested, and then individual component muscles examined in turn for weakness.

The precise location of the muscular weakness shows which organs are disordered, and can demonstrate the presence of food allergy (see below). Muscular imbalance is corrected (and normal organ and system function restored) by the use of touch and pressure on appropriate points, sometimes in combination with chiropractic manoeuvres.

Some chiropractors practise AK. More information about Touch for Health can be obtained from the Touch for Health Foundation.

Comment

A report by the Chairman of the Research Committee of the International College of AK (ICAK), Arizona, in April 1985 presented the

476

findings of some of the most recent research, backed by properly controlled clinical trials involving hundreds of people over several years.[132] Muscle testing has been found a reliable means of detecting food allergies, and can indicate specific problem substances in affected patients. Even 'hidden stressors' (foods that do not appear to affect muscle strength adversely) can now be identified by a new test which patients can be taught to perform for themselves.

Other tests are now available to show lymphatic congestion, and easy methods have been devised to relieve poor circulation in both left and right lymphatic ducts, with subsequent improvement in conditions such as lumpy breast tissue and hyperactivity. AK has also been used with benefit in dyslexia.

EXERCISE AND MOVEMENT THERAPIES

There is no doubt about our need for regular exercise. Directly related to what has been called our 'hypokinetic' lifestyle (i.e. one characterized by too little movement) are obesity, heart disease, hardening of the arteries, varicose veins, piles, osteoporosis, osteoarthritis, fibrositis, muscular rheumatism and chronic low-back pain. Much is currently being written in the popular press and in specialist journals about the musculoskeletal, metabolic and psychological benefits of becoming more active—often with particular emphasis upon the advantages of aerobic activity.

These advantages are numerous. But it is foolish to attempt to take up any type of strenuous activity when physically very unfit: strained tendons, torn muscles and worsened backache are among the milder problems that might ensue. It is vital to help our bodies adapt to the greater demands we intend to make upon them. An excellent way of accomplishing this is to take up a form of 'exercise therapy' which you can practise in your own home whenever you wish to. These therapeutic exercises reaccustom the body *gradually* to the feeling of exertion; and are highly beneficial, too, in a number of disorders.

YOGA

Yoga can greatly benefit both mind and body. Meditation is an inseparable part of most forms of yoga, but here we are largely concerned with the exercise aspect (Hatha yoga). (Meditation is treated separately on page 488.)

Yoga is a valuable movement therapy with remarkable physical, mental and spiritual benefits. It is believed to have originated more than 4,000 years BC in India and, according to its age-old philosophy, its objective is the uniting of the 'self' with higher consciousness through the harmonizing of body, mind and spirit. In the UK, although it had been studied by some as a curiosity, interest in yoga was not really established until the 1960s. During the 1970s yoga groups started to spread,[133] many of them emphasizing the physical appeal of yoga practice and steering away from the spiritual and mystical aspects.

Most yoga teachers will emphasize that the basic aim of yoga is to bring into balance and harmony both mind and body: good, or greatly improved, health naturally follows this achievement. Yoga exercise improves both posture and breathing; this benefits the circulation and the body's intake and utilization of oxygen. An additional bonus is an increase in the rate and efficiency with which waste materials are excreted from the body. The nervous and hormonal systems also function better. Yoga is also an excellent means of regaining lost flexibility and muscle tone, and of reintroducing the habits of stretching and bending after, perhaps, years of a sedentary way of life.

Form of exercise

Unlike aerobic workout classes and dance-therapy sessions, music is very unlikely to be played during the yoga exercise class. The object is to bring the mind and body into harmony with one another, and concentration is needed to achieve this.

In beginner classes the simplest exercises ('postures' or 'asanas') are taught. A popular one to start off with, since practically every pupil is capable of it, is the Corpse asana. (All asanas have Indian names, and most now have English equivalents. The name is suggestive of the shape your body takes in achieving it; e.g. the Coil, the Cobra, the Plough.) The Corpse is simplest of all because it consists of merely lying flat on your back, arms and hands by your sides, and legs straight out in front, parted slightly at the ankles. This position is usually chosen for beginning and ending a session, as it stills the mind and helps focus the attention as you start and, at the end, the few minutes spent in the Corpse position give you a chance to relax fully before finally concentrating again upon everyday affairs.

All the asanas are assumed slowly and smoothly, without rush or strain. Each is maintained for a few minutes (or however long is comfortable) and then gently released and followed by a brief spell of relaxation before the next asana is taken up. At all times you will be reminded of the importance of concentration and very likely shown how to breathe slowly, regularly and deeply in a manner that coordinates with the type of asana being used. (There are also specific yoga breathing techniques which are taught as independent exercises; e.g. 'alternate nostril breathing'.)

Most of the asanas are better demonstrated than described. Some are bound to be uncomfortable at first, but it is surprising how quickly many plump, unfit stiff-jointed people become competent. A yoga instruction manual written 1,300 years ago states that an asana has been perfectly learned when there is no longer any effort expended in achieving it.

Comment

Interest in the therapeutic benefits of yoga is now worldwide, and considerable research has been—and is being—carried out into its effects. It has been found, for example, that carrying out the Headstand asana reduces the inhalation of oxygen by 10 per cent and increases the blood's utilization of oxygen by 33 per cent.[134] Yoga is also especially beneficial in stress-related complaints such as peptic ulceration, spastic colon, hypertension, asthma and chronic backache.

Yoga is often included among the subjects offered by evening-class institutes.

T'AI CHI (T'AI CHI CHUAN)

This is a system of exercise consisting essentially of smoothly flowing circular movements performed in a prescribed sequence. It is Chinese in origin, and is thought to have been developed centuries ago from the martial arts. It was probably designed to help convalescent patients regain their strength, and is still recommended for this purpose. It is also practised as a form of preventive health care, since 20 minutes of T'ai chi daily over a period of years 'can prolong youthful vigor and rejuvenate the body'.[135]

Form of exercise

T'ai chi exercises every part of the body, yet is highly conservative of energy expenditure since no motion is superfluous. The 108 basic movements are carried out in a slow, calm manner in one of two possible sequences—one containing over 100 postures and the other 30–40. Although this sounds quite demanding, pupils rarely complain of fatigue during or after a session; they are more likely to feel they have *more* energy after than before! One of T'ai chi's most appealing features is that it is equally suitable for practice by the fittest and the least fit.

The movements are carried out ritualistically, each having symbolic significance and bearing a title (such as Golden Cock Stands on One Leg). The body-weight is frequently shifted from one leg to another, and carrying out the smooth, flowing actions has been described as 'feeling as though you were moving in water'. It is equally popular with children; Ruth West and Brian Inglis mention in their discussion of T'ai chi[136] that it may indeed have been developed in Taoist institutions as a game for children, to keep them occupied.

The emphasis in T'ai chi is upon developing a balanced harmony within the self, first of all at a physical level and then psychologically and spiritually. In teaching the harmonious use of the muscles, joints and tendons, it enhances the individual's inner vitality (*Ch'i*, as in acupuncture), and then trains him or her to expend some of this stored energy in a therapeutic and controlled fashion.

Comment

T'ai chi is a form of exercise that imposes no stress upon the heart, and for this reason is recommended by many heart specialists. Its particular benefits for sufferers from heart disorders, hypertension, coronary arterial disease and similar conditions is that it provides much-needed exercise safely, and increases their feeling of vitality and well-being. It also has a tranquillizing effect upon the mind and emotions, and is excellent for people who become stressed very easily. It is therefore an obvious choice for people with type-A personalities (see pages 242–3).

DANCE THERAPY

Dance therapy has two main healing aspects. Firstly, it exercises the body, improving posture, muscle control, and—when aerobic—heart and lung function. Secondly, it releases repressed inner tensions and conflicts in people afflicted by mental and emotional problems, thereby bringing these into conscious awareness and reducing their harmful influence.

Many examples of the curative use of dance exist in history and in diverse cultures today. Often chanting has been or is an essential element, as when groups of primitive people dance together to achieve a mutual aim or to encourage a witch doctor's patient to dance to the point of collapse and unconsciousness (which gives healing spirits the chance to enter the patient's body and cure it). And there is no doubt that when music is used, as it is in some types of dance therapy today, it exerts a strong effect on mind and emotions: this effect can be tranquillizing or provocative of violent activity.

Form of exercise

The object of dance therapy is to put people in touch with their emotions by getting them to express themselves through bodily movement. This translates these emotions into something more tangible than 'just thoughts', and makes people face and deal with inner turmoil. Individual needs are, therefore, of prime importance, and classes are usually small enough for each person's problems to be dealt with adequately. Most teachers begin with limbering-up exercises, and many choose to group their students in a ring as this—plus the act of holding hands—increases the awareness of being part of a whole and of communicating at a physical level.

The participants' natural rhythm is brought out by getting them to move as they feel they want to, attention being paid to the use of all parts of the body in turn so that the physical benefits are total. In some classes suggestions are made to the group such as 'jump up and down as you dance along' or 'curl up in a tight ball on the floor when the music next stops'. These ideas will often be elaborated in a natural way by individuals to express inner repressed desires—such as jumping up and down with anxiety or rage, or assuming the foetal position.

Comment

Dance therapy is a good way of getting rid of stress reactions and inner tension and, like yoga, can be very beneficial to people wishing to take up exercise again after years of inactivity. It can be very helpful in neurotic illnesses, especially depression, where withdrawal of 'self' from contact with the surrounding environment can be partly countered by both rousing music and physical movement. Dance therapy is also used beneficially with groups of mentally retarded children and adolescents, including those suffering from Down's syndrome; with autistic children, in whom, among other things, it helps to develop body awareness; with institutionalized people who have lost much of their sense of identity through being in a mental hospital for many years; and in individuals recouping from strokes, long illnesses, accidents, major operations and nervous breakdowns.[137]

Therapies of the Mind

The following therapies are directed primarily at relieving mental and emotional disorders. However, since the body, mind and soul are indivisible parts of an integral whole, effective treatment of mental problems almost inevitably results in an increased sense of physical well-being and improved 'spirits'. This is true whether the meaning of 'spirits' is taken at its most mundane or its most mystical.

PSYCHOTHERAPY

Psychotherapy began in earnest with Sigmund Freud. When he explored his patients' minds under hypnotic trance he discovered that reliving a traumatic experience which their conscious minds had 'forgotten about' (i.e. repressed) in many cases cured their neurotic illnesses (see pages 403–6). Later Freud evolved a method of bringing repressed experiences into his patients' conscious without the use of hypnosis. He found that encouraging patients to recognize their own underlying problems partly by their own efforts was often more effective in the long run. The method he employed, psychoanalysis, is used extensively to this day.

Both orthodox psychiatrists and lay psychotherapists practise psychoanalysis and the type of psychotherapy often associated with it (i.e. that based largely upon Freudian principles). Both are situated on the sometimes indistinct dividing line between orthodox and alternative medicine, and, as with a number of such therapies, orthodox doctors feel that only they should be permitted to practise the art. However, under the NHS full-scale psychoanalysis, which is very time-consuming, is practically nonexistent, and psychotherapy has only limited availability and, even when available, is often inadequately so.

Provided, therefore, that properly trained therapists are consulted there is every reason why 'lay' psychotherapists and hypnotherapists should be permitted to see and treat patients. There is every reason, too, why many overworked GPs and psychiatrists should feel grateful to them for the workload they take on and the need they fulfil.

Method of treatment

There is no prescribed timespan for psychoanalysis: some people undergo it for years. Several sessions per week are usually considered necessary, and patients who can afford it often opt for five per week.

The patient sits or lies comfortably on a couch (with the analyst sitting behind his or her head, just out of sight) and is asked to say whatever comes into his or her mind for an hour at a time.

The analyst interprets what the patient says in the light of both the principles of psychoanalytic psychology and the symptoms present. The whole session is conducted in a comfortable, relatively informal and relaxed way, since this encourages patients to 'regress' more easily to a previous stage in their life and to recollect earlier forgotten experiences, and for a therapeutic rapport to be struck between therapist and patient.

'Analytic psychotherapy' is the term now used[138] to describe the commonest modification of psychoanalysis, in which the sessions are reduced in number to three, two or one weekly.

For either type of analysis, to be therapeutic, patients must have some insight into their own problems. This means they must recognize that these come at least partly from within and that they may need to rethink entrenched attitudes and to modify their attitude in a number of ways.

Patients are helped gradually to do this by the therapist's interpretations and comments, and by the slowly growing awareness of the different levels of their experience of themselves and others. They come to see the extent to which past experiences continue to influence the present,[139] to recognize unconscious wishes and fears, and to understand the defences they have built within themselves against the pain all these can cause.

Communication may be very difficult for patients, especially at first. They may also find the reliving of past experiences and the necessity of coming face to face with the 'devil within' (their own psychopathology) extremely painful and perhaps humiliating. They also have to think hard about the sessions between appointments, and to work out new, better ways of dealing with threats and opportunities.

In this way, symptoms can be cured through patients gaining a more comprehensive and conflict-free experience of themselves and their relationships 'by deepening and extending his contact with alienated parts of himself, and so furthering his individual development. Both [classical psychoanalysis and analytic psychotherapy] involve a mutual exploration of the patient's problems within the developing relationship with the therapist.'[140]

Comment

The existence of psychosomatic illnesses and the growing awareness of the role of the mind and emotions in the generation of 'physical' disorders mean that the potential need for psychotherapy in one form or another is very great. Further details can be obtained from the British Association of Psychotherapists, the British Psycho-analytical Society, and the Association of Child Psychotherapists.

HYPNOTHERAPY

Hypnotherapy is the application of psychotherapy using the hypnotic trance as a valuable adjunct. Hypnotism still has a 'strange' image in some people's minds, but doctors are making increasing use of it, both by practising the art themselves and by referring suitable patients to 'lay' hypnotherapists. Some dentists use hypnosis instead of pain-killing injections.

Method of treatment

Hypnotherapy has two major applications: it can be used (a) to facilitate analysis ('hypnoanalysis') or (b) to enable therapeutic suggestions about the patient's underlying problem to reach the unconscious.

During the first consultation a complete case history is taken by the hypnotherapist, with particular reference to neurotic symptoms, length of time they have caused trouble, past medical history, etc. From this, the hypnotherapist will be able to assess whether he or she will be able to help the patient. The attitude of the patient towards hypnotherapy is then explored, as is his or her real desire to get well. The need for hard work on the patient's behalf is underlined, as many expect it to work miracles without effort on their behalf.

At this point the therapist would decide whether to use hypnotism for the purpose of analysis (if the neurotic problem seems complex and long-standing) or whether suggestion under hypnosis is likely to be the better choice. Whatever the course of treatment, the plan is sketched out to the patient, and—when possible—an idea is given of the possible length of the course of treatment. Normally, patients attend once a week—sometimes twice—for an hour: 3–4 sessions are usually enough to cure a habit such as smoking, provided no deep neurotic reasons underlie the habit, but for deep-seated depression or anxiety 20–30 sessions may be required.

The procedure is explained to the patient, and his or her suggestibility (ease with which he or she is likely to enter a trance) is tested. Hypnosis may or may not be used during the first session. Some patients are disappointed if it is not; but in those who have not experienced hypnotic trance before the trance induced on a first occasion will probably be very light.

484

Trance is induced by a wide variety of methods, the main feature being the distraction of the patient's attention while the therapist makes the suggestion that the patient is becoming more and more relaxed. The trance state itself is *not* a state of sleep—deep or otherwise: it has more in common with that state of drowsy semi-awareness one is in while waking up or going to sleep. The patient remains aware of the therapist's voice, and can generally remember afterwards everything that occurred while he or she was in trance.

The hypnotic trance cannot be used to get the patient to do anything that is contrary to his or her normal moral code; this is one of the fears patients have of hypnosis. Post-hypnotic suggestions *are* of course planted—e.g. acute anxiety can be gradually replaced with healthy feeling by the repeated effect of therapeutic post-hypnotic suggestion. However, few hypnotherapists are content nowadays merely to relieve troublesome symptoms without establishing why they came about in the first place. Simply suppressing symptoms by suggestion under hypnotic trance is unsatisfactory, and likely to prove of temporary benefit only. Much of the average hypnotherapist's time, therefore, is spent in counselling patients about their problems and in discussion of how these arose, with a view to establishing the real source and nature of the symptoms.

Comment

Certain patients are unsuitable for treatment by hypnotherapy. In particular, patients suffering from psychotic illnesses (manic-depressive psychosis, schizophrenia) must not be treated this way. It can prove very useful, however, in the treatment of nearly all forms of neurotic illness; in the removal of unwanted habits, such as nail-biting, overeating, smoking and the tendency to drink too much; and in reinforcing a patient's self-esteem. Hypnotherapy is also very useful in treating stress-related problems such as hypertension, migraine, spastic colon, bed-wetting, stammering, nervous tics and insomnia.

Further details and lists of practising hypnotherapists can be obtained by writing or telephoning the National Council of Psychotherapists.

Other types of psychological therapy deserve mention here, although space does not permit their being dealt with in detail.

Behaviour therapy is based upon conditioning the individual in such a way that desired behavioural responses are inculcated, very much as the production of saliva by 'conditioned reflex' was produced in dogs by Ivan Pavlov, upon whose work the theory of behaviourism rests.[141]

Behaviourists see neurotic illness as conditioned reflexes which can be unlearned. Simple examples of the application of behaviour therapy include the treatment of phobias by getting the patient gradually used to experiencing the object of the phobia; and aversion therapy for alcoholics, in whom the drug disulfiram (Antabuse) causes violent vomiting when alcohol is taken (this treatment is controversial).

Humanistic psychology is really a collective name for a number of psychological therapies, most of whose names are widely known. They include Rogerian therapy, transactional analysis, primal therapy (rebirthing) and gestalt therapy, and are derived eclectically from a number of traditional sources, including Jung and Freud. They help people not only to get rid of symptoms of neurotic illness but also to realize their full potential as complete human beings, physically, mentally and spiritually. They use nonverbal techniques rather than verbal ones. As a group they developed a great deal of strength during the 1960s' 'growth movement'.[142]

More can be learned about individual forms of humanistic psychology by contacting the Association for Humanistic Psychology in Britain.

RELAXATION METHODS

One of the most valuable features of relaxation methods is that they can be practised at home—and in some cases learned there as well.

Nowadays, when stress factors take such a heavy toll of our health, means of relaxing do in fact have to be learned. Many people believe that they know how to relax, and think that they are doing so simply because they sit down in front of the television for an hour or so each evening. But for real relaxation to take place, it is vital to 'switch off' our five senses so that we receive—for a prescribed interval each day—as *little sensory stimulation as possible*. For a short time, in fact, we can actually 'hear ourselves think'; adapt to the rhythms of the silent yet immensely potent life force within; and hopefully, with practice, transcend self-awareness and the *need* to think at all.

The most suitable setting for practising daily relaxation, is a quiet, comfortably warm, dimly lit room, containing an easy chair and no telephone.

There are several relaxation methods which are commonly prescribed. Each has its own variations and techniques, but all have much in common. All advocate setting aside a short time (perhaps 15 minutes to an hour) on a regular basis.

486

AUTOHYPNOSIS

The surest, safest way to learn autohypnosis (self-hypnosis) is from a qualified hypnotherapist. Tapes and books can teach the basic principles, but hypnotic trance does not suit everybody, and in certain individuals can be very traumatic. Should a person with psychotic tendencies or a vast store of repressed anger and guilt embark upon self-hypnosis and suddenly release a Pandora's box of uncontrollable rage or self-loathing, then clearly the results can be very hazardous. So, for safety, approach a qualified hypnotherapist if you wish to learn to relax through autohypnosis.

You will be taught to relax each muscle group slowly and deeply, often using an aid such as a candle-flame as a focus. When you are fully relaxed you should gradually begin to say to yourself something like: 'I am calm, relaxed and at peace, daily stresses no longer have the power to disturb my beautiful state of inner calm.' You will be taught how to surface gradually from this mild trance. There is no danger that you will be unable to leave the trance state: should any emergency arise you would simply come straight out of trance and be capable of dealing with the problem right away.

BIOFEEDBACK

The underlying principle in this relaxation method is that emotional changes produce physiological changes (i.e. that excitement, fear, anger, feelings of stress, etc., cause various functional changes in bodily organs). Everyone is aware of how the pulse beats faster, the mouth becomes dry and the desire to pass urine persists just before a driving test, job interview, or getting up to make a speech. Variations in mood also produce variations in the resistance of the skin to a small electric current.

In the 1960s, the potential application of this 'mind affects body' principle to treating and preventing diseases was realized by US scientists, in particular a neuropsychiatrist named Kamiya. He saw that, since brainwave activity and bodily changes are so closely linked, it should be possible to alter undesirable conditions in the organs and tissues by 'tuning in' to a different and more beneficial brainwave. The modern result is the biofeedback machine, which may be of one of two types. It can either indicate changes in brainwave type, in which case it works *via* an electrode strapped to your scalp; or it can be attached to the palms of your hands to indicate changes in skin resistance.[143] (Skin resistance and brainwave changes are chosen simply because they are reliable indicators of what is going on within.) When you are using relaxation techniques, therefore, you can use the machine to keep you aware of the changes that are taking place; this is the 'feedback' aspect of the procedure.

Another way of using the machines is to teach yourself how to modify your own brainwave patterns, and thus your mental state.

MEDITATION

Meditation is frequently practised as an aspect of yoga but can also be practised as a separate discipline. There are numerous approaches to meditation, and a variety of techniques exist; there is space here to discuss only one relatively simple one. (Other means of attaining the meditative state include physical exercise through yoga and T'ai chi, the relaxed state of which predisposes to meditation.)

Relax as much as you can, sit comfortably in an easy-chair, and look at a selected object (perhaps a candle-flame or a crystal or a gem-stone). Take slow, deep breaths that fill your lungs comfortably, and 'feel' the breath entering your body and leaving it again. Then say your mantra (see below) over to yourself, letting the syllables linger in your mind until it is filled only with the reverberation of those syllables.

A mantra word will be chosen for you by some teachers, especially if you attend yoga classes where meditation is a major feature. If you attend a course of transcendental meditation (TM) you will be given a mantra which you will be instructed to keep secret. Otherwise, if you choose one for yourself, give the matter sufficient thought before you make your decision. The object of the word is that it should beautify and tranquillize the mind and spirit by the nature of its structure and sound—thereby, of course, relaxing and tranquillizing the body as well. Typical words include 'tranquillity', 'transcendental', 'serendipity', 'pastoral' and 'relinquish', but it is best to choose a word that has particular appeal and suitability to you.

Meditation can be used to help cancer patients and people suffering from other potentially terminal conditions. The method is known as 'relaxation and mental imagery'.[144] This involves getting the patient to relax, breathing slowly and deeply, and then to picture the growth or disease together with the body's defence forces which are combating it. Healthy, powerful tissue cells may be pictured, for instance, rising up against the malignant cells, overcoming them in successful battle, and finally getting rid of them all. This method has had some strikingly successful results in seemingly hopeless cases.

AUTOGENIC TRAINING

This is an excellent aid to relaxation, since it is designed to combat the body's unnecessary use of its 'fight or flight' reaction in response to stress. Not only does it help to negate the stress response; its positive contribution to overall health is the fact that it switches on the beneficial response of relaxation and inner tranquillity.

You are likely to learn autogenics from a trained teacher, either privately or as a member of a group. You are shown how to settle in a really relaxed way in a chair and, when you have felt the tension flowing out of your body, how to enter a state of deep relaxation by a 'visualization' technique. You let every single fibre of yourself go absolutely floppy and loose, and then you take slow, deep breaths, counting each breath you draw, and noticing how each breath 'feels'. When you have mastered the art of concentrating entirely upon your breathing, and of feeling each breath enter and leave, you are in a very relaxed state, known as a state of 'passive concentration'.

You then picture yourself remaining equally calm and cool in the face of stress. Perhaps you see yourself driving sedately round the municipal car park, looking for a parking space and remaining cool, unruffled and relaxed. You see your face and body as they are when you are relaxed and unbothered, despite a possible deluge of stressful factors that might assault you. And you repeat to yourself three times some relevant suggestion such as 'My body and mind remain calm and relaxed'.

This state is very pleasant to experience, and the exercise, which takes 15–20 minutes, should be practised three times daily until the art of deep relaxation is mastered. Courses in autogenic training last 8–10 weeks, one session weekly.

Autogenic training works very well in the relief of many stress-related conditions. Many people find their autogenic training so beneficial that they continue to practise it three times daily for years on end.[145] The Centre for Autogenic Training offers group and individual training.

Therapies of the Soul

The most fundamental principle of holism is Man's tripartite nature. Body, mind and soul are united in an indivisible whole, and their remaining in a state of dynamic equilibrium is basic to the holistic concept of health.

The following therapies are directed at remedying health through methods directed primarily at the spiritual side of our nature.

SPIRITUAL HEALING

Spiritual healing has existed in one form or another for thousands of years and in all cultures. The true spiritual healer, then and now, is a spiritual person in tune with the life-force, both within Man and in its many manifestations throughout the Universe. Some refer to this life-force as a personified god, others think of it as the creative force that gives life to all things. The spiritual healer works by linking his or her patient to the god-forms, however they are conceived. The resultant triangle of harmony and attunement that develops between healer, patient and god permits the healing energies from the divine source to flow.

This type of healing aims at recreating the vital energy-flow throughout the whole of a person's being, including physical and mental as well as spiritual aspects. Spiritual healers, in common with other holistic therapists, view disease as the result of inner disharmony, and seek to restore the balance that is vital to total health, Man's richest gift.

More particularly, physical disease symptoms are viewed as resulting from fear and anxiety. Spiritual healers bring peace, too, to distressed minds and souls by explaining that many of the trials and tribulations we experience are sent to try us and do in fact have a purpose. This removes from many sufferers the overwhelming sense of purposelessness which is a common sign of a sick spirit. This state is often expressed by the term 'sick at heart'; a person who is truly sick at heart (as opposed to being mildly depressed or temporarily 'down in the dumps') not only unconsciously falls prey to physical and mental ills but also puts up barriers against eventual recovery.

The philosophy common to most spiritual healers is a down-to-earth commonsense one based on everyday observation of nature and the world around us. As the balance, symmetry and harmony of nature is apparent wherever one looks, so the harmonious, simple life, uncluttered by excessive materialistic strivings, is the most wholesome and the most conducive to health. Spiritual healers advocate simplicity and a natural approach in all things—from a wholefood diet based on humane principles (not necessarily vegetarian) to a lifestyle that respects the integral role we all play—plants, animals and inanimate objects included—in the divine scheme of things.

Particular emphasis is placed upon getting the patient to realize that to receive we have also to give; and that hatred and resentment, if stored up within, cause pain, disorder and instability to the person feeling these things. It should also be added that spiritual healers do not always see success in terms of the abatement of troublesome symptoms. As mediator between god and Man, the healer strives primarily to ensure that the sufferer be made whole and at peace, and strong enough to face whatever the future holds.

Frequently, disorders *do* greatly improve or disappear, and healing takes place as the sufferer in the first place requested. In other cases, it is the patient's lot to face the illness but perhaps not to recover from it; spiritual healing forces instead help him or her nevertheless to remain happy, at peace and contented.

Form of therapy

There are two main types of spiritual healing. In the first, known as the *laying on of hands* (also called contact healing, hand healing or touch healing) there is direct contact between the healer and the patient. In the second, *distant healing*, the healing is performed in the absence of the patient, with the therapist working in a state of meditation. Distant healers work alone or in a group, and attune their collective consciousness to the source of divine energy through prayer or meditation in order to 'beam' healing energies to the patient. Many animals are helped through absent healing, and it can also aid young children and babies.

A patient visiting a spiritual healer is helped to relax. The healer then lays his or her hands on or near the patient to allow the healing energy to flow. The sensation the patient experiences (if any) is a warmth or tingling, or a 'coolth'. Spiritual healing carried out over several sessions is almost bound to have *some* beneficial effects, psychologically and spiritually, and sometimes physically as well. There are no side-effects, and it can be used as an adjunct to any other type (or types) of treatment. Spiritual healing is welcomed by some doctors or therapists for their patients, and a cooperative liaison often exists, with the practitioner continuing to treat his patient as before and the spiritual healer concurrently working on a spiritual level.

Comment

Putting up a barrier of disbelief when receiving spiritual healing partly blocks the flow of spiritual energy; like all aspects of spiritual healing, this is impossible to prove conclusively. But, as is certainly true with meditation and visualization, a persevering and quietly confident attitude works wonders at all levels in a patient, while negativity and despair produce the opposite effect.

The National Federation of Spiritual Healers explains how spiritual healing works as follows: 'The Divine energies are transformed from the spiritual level by the agency of a trained healer so that they can induce a beneficial effect upon the patient's own energy field of personal life force and upon the person as a whole on levels of body, mind and spirit. In individual cases of illness or stress these energies can be directed and applied to a particular disease or imbalance in the life force within the person to stimulate natural recovery and to bring peace of mind.' Further details can be obtained from the National Federation of Spiritual Healers.

SOUL-DIRECTED THERAPY

This therapy arose with Louise Sand, a German doctor and psychotherapist who utilizes a mixture of psychology and psychic 'sight' in healing physical and mental disorders. To do this, she works together with a spiritualist medium, Inga Hooper, in a manner that seeks to loosen repressions in a comparable way to that taken in psychoanalysis or psychoanalytic psychotherapy.[146] The great difference in soul-directed therapy, however, is that the therapists work at an 'intuitive spiritual level' in a manner that gives full recognition to the human trinity of spirit, body and mind. Sand believes that disorders stem from the soul, which she describes as 'an indefinable but vital part of a person that gives charisma and is "a shining, loving spark"'. She feels that by directing curative techniques to the soul of a patient she is restoring full health and attacking and eradicating the problems' root cause—the exact opposite of attempting to get rid of only troublesome symptoms. While sharing much in common with the approach of Jung, Sand has extended the basic Jungian approach by delving more deeply into the spiritual aspects of the subject.

Form of therapy

Sand claims that, in most cases, a single session is sufficient to produce the same—or better—therapeutic effect than might result from two years of classical psychoanalysis. The sessions last for an intensive two hours, and start with Inga Hooper (who is strongly psychic) giving a clairvoyant reading about the patient. Hooper often gets mental pictures of the patient's childhood events, and sometimes of 'earlier incarnations'.

Then Sand discusses with the patient what has transpired, including the relevance and significance of any past events. This, she explains, often produces instant recognition in a patient, with a subsequent (healing) emotional reaction, during which 'forgotten' repressed feelings and fears are released so that they can cause no further harm (in the form of disease).

The treatment, when they are correct about the patient's past traumas, can be painful at the time but is 'totally curative', according to Sand. The patient remains in charge, and excellent results have been produced working with schizophrenic patients, attempted suicide cases, anxiety and depression, as well as with people suffering milder problems such as marital difficulties and a tendency to worry.

Comment

So far as the patient is concerned, it is vital to *want* to recover, as new (healthier, more harmonious) attitudes to life and circumstances are an inevitable result. Patients have also to be willing to be honest about themselves and their problems as they see them. The great emotional release that results in a totally curative effect has much in common with the classic 'abreaction' effect that Freud produced under hypnosis when patients relived under trance conditions past traumatic events that had affected them adversely. Further details of soul-directed therapy can be obtained from Dr Louise Sand (see Appendix).

MUSIC THERAPY

There is no doubting the therapeutic effect which music can exert upon us. It has been used for its relaxing effects as an adjunct to autogenic training, and it can prove most helpful in the treatment of depressive illness.[147] Music speaks to us through the sensory faculties and so to the soul. And, by revivifying a weakened or saddened soul, heartening a desolate one, or calming a stressed one disorders manifesting in the form of physical and/or psychological symptoms can be remedied at source.

Form of therapy

There are few music therapists, and they tend to have varying ideas —probably equally effective—regarding the procedure that ought to be adopted. The usual aim is to encourage the patient (often physically and/or mentally handicapped) to respond to the music and express some of his or her inner feeling in whatever manner comes naturally. In this situation, patients may dance, jump up and down, scream and shout, cry or laugh. Alternatively patients might simply have music played to them and be allowed to absorb its healing qualities without having to demonstrate how it affects them.

Comment

An alternative therapeutic use of music is to encourage patients with verbal-communication problems (speech difficulties, autism) to express themselves in other ways—i.e. to 'talk' through making musical notes rather than words.[148] The Association of Professional Music Therapists keeps a register of music therapists in the UK.

ART THERAPY

Art and music therapy have a common objective in seeking to provide alternative means of self-expression to distressed and disturbed patients who communicate—if at all—only with difficulty. Making a papier-mâché model or painting a picture with vivid poster paints can be highly therapeutic in that inner pent-up feelings which frustrate can be let free. The picture or model can in itself serve another purpose on behalf of the patient, since interpreting the symbology of the created work can yield further insight into the patient's emotional and spiritual state. This interpretation is largely a subjective judgement on behalf of the therapist, who has to use experience, knowledge of the patient as a whole, and a greater or lesser degree of intuition in making an assessment.

The study of a sequence of pictures or models produced by the same patient over a period of weeks or months of psychotherapeutic treatment can prove interesting and indicative of progress or regression. Patients often make illuminating remarks about their own work, too.

There exists a British Association of Art Therapists, which in 1981 became recognized as a 'Profession Supplementary to' medicine.

Form of therapy

As with music therapy, much of the procedure in art therapy stems from the theories held by individual therapists. Many feel that the disturbed patient should be 'let loose' with the art materials, encouraged to make a start, and allowed complete freedom of expression. Interpretation of the results will likewise depend upon the psychological school to which the therapist belongs, by training and by persuasion.

Putting feelings into tangible shape and colour can bring patients into closer confrontation than hitherto with their problems. They may react with violent emotion; but, as with the abreactive response, this can be highly therapeutic.

Encouraging patients to try representative art (drawing things as they really appear to them) can bring patients into closer contact with the world about them and their own relationship to it. Representative art can also speak volumes about the patient's interpretative powers, and this can help with the formulation of a working diagnosis.

Comment

Types of disorders which have been reported as responding well to art therapy include drug-dependence (including alcoholism), phobias, chronic anxiety and the neurotic illnesses in general. Further details are available from the British Association of Art Therapists.

COLOUR THERAPY

It is a tenable argument that, if Man receives sense impressions of light, colour, taste and sound with the bodily sense-organs, and perceives them within specialized areas of the brain, then he interprets them through the use of the mind and responds instinctually to them with the soul.

Some alternative therapists interested in the curative use of colour believe that we are drawn naturally towards certain colours and colour combinations because they enhance certain of our spiritual attributes, reinforcing them with energy at that particular wavelength. Conversely, we are repelled by certain colours because they 'clash' violently at wavelength level with our own. This working hypothesis fits in satisfactorily with the existence of the human aura.

The therapeutic use of colour is not a new idea. It can be traced thousands of years back to the ancient world, when the Egyptians, Chinese and Mesopotamians made use of it to cure the sick. Considerable interest has recently been shown again in its effects, especially upon our emotional reactions and intellectual function. The colour of our surrounding environment has been found to influence our concentration, arouse feelings of restlessness or tranquillity, and stimulate mentally handicapped children.

An interesting new form of colour therapy was reported in *Here's Health* in April 1984. Called Aurasoma, it is the invention of Vicky

Wall, an ex-pharmacist and chiropodist now practising as an alternative therapist in Buckinghamshire. Aurasoma combines aspects of herbal medicine, aromatherapy and mineral supplementation with colour therapy; and it originated when Wall observed that people with mental disturbances or emotional problems chose to purchase cloudy 'unsaleable' oil from an exhibition display stand in preference to the clear oils available.

Wall, like Sand's medium (see page 492), has been clairvoyant since childhood and can focus quite easily upon the human aura. She has noticed a close relationship between the coloured oils people choose and their auras, for people have a strong tendency to choose oils which match the colour of their personal energy field. They pick out oils relevant to themselves both in clarity (or cloudiness) and hue, the purpose of their attraction to a certain colour being their unconscious need for its reinforcing power within their own aura spectrum.

Form of therapy

The oils Wall uses (referred to as 'balances') consist of pairs of oils that form upper and lower layers within a set of bottles. Wall takes a few personal details from her patient, then lets them choose a balance. She gets the patient to shake the selected bottle, and she then reads the result, taking note of the speed or tardiness with which the oils separate into their respective layers, and of the form of the bubbles produced.

As Wall interprets it, patients' own energy fields set up minute waves of vibration within the oils in the bottle they handle. These oils are 'live' and highly sensitive, and so reflect the state of the person's field of vital force, healthy people producing oils that readily regain their respective layers and unhealthy people, who lack harmony and vital energy, producing a cloudy effect that takes some time to clear.

Another diagnostic use to which Wall puts the balances is to discover which part of the patient's body is sick. She takes the chosen bottle and she herself shakes it at different points over the patient's body surface within the sphere of their aura. She gains information about the various regions by seeing whether the oils separate or remain opaque.

Treatment consists of the patient looking at and absorbing the vital colour energy from his or her own particular balance—daily, at home, for however long Wall suggests. The oils can also be used as a massage for all over the body, before or after a bath, or just for the face, hands and scalp. In this way, the oils' vital properties—as well as those of the herbs and minerals they contain—can have maximum curative effect.

Comment

Andrew Stanway points out in *Alternative Medicine* (1982) that 'colour can be given to a patient by many methods and routes. Firstly, white sunlight can be used in a rather non-specific way. We all know how much better we feel when the sun shines and the psychological and physical benefits of reasonable exposure to sunlight are well known and hardly disputed. Colour therapists use colour in more controlled ways, too, and can focus simple sunlight using reflectors and other gadgets so as to expose specific areas of the body selectively. In certain diseases, physical massage with solar-chrome salts bags is advised. This involves a massage with coloured salt-containing cheesecloth bags which have been "charged up" by placing them in the sun or under a lamp for one hour before the massage.'

Further details about Aurasoma can be obtained from Vicky Wall (see Appendix).

ELECTROCRYSTAL THERAPY

Electrocrystal diagnosis (see pages 446–7) led to the expansion of this technique into electrocrystal therapy as a result of patients reporting a sense of well-being and of relief from symptoms after having had a diagnostic scan. It seems that the powerful electromagnetic signal 'reminds' the body's energy field of its normal, healthy strength. Harry Oldfield started to test the effects of various frequencies and waveforms, and discovered that certain frequency bands could be used to stimulate and strengthen the energy field, others to balance it, and yet others to calm it down.[149]

Oldfield then discovered that crystals and gem-stones, with their traditional powers of healing, produce a more powerful field when stimulated with an electromagnetic field of a given magnitude; it has thereby become possible to combine traditional gem-stone healing powers with the appropriate electromagnetic frequencies. Examples of gem-stones exerting a stimulating effect are garnet and ruby. Jade and emerald have a harmonizing and balancing effect, and sapphire and amethyst have a calming effect.

Form of therapy

The diagnostic scan is first performed, the electromagnetic probe being in contact with a series of small crystals enclosed in a test-tube containing brine to facilitate electrical conduction. When the scan has been carried out (see page 446) the test-tube containing the crystals is applied to the affected area. A severe migraine has been terminated in 10 minutes, and the acute pain of cystitis relieved within 7–8 minutes. The appropriate chakras (energy centres) are then treated, and a final scan is made to assess the extent to which the energy readings have been returned to normal.

Comment

The chakras are the energy centrea, or nuclei, situated in the mid-line of the body at various levels along the length of the brain and the spinal cord. The chakras clearly indicate where specific organs and body areas require further investigation and energy balancing.

It is interesting, in passing, to note that holding a crystal in the hand or wearing it as jewellery produces an effect that can be picked up on an EEG machine, used by neurologists to observe patients' brainwaves.

References

Parts One and Two

(1) Skousen, M. B.: *Aloe Vera: New Scientific Discoveries*, private publication, Aloe Vera Research Institute, 5103 Sequoia, Cypress, CA 90630, pages 8–33, 37–8, 73–4, 137

(2) Bricklin, M.: *The Practical Encyclopedia of Natural Healing*, Rodale Press, 1976, pages 77–8

(3) Mindell, E.: *The Vitamin Bible*, Arlington Books, 1982, page 65

(4) Dixon, A. St J.: 'Calcium supplements in the treatment of osteoporosis, part II', *Rheumatology in Practice*, April 1985, page 8

(5) Update, *Journal of Alternative Medicine*, October 1983

(6) Bord, J.: *Honey, Natural Food and Healer*, Science of Life Books (UK distributors Thorsons), 1972, page 20

(7) Bricklin, M.: *The Practical Encyclopedia of Natural Healing*, Rodale Press, 1976, page 310

(8) Taufiq Khan, M.: 'Marigold a cure for corns and callosities', *Journal of Alternative Medicine*, July 1985, pages 11–12

(9) Bord, J.: *Honey, Natural Food and Healer*, Science of Life Books (UK distributors Thorsons), 1972, page 19

(10) Bricklin, M.: *The Practical Encyclopedia of Natural Healing*, Rodale Press, 1976, pages 119–20

(11) Bricklin, M.: *The Practical Encyclopedia of Natural Healing*, Rodale Press, 1976, page 129

(12) Update, *Journal of Alternative Medicine*, May 1984, page 13

(13) Update, *Journal of Alternative Medicine*, March 1985, page 16

(14) Watson, J.: 'A GP view of glue sniffing', *Mims Magazine*, 1 May 1985, pages 79–82

(15) Hoffman, D.: 'How herbs help in benzodiazepine dependence', *Journal of Alternative Medicine*, April 1985, pages 10, 11, 27

(16) Wilson, D. E., Engel, J., and Wong, R.: 'Prostaglandin E-1 prevents alcohol-induced fatty liver', *Clin. Research* 21: 829, 1973

(17) Campbell, A., and MacEwen, C. G.: 'Systemic treatment of Sjogren's syndrome and the sicca syndrome with Efamol (Evening Primrose oil), vitamin C and pyridoxine', *The Clinical Uses of Essential Fatty Acids*, edited by David Horrobin, Eden Press, Quebec, 1982

(18) Blythe, P.: Letter to Editor of *Journal of Alternative Medicine*, July 1985, page 6

(19) Butler, B.: 'One Brain', *Journal of Alternative Medicine*, June 1985, page 22

(20) Letter to *New England Journal of Medicine*, vol. 3,114, 6, page 413

(21) Key, C. and G.: 'The natural way to health', *Here's Health*, May 1985, page 135

(22) Colquhoun, V., and Bunday, S.: 'A lack of essential fatty acids as a possible cause of hyperactivity in children', *Medical Hypotheses* 7: 681–6, 1981

(23) Kolars, J.: 'Yoghurt. An autodigesting source of lactose', *New England Journal of Medicine*, vol. 3, 10, 1–3

(24) Mindell, E.: *The Vitamin Bible*, Arlington Books, 1982, pages 74–5

(25) Update, *Journal of Alternative Medicine*, October 1984, page 13

(26) Chaitow, L.: 'Pain: there's no need to suffer in silence', *Here's Health*, August 1985, pages 36–9

(27) Pfeiffer, C. C.: *Mental and Elemental Nutrients*, Keats Publishing, 1975, page 95

(28) Sargent, L.: 'Natural way to health', *Here's Health*, January 1985, pages 71–2

(29) Blank, C. E.: letter in *Lancet*, 4 February, 1984, vol. 1, no. 8,371, page 291

(30) Binder, A., Parr, G., Hazelman, B.: 'PEF Therapy of Persistent Rotator Cuff Tendinitis', *Lancet*, 1984, vol. 1, no. 8,379, 695–8

(31) Chaitow, L.: 'Your Body's Unwelcome Guests', *Alternative Medicine Today*, no. 1, 1984, pages 14–16

(32) Chaitow, L.: 'The tendrils of disease', *Here's Health*, January 1985, pages 23–4

(33) Lawrence, E.: 'Heal your teeth naturally', *New Health*, May 1985, pages 24–8

(34) Mindell, E.: *The Vitamin Bible*, Arlington Books, 1982, page 192

(35) Horrobin D.: 'Alcohol—blessing and curse of mankind! New research leads to simple nutritional techniques for controlling the bad effects and exploiting the good ones', *Executive Health*, June 1981; 17(9): 1–6

(36) Ritchie, J. A., and Truelove, S. C.: 'Comparison of various treatments for inflammatory bowel syndrome', *British Medical Journal*, 1980, 281: 1317–19

(37) Dew, M. *et al.*: *British Journal of Clinical Practice*, vol. 38, pages 11–12, 394–8

(38) Bricklin, M.: *The Practical Encyclopedia of Natural Healing*, Rodale Press, 1976, page 223

(39) Lewith, G. T.: *Acupuncture—Its Place in Western Medical Science*, Thorsons, 1982, page 77

(40) Bord, J.: *Honey, Natural Food and Healer*, Science of Life Books (UK distributors Thorsons), 1972, page 19

(41) Austin, D.: 'Not to be sneezed at', *New Health*, January 1985, pages 33–5

(42) Burke, P.: 'Hayfever', *GP*, 24 May, 1985, pages 45–8

(43) Inglis, B. and West, R.: *The Alternative Health Guide*, Michael Joseph, 1983, pages 309–11

(44) Azuma, J. *et al.*: *Current Therapeutic Research*, 1983, 34: 543

(45) Felmore Newsletters (no. 29), Felmore Ltd. Health Publications, 1 Lamberts Road, PO Box 1, Tunbridge Wells, Kent

(46) Felmore Newsletters (no. 23), Felmore Ltd. Health Publications

(47) Felmore Newsletters (no. 10), Felmore Ltd. Health Publications

(48) Felmore Newsletters (no. 59), Felmore Ltd. Health Publications

(49) Felmore Newsletter (no. 64), Felmore Ltd. Health Publications

(50) Update, *Journal of Alternative Medicine*, December 1984, page 11

(51) Felmore Newsletter (no. 39), Felmore Ltd. Health Publications

(52) Chaitow, L.: 'Is chelation a real alternative in coronaries?', *Journal of Alternative Medicine*, December 1984, pages 8–9

(53) Felmore Newsletter (no. 16), Felmore Ltd. Health Publications

(54) Update, *Journal of Alternative Medicine*, June 1985, page 14

(55) Update, *Journal of Alternative Medicine*, September 1985, pages 11–12

(56) Update, *Journal of Alternative Medicine*, April 1985, page 18

(57) Hanssen, M.: *The Healing Power of Pollen*, Thorsons, 1979, pages 22–4

(58) Hanssen, M.: *The Healing Power of Pollen*, Thorsons 1979, pages 48–50

(59) Update, *Journal of Alternative Medicine*, February 1985, page 13

(60) Update, *Journal of Alternative Medicine*, September 1984, page 14

(61) Ohkawa, T. *et al.*: *Journal of Urology* (1983) vol. 129, no. 5, pages 1001–11

(62) *Carcinogenesis* (1984), vol. 5, no. 3, 423–5

(63) *Journal of the National Cancer Institute* (1983), vol. 70, no. 5, 1151–70

(64) Pashby, N. L., Mansel, R. E., Hughes, L. E., Hanslip, J., Preece, P. E.: 'A clinical study of evening primrose oil in mastalgia' (abstract), *British Journal of Surgery* (1981), 68(11): 1. Clinical Study

(65) Cramer, D. N. *et al.*: *Obstetrics and Gynaecology* (1984), vol. 63, 6, 833–8

(66) La Vecchia, C. *et al.*: *International Journal of Cancer* (1984), vol. 33, 5, 559–62

(67) Mandal, B. K.: 'Herpetic diseases', *The Physician*, April 1985, pages 201–6

(68) Chaitow, L.: 'Help for herpes?' *Here's Health*, November 1984, pages 85–7

(69) Brush, M. G.: 'Nutritional approaches to the treatment of premenstrual syndrome', *Nutrition and Health* (1983), 2: 203–9

(70) Padwick, M. and Whitehead, M.: 'Oestrogen deficiency: causes, consequences and management', Update, *Journal of Alternative Medicine*, August 1985, pages 275–84

(71) Chaitow, L.: 'Menopause', *Here's Health*, November 1983, pages 14–15

(72) Hanssen, M.: *The Healing Power of Pollen*, Thorsons, 1979, pages 31–3

(73) Chaitow, L.: 'Improve your fertility', *Here's Health*, February 1985, pages 55–7

(74) Chaitow, L.: 'Arthritis', *Here's Health*, October 1983, pages 29–31

(75) Bricklin, M.: *The Practical Encyclopedia of Natural Healing*, Rodale Press, 1979, pages 24–9

(76) Hanssen, M.: *Hanssen's Complete Cider Vinegar*, Thorsons, 1979, pages 38–42

(77) Bricklin, M.: *The Practical Encyclopedia of Natural Healing*, Rodale Press, 1979, page 171

(78) Cunliffe, W. J.: 'Acne vulgaris—a treatable disease', *The Postgraduate*, 1 December, 1983, pages 26–31

(79) Chaitow, L.: 'Acne', *Here's Health*, 1983, pages 38–40

(80) Fry, J.: 'Aids for AIDS', Update, *Journal of Alternative Medicine*, 15 June, 1985, pages 1179–81

(81) Wright, M.: 'The gentle touch to aid stroke patients', *Doctor*, 27 June, 1985

(82) 'Guidelines for the feverfew migraine "cure"', *Journal of Alternative Medicine*, October 1984, page 21

(83) Update, *Journal of Alternative Medicine*, July 1985, pages 15–16

(84) Swank, R. L.: *The Multiple Sclerosis Diet Book*, Doubleday, 1977

(85) Dworkin, R. H.: 'Linoleic acid and multiple sclerosis', *Lancet* 1: 1153–4, 1981

(86) Update, *Journal of Alternative Medicine*, October 1984, page 16

(87) Parsons, S.: 'Natural way to health', *Here's Health*, February 1984, page 70

(88) Chaitow, L.: 'The new approach to diabetes', *Here's Health*, September 1984, page 47

(89) Lockie, A.: 'Miasms and vaccines: the Vithoulkas view', *Journal of Alternative Medicine*, January 1985, page 8

(90) Brown, D., and Pedder, J.: *Introduction to Psychotherapy*, Tavistock, 1980, page 50

(91) Brown, D., and Pedder, J.: *Introduction to Psychotherapy*, Tavistock, 1980, pages 52–3

(92) Pusey, J.: 'What's driving us mad?', *Here's Health*, September 1984, pages 25–31

(93) Update, *Journal of Alternative Medicine*, January 1985, page 11

(94) Pfeiffer, C. C.: *Mental and Elemental Nutrients*, Keats Publishing, 1975, page 409

(95) Update, *Journal of Alternative Medicine*, October 1984, page 15

(96) Pfeiffer, C. C.: *Mental and Elemental Nutrients*, Keats Publishing, 1975, page 333

(97) Pfeiffer, C. C.: *Mental and Elemental Nutrients*, Keats Publishing, 1975, pages 413–5